Dyslexia:
The Pattern of Difficulties

Second edition

Dyslexia: The Pattern of Difficulties

Second edition

T. R. MILES
Professor Emeritus of Psychology
University of Wales, Bangor

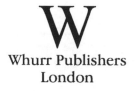

Whurr Publishers
London

© 1993 Whurr Publishers
19b Compton Terrace, London N1 2UN, England

First published in Great Britain by Granada Publishing 1983
Reprinted by Collins Professional and Technical Books 1986
Second edition published by Whurr Publishers Ltd 1993
Reprinted 1994 (twice)

British Library Cataloguing-in-Publication Data
A catalogue record for this book is available from the
British Library.

ISBN 1-870332-39-3

Photoset by Stephen Cary
Printed and bound in the UK by Athenæum Press Ltd,
Gateshead, Tyne & Wear

Preface to the Second Edition

It is over ten years since the first edition of this book appeared, and during this time there have been many exciting new developments. In particular the position on the theoretical side has changed considerably. The final chapter (24) of the first edition has therefore been discarded, not so much because it was erroneous but rather because it was scrappy and incomplete. In its place I have provided a brief account of those recent developments which seemed to me of special relevance to the main theme of the book. Eight fresh chapters have then been added. In Chapter 25 I try to show how an explanation in terms of a verbal labelling deficiency makes sense of the many interesting responses which the Bangor Dyslexia Test brought to light. The next five chapters are written in collaboration with colleagues. In Chapter 26 Dr Haslum, Professor Wheeler and I offer some norms for three items of the Bangor Dyslexia Test (Left–Right, Months Forwards, and Months Reversed) and by means of a suitable statistical technique we then show that these three items, along with the Recall of Digits item from the British Ability Scales, can be used to predict educational underachievement. In Chapter 27 Sula Ellis and I present data showing that dyslexics at two different age levels, 10 and 11 years and 13 and 14 years, had more 'pluses' (dyslexia-positive indicators) on the Bangor Dyslexia Test not merely than age-matched controls but than younger children matched for spelling age. In Chapter 28, which was written in collaboration with Andriana Kasviki, there is an account of what happened when the Bangor Dyslexia Test was translated into Greek and given to Greek children: here, too, younger spelling-age-matched children had more 'pluses' than older children whom we believed to be dyslexic. Chapter 29, written in collaboration with Claudia de Wall, reports on the use of a German version of the test where again there were similar results, while in Chapter 30, written in collaboration with Professor Jun Yamada and Mr Adam Banks, there is an account of what happened when some of the test items, adapted for use in Japan, were given to Japanese children. Chapter 31 contains data on 48 dyslexic adults and Chapter 32 offers some reflections on the book as a whole.

Some changes have been made to the end-of-chapter notes, and I have taken the opportunity to update the references. All notes will be found listed by chapter at the end of the book (pp.261–296). As the majority of dyslexics are male, the pronoun 'he' has been used throughout the book in general discussion.

I am grateful not only to the contributors to Chapters 26 to 30 but to many other friends and colleagues in addition. These include Dr R.L.Masland, Dr Isabelle Liberman (who, sadly, died last year), Dr P.G.Aaron, Dr Hugh Catts and Dr Thomas West, all from the USA, and Professor Gordon Stanley from Australia. Among those in the UK I should like to thank in particular Dr Uta Frith, Dr Alan Baddeley, Dr Stanton Newman, Dr Rod Nicolson and Dr Angela Fawcett, as well as my Bangor colleagues, Mrs Elaine Miles, Dr Nick Ellis, Dr Gordon Brown and Dr John Everatt. None of them is responsible for my views, but I have learned a great deal from all of them in the course of discussion.

T. R. Miles
Bangor, 1993

Preface to the First Edition (revised)

Since this book has been written for interested laymen as well as for specialists I have tried to keep technicalities to a minimum. The notation used in the Summary Chart in Chapter 6 will, I hope, be intelligible without too much effort on the reader's part, and I have made use of end-of-chapter notes in order to refer to specialist information which would have been something of an encumbrance in the main text. Statistical tables are relatively infrequent. This is partly because such tables tend to be somewhat indigestible when they appear en masse and partly because my concern in this book has been primarily to 'set the stage' for further quantification rather than make use of every opportunity for quantification which occurred.

I have made no attempt to write impersonally. It seemed preferable to include in the book an indication of the ways in which my ideas developed – how I reacted to the earlier literature, for instance, and how the dyslexia test, on which many of my conclusions are based, evolved into its present form. In an important sense, too, each assessment was an interaction between (usually) the child, the parents and myself, and there would have been some absurdity if I had tried to give the impression that I was merely a detached observer. My hope is that it has been possible to write in a personal way without thereby losing scientific objectivity.

It remains for me to thank the many people with whom I have been able to share ideas. These include Professor Oliver Zangwill, Dr Macdonald Critchley, Dr A. White Franklin, Mrs Sandhya Naidoo and Miss Gill Cotterell, all of whom were involved in the work of the Word Blind Centre in London in the 1960s. They also include Mrs Helen Arkell, Mrs Joy Pollock and Mrs Jill Playford, of the Helen Arkell Dyslexia Centre, Dr Bevé Hornsby, formerly of the Dyslexia Clinic at St. Bartholomew's Hospital and now Director of the Hornsby Centre in Wandsworth, Dr Harry Chasty, Mrs Wendy Fisher and Mr Guy Gray who have been associated with the Dyslexia Institute, Mrs Marion Welchman, Mrs Beryl Wattles and other members of the British Dyslexia

Association at both national and local level, and among my university colleagues Dr George Pavlidis, formerly of the University of Manchester and Drs Margaret Newton and Michael Thomson, formerly of the University of Aston. Coming nearer home, I should like to thank all those friends and colleagues who have worked with me in the dyslexia field at the University of Wales, Bangor. I have learned from my wife, Mrs Elaine Miles, not only some of the basic principles needed in teaching dyslexic children but also much about the essential rationality (despite appearances) of the English spelling system. I have also had the chance over many years to discuss assessment procedures with Mr Alun Waddon, and some of the central theoretical ideas in this book owe their origin to Dr Nick Ellis. Among former postgraduate students I should like to mention in particular the contributions of Dr (now Professor) Tim Wheeler, Dr Ann Williams, and Dr Caroline Dobson, and, more recently, those of Dr John Done, Mr Ian Pollard and, not least, Mr John Griffiths, whose wide experience as a teacher of mathematics has made him a particularly valuable member of the research team. Elaine Miles, Alun Waddon and Nick Ellis have all been kind enough to read an earlier draft of this book and have made many useful comments. I have also received some helpful suggestions from Dr A. D. Baddeley, Professor G. A. V. Morgan and Dr A. C. Wales. I am particularly grateful to Mrs Llio Ellis Williams for her patience in typing – and retyping – untidy pages of manuscript until the book reached its present form.

Finally, I should like to thank those to whom the book is dedicated – the dyslexics of all ages who have been willing over the years to talk to me about their problems. A special word of tribute is also due to the parents, since in many cases they had not only to contend with their child's difficulties but also to convince a sceptical world that these difficulties needed to be taken seriously. If I had not believed them to be in the right, this book would not have been written.

T. R. Miles
Bangor, 1982

Contents

Dedication

This book is dedicated to all those dyslexic children and adults whom I have met over the years and to the many concerned parents who were willing to talk to me about their children's problems.

Chapter 1
Background

During the last 30 years I have had the opportunity of meeting large numbers of dyslexic children and their parents and a smaller number of dyslexic adults. This book is first and foremost a record of what took place.

Unrelated facts, however, cannot from the nature of the case be of any special scientific significance; my policy has been to select those aspects of my subjects' behaviour which seemed to me to be important (Note 1.1). My task, as I have envisaged it, was not to function like a camera or tape-recorder which records everything that happened *as it happened*; nor have I tried to be like the student of unkind legend who is said to have conscientiously written down every word uttered by his lecturer, including 'um' and 'good morning'. The role which I have taken on is perhaps more like that of a portrait painter who purposely highlights certain features of what is before him in order to convey a particular message. Whether this message is important is for others to decide, and I do not believe that the issue can be resolved by any single knock-down argument. One can present evidence – and I shall do so – which indicates that those classified as 'dyslexic' behave differently in certain situations from otherwise comparable people not so classified, and one can specify the procedures for determining if a person is dyslexic, thereby showing that the word can be given a relatively precise meaning (Note 1.2). In the last resort, however, acceptance of the concept of dyslexia calls for a change of orientation; this is something which can come about only when a large body of evidence is recognised as being coherent and meaningful. My policy in what follows will in effect be to take the concept for granted and then show some of the things which can be done with it.

My starting-point was that a person should be called 'dyslexic' if a particular pattern of difficulties was present. The nature of this pattern and the variations which occur within it will be described in later chapters (Note 1.3).

When I came to study the relevant literature, I found many reports of children's difficulties which were remarkably similar to those which I myself was meeting. For example, Dr Pringle Morgan, writing in 1896, describes a 14-year-old boy called Percy who wrote his name as 'Precy' and 'did not notice his mistake until his attention was called to it more than once' (Note 1.4). Similarly Dr Hinshelwood gives some fascinating examples of children who despite adequate intelligence were extremely poor readers (Note 1.5).

Both writers emphasised the analogies between word-blindness (as they called it) which is acquired and word-blindness which is congenital, and Hinshelwood cited evidence in support of the view that the condition was more frequent in boys than in girls and that it ran in families (Note 1.6).

It seems, however, that in educational circles these ideas were largely ignored; it was again a medical man, Dr Orton, who in the 1920s and 1930s called attention to this group of difficulties (Note 1.7). It is widely agreed that Orton did more than any other early pioneer to put dyslexia 'on the map', and the society in the USA which is named after him is now recognised and respected internationally.

A further important influence on my thinking was a booklet by MacMeeken published in 1939 (Note 1.8). This reported a survey of 383 children in Scotland in which the author made a special study of those children whose reading performance lagged behind their intelligence level. She gives some interesting examples of what would now be regarded as typically 'dyslexic' mistakes, and she concludes that 'there can be no doubt whatever that we are here in touch with a pattern of difficulty *aphasic* in type' (Note 1.9).

For the next two decades, however (i.e. in the 1940s and 1950s), it appears that large-scale educational measurements were in fashion rather than the detailed study of individual cases. Surveys which gave figures for 'reading age', 'spelling age' and 'IQ' were plentiful, and in some cases the figures were subjected to elaborate statistical treatment. Although I do not dispute that such surveys can, in the right hands, produce useful information, I sometimes think to myself that it might have been better if the researchers had spent more time observing individual children.

Alongside the emphasis on educational measurement was a quite different approach to children with problems, namely an approach which emphasised the importance of family dynamics. According to this view, an effective way of helping children often involves the ability to understand and bring into the open those subtle forces which are necessarily present in every family even if they are not consciously recognised for what they are – feelings of inadequacy, resentment and jealousy, for instance, which sometimes hamper the growth of warm relationships. Such an approach can sometimes lead to the view that if a child is failing at reading and spelling, this must be because of fears or perverseness (or both) on his part or because of inappropriate pressures on the part of his parents; it follows that if child and parent, each with the aid of a suitably skilled therapist, are able to 'work through' their aggressive feelings, the child will learn to master reading and spelling as a matter of course. I am in no way disputing the value of what can be done by sensitive therapists with suitably selected families, but such a climate of opinion was not one in which the concept of dyslexia – a specific, constitutionally caused handicap – gained ready acceptance, and, as will be seen in Chapter 22, there is evidence, in the case of dyslexic children, of a certain *lack* of sensitivity among those who claim to have a psychodynamic orientation. If, in addition, one is told, without any detailed supporting evidence, that when a particular child reverses letters he is trying to attack his mother by 'turn(ing) the English taught at school into Hebrew by writing it backwards' (Note 1.10) one's lack of confidence in such an approach – at least as far as the dyslexic child is concerned – becomes even greater. In my experience the situation since the 1950s has changed considerably, but I suspect that misuse of psychodynamic notions is still not wholly dead.

The first occasion on which I was consciously aware that I was meeting someone with a dyslexic-type handicap was in the autumn of 1949. This was the girl, Brenda, whose difficulties I later described in a published paper (Note 1.11). She was aged 10 when I first met her, and her headmistress's description is one that has since become extremely familiar: 'appears very bright and is keen to answer in oral work, but... she is very slow at any written work – possibly she is a little afraid of making mistakes. Her entire inability to spell is her great weakness'. There was the opportunity to give teaching to Brenda on an individual basis, and some years later I gave similar teaching to Michael, a bright boy who was seriously handicapped at spelling. At the time I did not use the word 'dyslexia', but, following the lead of MacMeeken (see above), I spoke of 'developmental aphasia'.

Until the 1960s my work in the dyslexia field had been on a very limited scale. An important landmark was the year 1962 when, on the strength of my article about Brenda and Michael, I was invited to a conference on dyslexia in London organised by Dr A. White Franklin of the Invalid Children's Aid Association. This conference tended to be acrimonious at times: one speaker, for example, said that in using the word 'dyslexic' one was 'tying a ball and chain' round the teachers. (I believe that he was under the quite false impression that if a child was said to be dyslexic there was nothing one could do about it.) The outcome, however, was the setting up of the Word Blind Centre in London, and I was lucky enough during the next seven or eight years to be able to attend its committee meetings and discuss problems of dyslexia with the members. It was at this time that I first met Dr

Macdonald Critchley whose writings on dyslexia have been influential on a world-wide scale (Note 1.12), while shortly afterwards I met Mrs Naidoo whose book, published in 1972, contains a wealth of valuable comparisons between dyslexic and control subjects (Note 1.13).

From the early 1970s onwards, interest in dyslexia grew rapidly. Even the largely negative comments of the Tizard Report published in 1972 (Note 1.14), whose members did not draw the distinction between dyslexia and 'poor reading', and the sparse and inconsistent comments of the Bullock Report published in 1975 (Note 1.15) did little to stem the tide. More constructively, the Warnock Report (Note 1.16), published in 1978, paved the way for official recognition of dyslexia by its emphasis on the concept of 'special educational needs'. During this period a number of individuals already in the public eye admitted to being dyslexic and thereby demonstrated that the handicap does not necessarily prevent a successful career (Note 1.17). Another interesting occurrence was the emergence of a number of local 'Dyslexia Associations', whose aim was to increase public awareness of the problem and give help to dyslexic children and their parents in whatever ways they could. In 1972 a parent body, the British Dyslexia Association, was formed and there are now branches in almost every part of the UK. I have been impressed not only by the dedication of workers in this field but by the remarkable unanimity with which they have pursued their common objective; had 'dyslexia' been the poorly defined concept which some of its critics supposed, it is hard to see how this unanimity would have been possible.

As a result of my experiences in the 1960s, I was encouraged to write a short book, primarily on teaching methods, which I thought might be of help to parents and others. This was followed by a later book of the same kind, much of which was contributed by my wife (Note 1.18). Partly as a result of 'grape-vine' information and partly because of the increasing references to dyslexia in the press, the number of children coming to me for assessment was rapidly increasing; as a result I was able to try out a variety of methods for pinpointing specifically dyslexic weaknesses. These eventually led to the development of the Bangor Dyslexia Test as described in Chapter 3. By 1972 my assessment procedure had more or less stabilised; when, in 1978, I came to examine the files which had accumulated in my office, I found that it was possible to provide data on over 250 dyslexic subjects who had been tested in standard conditions. I therefore decided to look at the files of all those who had come for assessment within certain specified dates, namely the six-year period between April 1972 and March 1978. From these I selected a 'dyslexic population' as described in Chapter 4, and their behaviour will be described in Chapters 2–23.

During the early stages of the research my intention was primarily to get to know dyslexic children and their parents, to give myself the clinical 'feel' of what dyslexia was like and to find out from experience what difficulties to expect. Although my training had been as an experimental psychologist, it did not seem sensible to attempt systematic experiments in highly controlled conditions until I had a clear idea of what was worth investigating. The first requirement was to record systematically what happened at assessments.

Chapter 2
Assessment Procedures

At the start of the assessment the parents and child were invited in for a talk which lasted about 15 minutes. Next, I saw the child on his own for, say, an hour and a quarter to an hour and a half. Finally, after about a 20-minute break for scoring and interpreting the test results and studying the child's exercise books, I again saw the child and his parents together, explaining my findings and discussing with them the decisions which needed to be taken. This sometimes took a further hour or more, and the total time for most assessments was about three hours. Often, though not invariably, both parents accompanied the child and I did not object if brothers, sisters, or even friends of the family were present at the final discussion; this was a matter which depended on the parents' wishes and on the individual circumstances of each case. On a few occasions the child was brought by a teacher from his school and not by the parents, and in these cases the final discussion comprised a joint conversation between the teacher, the child and myself.

All the children and adults (264) whose numbers appear in the Summary Chart in Chapter 6 were seen by me personally. In many cases no-one else participated in the testing, though on some occasions I was helped by trainee postgraduate students, particularly with the administration of reading and spelling tests. I was involved in every case in both the evaluation of the evidence and the final interview. Occasionally results in the Summary Chart are given in brackets; this means that a particular test had already been given (usually within the last two months) and that I therefore thought it unnecessary to give it again. Asterisks in the Summary Chart indicate that the information is incomplete. This sometimes happened as a result of shortage of time and a deliberate decision to omit a particular item, though occasionally there was 'human error' in the sense that either I or a trainee unwittingly failed to follow the standardised procedure in exact detail. Data in respect of 34 children or adults whose records are incomplete are given at the end of the Summary Chart. These data do not regularly figure in the statistical calculations, but since the diagnosis was unaffected by minor gaps in the record I have referred to these cases, when it seemed appropriate, in some of the discussions.

One of my first tasks at the initial interview was to try to put the subject at his ease, particularly in the case of younger children. Most of them were carrying a long history of failure, and some were reported by their parents as having been anxious or apprehensive as to what I might do to them. Indeed, since their poor performance at reading and spelling had often been a source of rebuke in the past, they may well have expected that their weaknesses would be exposed yet further by me. In the case of younger children in particular, I therefore made clear that I had seen plenty of people who had difficulties over reading and spelling and that they were not to worry if they could not do some of the things which I asked them to do. I then explained that it was of special help to me to know what they could not do since we could then set about putting things right. Early in our talk the parents often described their struggles in getting anyone to recognise that there was a specific problem. Many reported that they had been told, in connection with the child's reading and spelling, 'Don't worry; it will come', but had found that this was not the case. These points were noted down and will be discussed in Chapter 22. I also asked if there were any specific areas where advice might be helpful, e.g. over whether to make a change of school or over choice of courses, and I indicated that this would help me in carrying out the assessment (Note 2.1).

When the parents went out I had a brief talk with the child, after which I gave him a reading test, a spelling test, the dyslexia test and an intelligence test, usually in that order. To determine his standard of reading I decided to use the Schonell R_1 word-recognition test (Note 2.2). The great advantage of this test is that words are presented out of context and there is therefore no opportunity for clever guessing. There is the further advantage that the test is suitable for persons of all ages from 5 upwards, and as a result it was possible both to compare my subjects with each other and to determine the position of any particular subject in relation to the norm for his age. The figure under the heading 'R_1' in the Summary Chart indicates, for each subject, the number of words read correctly, out of a maximum of 100, and against each age-level will be found the expected score in accordance with the original norms provided (Note 2.3); for example, subjects between the ages of 10 and 11 are expected, according to these norms, to read between 50 and 60 words correctly. If any of my subjects were within 80% of the norm a line has been placed under their score. This is a reminder that, as far as untimed word-recognition is concerned – and with intelligence level not taken into account – the subject is not grossly different from an average child of his age. This does not, of course, exclude a diagnosis of dyslexia; there may still have been a history of earlier difficulty in learning to read (compare Chapter 8), and in any case it is necessary to look at the total picture, not at the result of a single test taken in isolation.

To obtain an indication of the subject's spelling level the Schonell S_1 spelling test (Note 2.4) was used. Like the R_1 word-recognition test it is suitable for all ages from 5 upwards, and under the heading 'S_1' in the Summary Chart I have again indicated the number of words spelled correctly by each subject. As in the case of the R_1 test the maximum possible score is 100 and the same norms are applicable; thus 50 words spelled correctly on the S_1 test represents a 'spelling age' of 10, just as 50 words read correctly on the R_1 test represents a 'reading age' of 10. Scores within 80% of the norm were again underlined.

It will be seen from the Summary Chart that for 40 out of the 223 subjects there was underlining in the case of both reading and spelling scores. This may seem surprising: even if it is agreed that a person whose reading is somewhere near the norm for his age can still be dyslexic, is there not some absurdity in classifying a subject as dyslexic if neither his reading nor his spelling present him with any major prob-lem? This was my view at the start of the research. When, however, I examined the records of the 40 subjects in question, the evidence left me in no doubt that they *were* dyslexic, even though they had learned to read and spell not too badly. The situation as I see it is that reading and spelling are important as social skills, whereas other signs of dyslexia, for example, the inability to repeat strings of digits correctly, are less crippling. This, however, is not a justification for giving any particular test a privileged position as a diagnostic indicator; it is the consistent absence of 'positive' indicators over a *variety* of tests which justifies a negative diagnosis.

In the case of the R_1 test, accurate pronunciation was required if the word was to count as having been read correctly (for example if the subject said 'cánary' as opposed to 'canáry' this was scored as wrong); in the case of the S_1 test, words in which 'b' was substituted for 'd' and vice versa were scored as incorrect (Note 2.5), though no account was taken of whether the subject used capital or lower-case letters. Many of us are aware of the feeling that it is more 'charitable' to score a response as correct than to score it as incorrect, but there is, of course, nothing charitable in purveying incorrect information about a subject's performance (Note 2.6).

The problems which arise in assessing the intelligence of a dyslexic subject are very complex and I shall not attempt to discuss the issue exhaustively. Briefly, however, one of the central difficulties was this. Almost all intelligence test items involve a variety of component skills and some of these skills – at times seemingly irrelevant ones – may be lacking in a dyslexic subject. For example, there is a series of items in the Terman–Merrill intelligence test (Note 2.7) which involve awareness of direction, for example, 'If you are going *west* and then turn *right*, in what direction are you going now? ' Now I have met subjects who have marked out the points of the compass on a piece of paper and have clearly grasped what is needed but, as they say the word 'right', have turned their pencil to the left and hence incorrectly given the answer as 'south'. (For further details see Chapter 11.) Similarly there may be failure at the Terman–Merrill 'ingenuity' items, which involve complex problems of filling and emptying cans of water with the correct number of pints, and this failure may arise not because they do not understand what is needed but because they do not know that $9 + 4 = 13$. (For further details see Chapter 15.) If, therefore, a subject has grasped the necessary reasoning but makes an error over calculation, one has either to score the response as wrong – and hence underestimate his reasoning power – or depart from the standardised instructions by allowing pencil and paper or suggesting that he should check his calculations (Note 2.8).

There are similar difficulties with the Wechsler Intelligence Scale for Children (Note 2.9). It is now well established that dyslexic subjects have difficulty with some of the sub-tests of this scale and not others (Note 2.10). In particular they regularly obtain low scores on the Digit Span sub-test (where the tester reads out strings of numbers of increasing length and the subject has to repeat them either as they were said or in reverse order), the Information sub-test (which is a series of items on general knowledge), the Arithmetic sub-test (which involves a number of arithmetical items and in the later stages calls for a knowledge of tables) and the Coding sub-test (which is a timed test involving the reading of numerals and the writing of the appropriate 'code-mark' against each numeral). The overall IQ figure is obtained (after various mathematical transformations) by combining the different sub-test scores. For the dyslexic subject, however, the resultant figure may be a composite of widely differing sub-test scores and may therefore not represent an overall score for 'general intelligence' – which is what IQ is assumed to be. The alternative, however, is to ignore those sub-test scores which represent the weakest part of the subject's performance and base an IQ figure on the remainder; this, too, seems a highly questionable procedure. Unfortunately, once one departs from standardised procedures at all, one is on the first stages of a slippery slope.

At the upper parts of this slope one need not be too unhappy. As has been pointed out already, there appears to be no particular difficulty in asking what is a person's reasoning power independently of his ability to read instructions. Nor does there seem any absurdity in trying to assess the reasoning power of a person who sometimes muddles up left and right. Ability to remember strings of digits, however, has traditionally been regarded as a component of 'intelligence', and it is starting to become uncomfortable if one asks what a person's intelligence level would have been had he been able to remember digits better. It is even more uncomfortable to ask what his intelligence level would have been had he been able to carry out the operations of adding, subtracting, multiplying and dividing; in particular, one should surely be unhappy about the question, 'What would his intelligence level have been if he had not been dyslexic?' This seems almost like asking, 'What sort of a person would he have been if he had been different?' I do not myself believe that one need be committed to this degree of absurdity. Whatever else an IQ figure represents – if indeed anything else at all – it can be taken to be a reasonably good predictor of academic success in children of similar backgrounds provided other things are equal in terms of environment, opportunity etc. Now for a dyslexic child other things are *not* equal; in particular, unless he acquires the necessary standards of literacy his prospects of academic success are appreciably less. It makes perfectly good sense, however, to make a prediction as to what his success is likely to be if these standards are attained. Such predictions may be difficult in practice in the case of the dyslexic, and it is important to make clear to parents and teachers the extent of the uncertainty; but at least the results of an intelligence test reduce the uncertainty to some extent. Often, indeed, they serve as confirmation of views reached by parents and teachers on independent grounds, namely that in some respects the child is extremely bright. In this context, too, of course, they can be used as a source of encouragement which is recognised by all those concerned as being realistic. In contrast, if one gives a conventional IQ figure based on the results of a battery of tests which includes items where dyslexic subjects are known to perform badly, one is making an underestimate; this is no way to handle a person who has in all probability seriously underestimated himself already.

The practical problems arising from these difficulties were not, on the whole, all that difficult to solve. When I cited IQ figures to parents I was as careful as possible to add the necessary reservations and qualifications, and I emphasised that at best the figure was a rough guide. In some cases I called the subject's attention, and that of his parents, to a particularly difficult test item – one which we could all see to be difficult – where he had been successful. Sometimes, after showing some of the details on the test-form, I would simply say, 'It looks from the evidence as though you shouldn't set your sights too low'. With these and similar remarks it was possible to be encouraging without committing myself to giving an exact IQ figure (Note 2.11).

A more difficult problem was that of devising a notation which would indicate the subject's intelligence level in the Summary Chart but would not at the same time invite inappropriate statistical procedures. An IQ figure, though having the merit of brevity, was clearly unsatisfactory in this respect, since it would have been based on the cumulative effect of sub-test scores that were sometimes very divergent. If, in addition, the procedure laid down in the manual had been only partially followed, an unqualified IQ figure would have been dishonest and misleading. At quite an early stage of the research, I decided to exclude the Digit Span sub-test from the items designed to measure intelligence and instead to use it diagnostically as part of the dyslexia test. I also decided that if one specified particular test items in advance and had good reason, in the context of assessing for dyslexia, for picking on these particular items, it was legitimate to think in terms of a 'selected IQ', i.e. a figure based on selected test items, which could then be contrasted with a 'composite IQ', i.e. one which represented a composite of the results on all the sub-test items specified in the manual. The selected IQ would reflect performance on items which were not 'dyslexia-laden', that is, did not present distinctive difficulty to the dyslexic person. Such a procedure would not be misleading provided (1) that one made clear what one was doing, and (2) that one specified the items in advance of giving the test. On this basis I decided to use the Similarities, Vocabulary and Comprehension sub-tests from the so-called 'verbal' scale of the Wechsler test, and the Picture Completion, Block Design and Object Assembly sub-tests from the 'performance' scale (Note 2.12).

In the case of the Terman–Merrill test, I selected the Vocabulary, Ingenuity, Direction, Similarities, Abstract Words, Enclosed Boxes, Proverbs and the 'tree' item. I departed from the strict rules of the manual in permitting the use of pencil and paper if the subject found this helpful, and if there was an obvious slip over 'left' and 'right' in the Direction items or a blatant error of calculation in the 'tree' item I sometimes allowed myself a comment such as 'Are you sure?'. My usual policy was to give the Terman–Merrill test to older subjects (from about age 11 upwards) and the WISC to younger ones. There is, of course, more variety in the WISC; but I found it somewhat incongruous to give 'jig-saw' items (particularly the Object Assembly sub-test) to bright 13-year-olds, the more so as it was a central part of my policy to talk to my subjects as their intelligence merited and avoid any suggestion of asking them to carry out tasks which might seem childish. In addition I have always found many of the later Terman–Merrill items particularly interesting and challenging and it is an important principle that testers should use tests which suit their personal style.

In a small number of cases I gave the Advanced Progressive Matrices (Note 2.13), since experience showed that this was a test on which older dyslexic subjects sometimes obtained strikingly high scores (see also Chapter 31). On the basis of the subjects' performance on the Wechsler or Terman–Merrill tests, it was possible to calculate a 'selected' IQ for each of them. Since a precise figure, however, would have

implied an accuracy level which was spurious, I decided to limit myself
to six categories rather than the far larger number which the traditional
concept of IQ makes available. The letters used, Z to U (Note 2.14),
represent a rank order in accordance with the following conversion
table:

Table 2.1 Selected IQ rank order	
Selected IQ	*Grade*
140 or above	Z
130–139	Y
120–129	X
110–119	W
100–109	V
90–99	U

Subjects with a selected IQ of below 90 were assigned to a further group, namely Group III (see Chapter 4).

As a very rough approximation one can say that a selected IQ comes
out about 10–15 points higher than a composite IQ (Note 2.15). In the
Summary Chart I have used the above grade labels rather than figures
for selected IQ. This was in part a 'safety device' designed to prevent
myself – or an unwary reader – from confusing selected IQ with composite IQ and in part a way of emphasising the approximate nature of
the gradings. I have also converted the scores on the Advanced Matrices
test into letter grades which, once again, give very approximate comparability (Note 2.16). The following are the conversion figures:

Table 2.2 Conversion of Advanced Matrices Score	
Score on advanced matrices	*Grade*
26 or above	Z
22–25	Y
17–21	X

This procedure, though rough and ready, ensures that the grades U
to Z represent a rank-order of intelligence level and that anyone who
achieves grade U is within the average range. It also makes possible the
matching of intelligence grades between dyslexic and control subjects
(see Chapter 7) and establishes that the difficulties shown by many of
my subjects on the dyslexia test items could not have been simply the
result of low intelligence.

A further important consideration is this. If one is looking for evidence of the kind of reasoning powers that are necessary for academic success, the fact that the subject passed *any items at all* at the difficult end of the scale must surely be relevant. An important device, therefore, which I decided to use was to present two figures for each subject indicating what he did at the 'top' end of the scale. In the case of the Terman–Merrill test I have recorded the level of 'mental age' where the subject obtained his two highest passes (Note 2.17), while in the case of the Wechsler test I have recorded the highest two sub-test scores. Suitable levels are sufficient on their own to exclude any possibility of dullness and can be made the basis for discussion, since one has confirmed that there are some difficult reasoning items which the subject *can* do.

To sum up, nearly all the subjects in this study were given either (1) selected items from the Terman–Merrill test (with use of pencil and paper sometimes permitted even where the instructions indicate the contrary), or (2) selected items from the Wechsler Intelligence Scale for Children, or (3) the Advanced Raven Matrices. In a few cases, where the Wechsler test had already been administered, an IQ figure is given in brackets in the Summary Chart and the grade letter is adjusted so as to be one grade higher than that given in the conversion table.

Central to my argument is the claim that the difficulties of the dyslexic person are incongruous; in other words they are at variance with what one might expect in view of his age and the other skills which he possesses. The results of testing showed that my subjects *did* possess other skills, and the items in the Summary Chart marked 'int.' (intelligence) and 'limits' are evidence that this was the case.

Chapter 3
The Dyslexia Test

Details of the dyslexia test are given in Appendix I. In this chapter I shall say something about the way in which it evolved and how the decisions on scoring it were reached.

In the early stages of the research it was necessary to try out particular items without knowing in advance whether they would present any special difficulty to a dyslexic subject. By reading the literature, however, by talking to other workers in the field and above all by letting my subjects talk to me, I was able to choose items which seemed at first sight as though they might be of interest. The procedure was neither based on firm evidence on the one hand nor totally random on the other, but something in between. Thus I knew – or thought I knew – that dyslexic subjects had unusual problems over 'left' and 'right', and it was clearly useful to ask the subject in the first place if he could show me his right hand. I came to realise that slight hesitations and pauses might be significant, and soon afterwards I decided to add the supplementary question, 'Did you have any difficulty when you were younger?' This gave the subject a chance, if he so wished, to tell me about earlier problems or the use of compensatory strategies. I wondered if the 'double' command, 'Touch your right ear with your left hand' would present any extra difficulty compared with the single one, and common sense suggested that the 'inverted' command by which the subject had to say which was my right hand would be more difficult still. At a later stage I noticed that some subjects turned in their seats in order to answer this question. I do not even now know for sure whether this response is more common in dyslexic subjects than in controls, but at least it seemed significant enough to be taken seriously and to be noted for purposes of scoring. To increase the difficulty I combined a 'double' command with an 'inverted' command, for example, 'Touch my right hand with your left hand'; finally, since a correct response to a single item does not guarantee that the subject will consistently give the right answers, I drew up a series of variant items involving the subject's left and right hands and my own right and left hands, eyes, and ears.

It was also obvious at a fairly early stage that my subjects tended to be weak at digit span items when these occurred in the Terman–Merrill and Wechsler intelligence tests. I therefore discontinued using the 'digit span' items as possible measures of intelligence (compare Chapter 2) and included them in the dyslexia test as diagnostic indicators.

On one occasion I was told that a boy who was due to come to me for tuition in reading and spelling had also showed considerable difficulty in learning his tables. Without attaching any special significance to the matter, I agreed to try to help with the tables as well as with the reading and spelling. It immediately became apparent that this boy's difficulty with his tables was no accident; on the contrary, it was obviously part of the overall dyslexic picture. From that moment onwards I asked all my subjects to recite their tables, with results that never cease to amaze me (compare Chapter 16).

After I had administered the Schonell R_1 word-recognition test on a number of occasions to older subjects, it occurred to me that many of them were stumbling over the word 'preliminary'; discussion with friends and colleagues at the Word Blind Centre in London confirmed that dyslexic children were quite frequently liable to become 'tied up' in saying words, e.g. 'par cark' for 'car park'. I therefore included a series of such items. 'Anemone' seemed a good word because of possible complications over the 'm' and 'n' and 'statistical' contains a complicated arrangement of s's and t's. 'Contemporaneous' was included because of its length, though I suspect that length of word on its own is not a decisive factor. Finally, the mother of three dyslexic boys who were coming for tuition told me that their father was also dyslexic and that when he tried to say that he wanted to be philosophical about the matter he had become 'tied up' over the word 'philosophical'! Into the list, therefore, went the word 'philosophical'. The original dyslexia test also included the word 'competition', but this word was omitted when it became plain that neither dyslexic nor control subjects were having difficulty with it.

I also came on some children – and in at least one case a highly intelligent dyslexic adult – who needed to use their fingers for simple addition and subtraction. I therefore included some subtraction tests of graded difficulty. I suspected that taking away small numbers (less than about 5) might be relatively easy and I thought it might be interesting to compare '9 – 2' and '24 – 2' because the latter was at a higher point in the number scale. I also thought that if a larger number had to be subtracted and/or if it was necessary in calculation to pass a 'ten barrier' (e.g. '44 – 7') there would be more difficulty. Why I included '6 – 3' I do not remember!

Nor do I remember exactly how I came on the idea that dyslexic subjects might have difficulty in saying the months of the year, but presumably some intelligent subject whom I believed to be dyslexic surprised me by the difficulty which he showed. Certainly when a BBC camera team came to film the behaviour of a dyslexic boy and a control, the dyslexic boy named only a few of the months – and even these were in the wrong order – whereas the control, who had been less successful on two intelligence test items, gave all 12 in the correct order with no difficulty.

At one stage I included tests for finger agnosia. For example, the subject would be told to shut his eyes and I would touch, say, two or three of his fingers and ask, 'How many fingers am I touching?' or 'How many fingers are there in between?' I did not continue with this test, however, as I had some doubts as to what it was achieving. Even now I do not know if any significant number of dyslexic subjects would find it distinctively difficult.

A small number of children were also failing at the 'rhymes' item in the Terman–Merrill test. This is set at age 9 and the subject is asked to give 'a number that rhymes with "tree"', 'a flower that rhymes with "nose"', etc. At one stage, therefore, I gave this item routinely and I have collected a small quantity of data (see Chapter 18), though I have not used the results in the Summary Chart in Chapter 6. I have also collected some data on 'memory for sentences' using three items of graded difficulty from the Terman–Merrill test (again see Chapter 18).

Originally I found myself trying out items in a somewhat unsystematic way, without necessarily giving each subject the same item. I soon decided, however, that it would be helpful to use prepared and standardised material; when a number of copies were run off on a stencil this in effect marked the birth of the dyslexia test. It has been modified over the years but most of the items in it have remained the same.

After having given the test on a number of occasions, I became increasingly convinced that the idea of dyslexia from which I had started was basically correct. A recognisable pattern of difficulties was clearly emerging: in particular the spelling of many subjects seemed bizarre; many of them continued to confuse 'b' and 'd' at a relatively advanced age; and they were regularly showing some or all of the difficulties mentioned above – problems over left–right, over repeating polysyllables, over subtraction and tables, and over repeating the months of the year and strings of digits. I was also confronted with clear evidence that the condition sometimes runs in families. Confirmation of these ideas came not only from discussions with colleagues and a study of the relevant literature, but from the fact that what I said was clearly making sense both to the children and to their parents.

Provisionally, therefore, I decided to classify a person as dyslexic if his performance at reading and/or spelling was discrepant with his intelligence level and if enough of the above signs were present. I had at this stage to leave in abeyance the question of what exactly constituted 'enough': there was clearly a difference between a dyslexic and a non-dyslexic person in straightforward cases, and I was not unduly troubled by the fact that from time to time I came on doubtful or marginal cases. I also came to realise that no *one* of the criteria listed above was a necessary or sufficient condition for a diagnosis of dyslexia. Even in the case of reading and spelling a *history* of early difficulty seemed more important than the subject's score at the time of testing (compare Chapter 8). I did not doubt that people could be found who were weak at reading and spelling for reasons other than dyslexia, in particular lack of opportunity or, for all I knew, unhappy personal circumstances. In these cases, however, I believed that there would be no reason to expect the distinctively dyslexic pattern of difficulties (Note 3.1). I also realised that there would be subjects for whom the items in the dyslexia test were too difficult, namely those aged under about 8 and those older subjects who were of limited ability. In general, however, it seemed to me that I could usefully pick out a relatively homogeneous population of children, who coincided fairly well with those whom others had designated as 'dyslexic', by looking for past or present problems over reading and spelling of a kind that were incongruous with the subject's intelligence level, in a context where there were a number of distinctive difficulties over items in the dyslexia test.

It has sometimes been said that the grounds for a diagnosis of dyslexia are negative, or, in other words, that one diagnoses dyslexia when one cannot find any other explanation for the literacy problems. This has never been my view. For all I know, there may be children whose reading and spelling is poor relative to their intelligence level for no obvious reason, but unless they responded in characteristic fashion to some or all of the items in the dyslexia test it was not my policy to class them as dyslexic. This is quite different from saying that they are dyslexic because no other cause of their difficulties can be found.

Now I was fairly confident, after a small amount of investigation, that it was possible to diagnose someone as dyslexic on 'clinical' grounds, that is, by the 'feel' of the case even in the absence of convincing statistical evidence. When people claim to be making a clinical judgement, however, I suspect that they are in effect using a large number of 'cues' or signs of which they are not always explicitly aware. I myself have sometimes been tempted to say that it does (or does not) 'feel' like a case of dyslexia. To carry conviction, however, it is clearly necessary for the investigator who claims to be relying on 'feel' to specify the signs or cues on which he is basing his conclusion. In the case of the dyslexia test I found that I could draw inferences from the fact that my subjects used unusual strategies, for instance, or showed unusual hesitations even though they ended up with the correct answer. I therefore decided to try to devise a scoring system which took such things into account.

Some years ago I delivered a paper on this topic which I entitled, 'How do I score the "crikey"?' The situation which I envisaged was one in which a bright 11-year-old is asked to recite the months of the year and in reply says, 'Oh, crikey!', in a tone of voice suggesting that it is a difficult task, yet after something of a struggle gives the correct answer. If one fails to score the 'crikey' at all one is throwing away potentially useful data (since the fact that the task is difficult is clearly important), yet if one says 'I took the "crikey" into account clinically but I did not score it' one is losing objectivity. I suggested as a solution that factors other than correctness of response could be taken into account – for example exclamations or pauses – provided these were specified with enough precision to be identifiable. By this procedure one could take into account the clinical 'feel' of the case and yet record what happened in a way that could be quantified.

At about the same time I had become convinced that dyslexia involved some kind of limitation of immediate memory (Note 3.2); this led to the thought that dyslexic subjects might need more 'props' for memory than did controls. Now one such 'prop' is to ask for the question to be repeated, and a further prop is to say the instruction over to oneself while one is thinking out the answer. Thirdly there was the response-characteristic for which I took over the grammarians' term *epanalepsis*, that is, the taking up of something which has been said just before; for example if a child is in difficulty over 'seven eights' he may re-orientate himself by going back to 'five eights are forty', and by giving himself a fresh start may then come up with the right answer. Successful memorising often seems to depend on becoming 'cued in' (Note 3.3). I therefore devised the following symbols for recording on the subject's response sheet:

RR = the subject requested that the question be repeated
EQ = the subject echoed the question, i.e. said it to himself as a 'prompt'
EP = the subject 'cued' himself in by repeating what he had said before (epanalepsis)

These symbols, along with the symbol 'hes' to indicate that the subject hesitated, are included in the instructions for scoring the dyslexia test given in Appendix II.

Basically what was needed was a notation which summarised relevant aspects of the situation in such a way that it indicated whether or not the subject was producing responses that were typically 'dyslexic'. It seemed, therefore, that the most helpful procedure would be to specify certain kinds of responses as 'dyslexia-positive' and other kinds as 'dyslexia-negative'. A single 'dyslexia-positive' response, or indeed a single 'dyslexia-negative' response, would be of little significance on its own, but if, in the appropriate context as regards age, opportunity and intelligence level, a cluster of 'dyslexia-positive' responses were found, then in combination they would be evidence that further dyslexic-type responses were likely. In practice I also found it convenient to have an intermediate classification for those responses which were neither unambiguously dyslexia-positive nor unambiguously dyslexia-negative. Correct responses, if given without hesitation and without any compensatory strategy, would be scored as dyslexia-negative, whereas incorrect responses and responses which, though correct, were made only after hesitation or as a result of compensatory strategies would be scored as dyslexia-positive.

The obvious notation in this context was to label as '+' a dyslexia-positive response, to label as ' − ' a dyslexia-negative response and to label intermediate responses as '0'. In what follows, therefore, I shall speak of dyslexia-positive responses as 'pluses', dyslexia-negative responses as 'minuses' and intermediate responses as 'zeros'.

Full details of what responses should be scored as 'plus', 'zero' and 'minus' are given in Appendix II; in the present chapter I shall limit myself to giving some brief indications as to how particular decisions were reached.

This is an area where further investigation and further statistical treatment of the data are likely to lead to greater accuracy. How to score the items so that they would best differentiate dyslexic subjects from controls was to some extent a matter of guesswork. In a sense I had to begin by begging the question: I had some idea of the ways in which the subjects whom I called 'dyslexic' would behave differently from most other children of the same age, experience and intellectual level, and by suitably modifying my criteria I hoped to define the two groups with greater precision. I was helped at this stage of my enquiry by having available the data which had been collected in ordinary schools in the Manchester area by my friend and former pupil, Ian Pollard. These data had not at this time been scored, but they helped me to determine what might be expected of a typical non-dyslexic child in the age range 9–12 and they influenced my choice of what exactly should count as 'plus', 'zero' and 'minus'. For example, a single error on the subtraction tasks was scored as 'minus'; this was necessary because at this item very few of the controls were error-free and one clearly cannot use as an indicator of dyslexia a criterion which is satisfied by dyslexic and control subjects alike (Note 3.4).

The following further comments on the scoring of individual items are perhaps worth recording. For convenience I have set these out in the order in which they appear in the Summary Chart.

Digits Forwards and Digits Reversed

In view of the inconsistent performance of dyslexic subjects, I thought it would be helpful to record the lowest number of digits at which there was a failure as well as the highest number at which there was a success; hence for each name in the Summary Chart there are two entries for Digits Forwards and two entries for Digits Reversed. The first entry indicates the highest number passed, the second the lowest number failed. In the normal way the highest number passed is sufficient for scoring the result as 'plus' or 'minus'. In the case of a 'double inversion', however (where the first entry is greater by 2 than the second – for example if there is a pass at '7 digits forwards' but a failure at '5 digits forwards'), the result is scored as 'plus', since this appears to reflect unevenness of performance. (The only exception is if a weaker performance, for instance '65' in the above example, would have counted as 'minus', in which case the response is scored as 'minus' (Note 3.5).) Moreover, for the 9-year-olds and upwards, any failure at 'three digits reversed' was striking enough to merit a 'plus'.

Left–Right (body parts)

I was not convinced that the *number* of errors in this test was a valid measure, but it seemed reasonable to say that a person was having some degree of difficulty if he made a single error (this was scored as 'zero') and was having appreciable difficulty if he made two or more errors (this was scored as 'plus'). Some intelligent dyslexic children consistently gave me the mirror-image of the correct answer, and some of them turned in their seats (or made slight movements of pretending to turn) in order to work out which were the right and left sides of the tester's body. All such responses were scored as 'plus'. Reports of earlier difficulty over left and right seemed to me less convincing than the evidence of my own eyes; in general I tended to score reported difficulties (including difficulties over 'b' and 'd' and hearsay evidence of dyslexia in other members of the family) as 'zero' in contrast with actually observed difficulties which were scored as 'plus'. Where the subject had worked out compensatory strategies, his response was scored as 'zero' (though it did not count as two separate 'zeros' if he both reported earlier difficulty and had worked out a compensatory strategy). Hesitations, corrections, requests for the question to be repeated and echoing the question, if they occurred on at least two occasions, were all scored as 'zero', and if more than one condition for a 'zero' was satisfied the two 'zeros' counted in conjunction as a 'plus' (This was also true in the case of Subtraction, Tables, Months Forwards and Months Reversed.) A single hesitation in conjunction with a single correction would also be scored as 'zero'. I have not so far defined what exactly counts as a hesitation and there is therefore still some degree of inexactitude on this point. It would be helpful in the future if the subjects' responses could be timed by means of apparatus having suitable precision and, if possible, apparatus which recorded slight movements in the muscles of the *wrong* hand even when the correct hand was used.

Repeating Polysyllabic Words

A sympathetic headmaster tried out, in my presence, some of the members of his 8-year-old class on the word 'preliminary'. Only a relatively small number could say it, and in a pilot study by one of my undergraduate students (Note 3.6) a 'nil' success rate with this particular word was reported. I therefore decided that the responses of children under 9 should not be scored as 'plus' unless there were four or five errors. At the other end of the age range it seemed to me that even a single error in anyone aged 15 or over was worth a 'zero' and that two errors were worth a 'plus'. Some approximate interpolations then gave me the rest of the table.

Subtraction

The scoring here is mostly self-explanatory. Use of fingers or marks on paper was an automatic 'plus'. Also I had the suspicion that it was no accident when a subject suspected on other grounds of being dyslexic used unusual strategies, for example, in the case of 44 – 7, breaking the 7 into 4 and 3 and counting backwards from 40; any strategy which seemed to me 'unusual' (in an admittedly ill-defined sense) was scored as 'zero'. Inspection of Pollard's data indicated that a large number of the control subjects made at least one error, and I therefore set the standard for a 'plus' as three errors and the standard for a 'zero' as two errors.

Tables

All kinds of interesting responses occurred in this test. Any response of the form 'Where have I got to?' was scored as 'plus', and I was interested in the fact that some of my subjects had learned to avoid this kind of difficulty by omitting the 'preamble' (e.g. 'One six is ...', 'Two sixes are ...' etc.). I thought it likely that slower children would make the simple response that they 'couldn't do it' whereas dyslexic children, even after going wrong, might still try to apply rules; for this reason I scored as 'plus' any 'consistent' error – for example, if, having said that six threes were twenty, the subject – consistently with this mistaken assumption – said that seven threes were twenty-three. In addition, breaking into the 'wrong' table (e.g. 'Six sevens are forty-two, seven sevens are forty-nine, eight eights are sixty-four') seemed to be another example of 'losing the place' and was therefore scored as 'plus'. Any attempt by the subject to 'cue' himself in by repeating an earlier product (epanalepsis) was scored as zero, and on the basis of not wholly arbitrary guesses, three pauses, two 'slips', whether corrected or not (e.g. 'eight eighties, I mean eight eights') and one 'skip' (e.g. from six eights to eight eights), were scored as 'zero'. All such responses seemed to me to be possible – though not fully certain – indicators of memory overload and therefore, in the right context, confirmatory evidence for dyslexia.

Months Forwards

Occasional errors were made by the control subjects, and I therefore decided that at least two omissions or inversions were necessary for a 'plus'. Uncertainty over where to start was also scored as 'plus', as was any question as to whether they should be said 'in order'. The fact that an intelligent subject of suitable age should be unsure as to whether the order mattered seemed to me sufficiently anomalous to justify counting the response as 'plus'. In accordance with policy in other parts of the test, evidence of earlier difficulty was scored as zero.

Months Reversed

Here, too, two omissions or inversions were needed for a 'plus', a single omission or inversion counting as 'zero'. Both in this item and Months Forwards a single correction was scored as 'minus' on the grounds that single corrected errors are sufficiently common to be regarded as insignificant.

b–d confusion

First-hand evidence was scored as 'plus', for example if the subject, in reading, said 'done' for *bun* or if his exercise books or his spelling test contained 'b's for 'd's or vice versa. Second-hand evidence, when such confusions were reported but not observed by me personally, were scored as zero (Note 3.7).

Familial incidence

If I had myself assessed two or more members of the same family and found them to be dyslexic or if a diagnosis had been made by one of my colleagues using similar criteria, I scored this item as 'plus'. The difficult point for decision was to determine how weak the evidence had to be before one scored it as 'minus'. The statement 'Uncle Jack was a poor speller', on its own, is by no means decisively significant! Approximate guide-lines are given in Appendix II.

Finally, administration of the tests for handedness and eyedness, as given in Appendix I, is self-explanatory. If the subject consistently used his right hand for writing, cleaning his teeth and throwing a ball he was scored as R (= right) in the first column, representing handedness; if he consistently brought the paper to his right eye when asked to 'spy' a pencil through the hole he was scored as R (= right) in the second column, representing eyedness. Consistent use of the left hand was similarly scored as L in the first column and consistent use of the left eye as L in the second column. Any inconsistency in the 'handedness' items was scored as M (= 'mixed') in the first column and any inconsistency in the eyedness items was scored as M (= 'mixed') in the second column. This gives the nine possibilities RR, LR, RL, LL, MR, ML, MM, RM, and LM. Administration of the 'memory for sentences' and 'rhymes' tests is also self-explanatory. The procedure for scoring the responses to the ten items used in the Summary Chart is given in Appendix II (Note 3.8).

It is thus possible to determine the 'index-figure' for each subject, that is, the number of 'dyslexia-positive' responses out of a possible ten. My intention was to use this 'index-figure' not so much as a measure of the severity of the subject's dyslexia – as though there were some kind of 'dyslexia continuum', which is perhaps a doubtful notion – but rather as a guide to clinical diagnosis. I have never claimed, and do not wish to claim, that a subject with, say, seven 'pluses' is in some way 'more dyslexic' than a subject with, say, five 'pluses'; still less do I want to stipulate that a person should be defined as (or 'deemed') dyslexic if he scores over a certain number of 'pluses' (Note 3.9). The position seems to me rather that the subject's score can legitimately be taken into account in deciding whether the total picture is one of specific handicap. A high score, in the right context, can increase one's confidence that such a handicap is present; since there is little possibility at present of adequate confirmation from direct neurological evidence, a diagnosis of dyslexia is in a sense a 'bet' that other manifestations of dyslexia will be present (Note 3.10). This is a point to which I shall return at the end of Chapter 4.

Chapter 4
Selection of Subjects

When I came to take stock of the data which I had collected, I decided to make my first task an examination of the files of all those whom I had assessed during a given period of time. The period chosen was between April 1972 and March 1978 and the number of usable files turned out to be 291 (Note 4.1).

Now clearly in any educational survey one can expect to find a large number of children who show no particular difficulties in either reading or spelling. For obvious reasons few such children could be expected to be referred to me for assessment, though in fact there were three subjects among the 291 who seemed to me to have very little the matter with them from an educational point of view. From an initial inspection of the files I decided that it would be helpful to distinguish those who were undoubtedly dyslexic from those who were either very slightly dyslexic or about whose dyslexia there was any appreciable doubt. Dr Critchley and his wife have indicated that there can be 'formes frustes' – variants of dyslexia where some of the signs are present but only to a limited degree (Note 4.2), and in the years before 1972 I myself had come on a few boys, known to have dyslexic relatives, who were not grossly weak spellers and whose performance on the dyslexia test was not fully typical of the dyslexic person but who showed slight or occasional dyslexic signs. I decided therefore to implement this distinction by assigning to Group I those who were clearly and unambiguously dyslexic and to Group II those who were marginally or slightly dyslexic. I also decided to have a third category, Group III, which I provisionally called 'contaminated cases', i.e. cases where there were other major contaminating factors. Even, therefore, if they scored 'pluses' on some of the dyslexia-test items the subjects in this group could not be classified as pure or typical cases of dyslexia. These three groups, along with Group IV, those with no appreciable educational problems, were so defined that one or other of them would fit every child who might be studied in any large-scale survey. Clearly those in Group III would comprise a wide variety of children who for other purposes might need some more accurate classification; but for present purposes the important point was that, because of contaminating factors, none of them be classified as a 'pure' or standard case of dyslexia.

I decided that 24 subjects qualified for Group III. Their details have not been included in the Summary Chart in Chapter 6, but it may illuminate the concept of dyslexia if I indicate the kinds of reason which led to their exclusion.

From the point of view of research it seemed desirable to assume that low IQ, even on its own, was a contaminating factor; for this reason I excluded from Groups I and II anyone with a 'selected' IQ of below 90. This is not, of course, because I believe that those with a 'selected' IQ of below 90 can never be dyslexic; on the contrary it seems to me likely from the nature of the dyslexic handicap that it can fall on anyone, regardless of ability. With slower children, however, it is hard to be sure that one is seeing a pure or typical case, since many of the items in the dyslexia test may be too difficult for them independently of any dyslexic handicap. The decision was purely one of convenience in view of the purpose of this book: if I had included in my dyslexic population those of lower ability there would have been a risk of contaminating the data by an unknown amount and no compensating gain. This accounted for nine cases out of the 24.

It was not my intention to exclude anyone from Group I simply because he was known to have had psychiatric problems. In three cases, however, the psychiatric problems were too severe to enable adequate testing to be carried out (Note 4.3). In ten further cases there was a history of autism, non-communication, suspected brain damage or the like; although the justification for any of these expressions is to some extent controversial, it was at least clear that these were not true or typical cases of dyslexia. In the remaining two cases I was somewhat unsure of the diagnosis; one appeared to have a visual problem and one a hearing problem but neither showed unambiguous dyslexic signs. For present purposes the significance of those in Group III is not that they were in any way a homogeneous group but simply that none of them was straightforwardly dyslexic (Note 4.4).

It is also worth recording that of the 24 subjects in Group III, 12 were male and 12 were female. Since there is clear evidence of a male to female ratio in dyslexia of about 3:1 (Note 4.5) this supports the view that the members of Group III did not constitute a typical dyslexic population. In contrast, of the 223 Group I cases 182 were male and 41 were female, which gives a ratio of 4.4:1. As a matter of interest, cases 224–257 may also be compared. These were all subjects whom I had diagnosed as dyslexic but for whom the data were not fully complete. Here there were 26 males to 8 females, a ratio of over 3:1, which again suggests a genuinely dyslexic population.

The Summary Chart shows that seven cases were eventually assigned to Group II, i.e. those who were marginally or slightly dyslexic. In my earlier attempts at classification I had supposed it wise to 'play safe' by including in this group anyone about whom there could be any serious degree of doubt. When I came to re-examine about 20 such cases, however, I became increasingly convinced that in all of them there was a genuine dyslexic problem. This accounts for the fact that in the Summary Chart subjects are to be found in Group I having three 'pluses' or fewer on the dyslexia test. In these cases there was enough independent evidence of dyslexia despite the relatively small number of 'pluses'. If one regards a diagnosis of dyslexia as a kind of 'bet' that other dyslexic manifestations will be found (see Chapter 3), there is nothing inconsistent in making such a bet about a bright subject with three pluses and being unwilling to make it about a less bright subject with four pluses since there may be independent confirmatory evidence in the one case and not in the other (Note 4.6).

In a few cases the entry in the Summary Chart has been marked by an asterisk. This has been done where the information is incomplete but where the total number of 'pluses' is not affected. Where there was a definite 'gap' in the information the subjects were assigned to a separate place in the Summary Chart (nos. 224–257). I shall refer to some of these cases in later chapters but most of my statistical calculations relate only to subjects 1–223.

The final figures can therefore be summarised as follows:

Table 4.1 Grouping of subjects	
Group I	223
Group II	7
Group III	24
Group IV	3
Incomplete records	34
TOTAL	291

As a result of the above classification I believed myself to have a 'pool' of 223 subjects who could be regarded as pure or typical cases of dyslexia (Note 4.7). These are the subjects whose behaviour will be described in the chapters which follow.

Chapter 5
Sample Case Histories

In this chapter I present four case histories. My purpose in so doing is threefold: first to give the reader an indication of my sources of evidence; secondly to illustrate the scoring of responses as 'plus', 'zero', and 'minus' on the Summary Chart in Chapter 6, and thirdly – and perhaps most important – to call attention to the fact that those whose responses are recorded in this way were real people, each with his or her own distinctive life-style. Without such descriptions there is a risk that awareness of the individual *as an individual* may be overlooked; although the material in the Summary Chart is of course central to the arguments in this book (since adequate generalisations would be impossible without it), it should never be forgotten that the impersonal symbol '+' represents a human being struggling against a handicap. He may, for instance, have endured years of anguish in trying to learn his tables and still be relatively unsuccessful. Before making any generalisations, therefore, I decided that it would be helpful to introduce the reader to some of the people about whose behaviour the generalisations were made.

The four cases which I have selected were taken more or less at random, though with the constraint that they should belong to different age levels. Any other selection would, I am sure, have illustrated similar basic difficulties. All names have been changed.

S7: John

A letter from John's mother ran as follows:

> We are anxiously seeking advice and diagnosis as it would seem that John could be dyslexic to some degree. John will be eight years old next birthday. A brief resumé of his achievements and difficulties so far might be of help. I hope you don't find them too tedious and beg forgiveness in advance .

Further extracts from her letter are given in Chapter 8. The gist was that from the age of 5 John had encountered severe difficulties in reading and writing and had become withdrawn. 'A *very* occasional bed-wetter before this, he now reverted to this every night.' ITA (initial teaching alphabet) had been of no help to him, and although teachers had, in the main, been sympathetic, he nonetheless had a real sense of failure. At the age of 7 he had been given the WISC.

> John is very bright indeed and much above average. Remedial reading work suggested with the Remedial Reading teacher attached to the Child Guidance Clinic. A colleague of mine took John daily for reading; he enjoyed the sessions with a one-to-one relationship ... quickly progressed through the Schonell Happy Venture series ... showed difficulty in remembering any phonetic combinations but got along fast by reading content ... Discharged (age seven and three quarters) ... quite able to read the meaning by going for the content of the reading matter ...
>
> Dyslexia occurred to me in the early months of John's school difficulties three years ago, but as his traumas got worse we increasingly cast around for reasons within the context of our family life and John's emotional experiences ... his father's unavoidable adsence (sic) from home on business; having a clever elder sister, and of course, ITA ... I now realise we need proper diagnostic help ... There is so much more we need to know before we can help John. I wonder if there are degrees of dyslexic disability, how badly or otherwise John is affected, if at all. Whether he is by IQ ability managing to overcome dyslexia; whether he is now likely to achieve his potential without specialised help? Where this help should come from and what form it should take. Whether we should try and persuade a local prep. school with small classes to take him on, or whether I should do remedial work with him and how I could be trained in order to do this?
>
> Yours very sincerely ...'

John was in fact 7 years 11 months when I first met him. He read 32 words on the Schonell R_1 word recognition test correctly, which according to the original norms give him a 'reading age' of 8 years 2 months (slightly above his chronological age) but he spelled only five words correctly on the Schonell S_1 spelling test which gives him a spelling age of 5 years 6 months. I had managed to obtain the results of his intelligence test: with all items taken into account (apart from Picture Arrangement, for which no score was given) his overall IQ figure had been found to be 128; on the basis of the 'selected' items only (see Chapter 3) the figure came out as 142, which gives a Z on my notation.

A piece of his spontaneous writing was shown to me as follows:

> Im going to flangr to morow, becoes a man is inerasitb in me I am gowing bie car I am going to sta if scool and Elesebth is going to scool And rapre is loking aftr the boq colb tesr

(Elisabeth was his sister, and the last sentence, so I was told, was an attempt to write, 'Grandpa is looking after the dog called Tessa'.)

When I asked him to show me his right hand he did so correctly, but when I asked him which was my right hand he pointed to my left hand, and in all subsequent items, e.g. 'Touch my left hand with your right hand' he got *his own* side right but my side systematically wrong. On the method of scoring given in Appendix II this counts as 'plus'.

He could not repeat the words 'preliminary' and 'statistical' but managed the other words. At the age of 7 this is insufficient evidence to be scored as 'plus' or 'zero' and therefore counts as 'minus'.

He failed one of the two trials when asked to repeat five digits, and when the series-length was increased to six he failed both trials. This counts as a 'plus'. In the case of Digits Reversed the results were:

Stimulus	His response
927	279
25	52
574	759
259	592

This also counts as 'plus'.

When asked '9 take away 2' he paused and then said 'six'. Asked to explain, he said, 'I just go nine, eight, seven, six'. '6 take away 3' was answered correctly, as was '24 take away 2'; but '19 take away 7' was given as 'fourteen': 'I started to think nineteen, eighteen, seventeen, sixteen counting in my head how many numbers I took away'. This result is also a 'plus' .

Asked to say the months of the year he said, 'November, December, October, November, December, March, April, May, June, July, November, December'. This, and Months Reversed, were both scored as 'plus'.

Asked to say his 2 x table he replied, 'Once two is two; two twos are four; ... three' (as if about to say 'three twos') ... 'two twos are four' (reorientating himself); 'three twos are six; seven ... four twos are eight; five twos are ten; six twos are twelve; seven twos are fourteen; eight twos are sixteen; nine twos are twenty; ten twos are thirty'. When I started him off on the 3 x by saying 'Once three is three', he said 'Once three is three; two threes are six; four threes are nine; three twos ... four twos are ... five threes are (long pause) fifteen'. He explained that he went 'one–two–three; four–five–six; seven–eight–nine; ten–eleven–twelve; thirteen–fourteen–fifteen'. His performance on 'tables' was clearly 'plus'. As judged by the tests described in Chapter 3 John was right-handed and right-eyed.

John's father said that he himself was a very poor speller, and his mother said that she herself still used her fingers for arithmetical calculation. My suspicion is that both parents are dyslexic. The 'plus', under 'familial', in the Summary Chart, however, arises not from discussion with John's parents (since such evidence would at most be scored as 'zero') but from the fact that they afterwards asked me to assess John's sister, S74, whose dyslexia – as they afterwards realised – had been masked by high intelligence and adequate reading skill. Father said that many of the family had been architects, and I suspect – though I have not the figures – that this is often a suitable occupation for those with high ability who are handicapped by dyslexic tendencies.

In my report on John I wrote as follows:

> I confirm the earlier finding that he is an extremely bright boy with a special learning problem – one which affects reading, spelling, number work, and various other memory-tasks involving orientation and sequencing. This group of difficulties (often referred to as dyslexia) appears to be constitutional in origin; and it is therefore incorrect to attribute John's failure to any of the traditional educational scapegoats (poor teaching, the i.t.a., parental pressure etc.). It seems right, instead, to think of a specific *handicap*, which is affecting John in a few special areas. It therefore seems important that all his teachers should *know of* his handicap and adjust their standards accordingly; dyslexic children often give the appearance of being careless or lazy when in fact their pathetic attempts to get things down on paper are the result of an enormous effort.

This is not a book about the practical handling of dyslexic children, and in general I shall not be citing from the reports which I wrote. The present report, however, is reasonably typical: the problem both in John's case and many others was not so much in making the diagnosis as in ensuring that, once it was made, appropriate help was forthcoming. In some cases it is helpful if one or other parent learns the special teaching techniques that are needed, and this was the obvious answer in John's case.

Two months after the assessment John's mother wrote reporting progress and saying that 'the future seems much brighter'. Seven months after that I received a letter from an educational psychologist saying that he had met John during his training; and the following are extracts from his report:

> He read fluently, paid attention to punctuation marks and obviously enjoyed reading for me... His spelling has also improved though he has still some way to go in this area. His spelling age is 7.4 years on the Schonell Spelling Test and this compares with a spelling age of less than 6 years when he was seen by Professor Miles. Spelling is still a great struggle for him and on every word he had to think very hard before writing it down... John's number work is still behind. He take a long time to work out very simple additions and subtractions and unless he used his fingers he frequently made errors when adding single digit numbers... his handwriting is fairly neat and legible... However, reversals are still common, particularly the letters d and b, and the number 5. He is starting to write in cursive script which will, I think, help him to orientate his letters. Mr — is relatively pleased with the way John is progressing in school.

S95: Brian

I received through the post a letter from Brian's mother which included the following:

> I have been planning to write to you for some time, to seek your advice about my eleven year old son, Brian.
>
> As a result of hearing several discussions about dyslexia on the radio and television, I sent a description of my son's learning problems to the British Dyslexia Association... An educational psychologist... who said she was not an expert on dyslexia felt that Brian was probably not dyslexic. She felt that because Brian could read another explanation was more likely, in his case nervous tension.
>
> However, his remedial teacher after a year's work with my son believes that he reads almost entirely by remembering the shape of words... His handwriting is very poor for his age, slow, cramped and wobbly... his spelling, although showing some improvement as a result of his remedial work is still sub-standard. He does seem to have corrected the b–d confusion recently, but often leaves words out and transposes letters. He still shows occasional confusion between left and right but will work it out if given time. He finds arithmetical tables extremely difficult to learn and tends to lose his place when reciting them. He seems to have a reasonable concept of figures, however, for example when asked – How many minutes in two hours? – worked it out as follows:
>
> > 1 hour = 60 min
> > 60 = 50 + 10
> > 2 hours = (50 x 2) + (10 x 2)
> > = 100 + 20
> > 2 hours = 120 min
>
> This is a typical approach to his arithmetical work, compensating for not knowing his tables.
>
> On the other hand his maths teacher finds he has a fine analytical mind, able to accept, understand and implement new concepts, often before any other member of his class. He was a late speaker. When he was younger he was very clumsy.
>
> ...If you feel that because Brian can read, he cannot be dyslexic, then I will accept your advice and simply try to help my son over his difficulties as best I can.
>
> Yours faithfully...

Brian was aged 11 years 3 months when he came to see me. He read 60 words correctly from the Schonell R_1 word recognition test, which by the old norms gave him a 'reading age' of 11 years 0 months, and he spelled 21 words correctly on the Schonell S_1 test which gave him a 'spelling age' of 7 years 1 month. He passed all four items in the Terman–Merrill intelligence test at the xiii year level and all four items at the xiv year level. He placed 'east' and 'west' the wrong way round, however, and used 'concrete aids' (marks on paper) in order to solve the two more complicated 'cans-of-water' items. Asked how 'beginning' and 'end' were alike he immediately said 'Both are places'. I arrived at a 'selected IQ' figure of 130, which places him in category Y in the Summary Chart.

One of the interesting points which emerged, particularly when I gave him the dyslexia test, was his ability to be explicit about his compensatory strategies. Thus, when I said 'Touch my left hand with your right hand', he repeated the question to himself, gave the correct answer, and cryptically explained, 'You twist round – your right hand changes'.

The running commentary as he struggled with his 7 × table is worth quoting in full. After going correctly to 'five sevens are thirty-five' he said, 'I usually say five sevens are thirty-six. What's next? That's five sixes. Six sevens are forty-two; eight sevens... now, let's see... ah! it's fifty-six. Five – six – seven – eight so seven eights are fifty-six. Where am I? I've forgotten where I am; I was on seven. Five, six, seven, eight: seven nines are sixty-three; seven sev-, no, seven tens are seventy; seven elevens are seventy-seven and seventy twelves... seven twelves... no wonder I'm getting all confused... are... fourteen, eighty-four using the same system' (I think this means that he knew 7 × 10 = 70, and that the reference to 'fourteen' was a way of arriving at 7 × 12 since twice seven needed to be added).

He repeated six digits forwards correctly but failed in two out of his three attempts at saying three digits in reverse order. With slight corrections he just about managed to say the months of the year, but used his fingers to check that he had not left any out. There was no evidence of any close relative being similarly affected, though his mother spoke of a first cousin who had 'educational problems'. (This evidence seemed to me insufficient for a 'zero' and was scored as 'nk' – 'not known', though one certainly could not claim that one had *excluded* dyslexia in other members of the family.)

Brian's tally of 'pluses' was in fact 7, which is, of course, well outside normal limits for a boy of his age and ability.

His comments on how he tried to read words by examining their shape are referred to in Chapter 8.

He said that he wanted to be a radio engineer, and I confirmed with his parents that this seemed to me a perfectly realistic ambition. A letter from an educational psychologist 27 months later reported 'considerable progress' despite his still having difficulties with handwriting and spelling, while an informal conversation with his sister also gave grounds for optimism. Many years later he wrote to me saying that he *had* succeeded in becoming a radio engineer (see Chapter 23).

I end by recording something which he typed shortly before the assessment:

Homewrk

Haw to do you,r ti

Fist put you'r ti under you'r Coler then mack the fat bit longer than the shot bit. Put the long bit *(crossings out)* The sort bit and go raond twice. Now btween you'r neck and wer the bit that go's rand yor'r Neck gone up you put the fat bit through the tip of upside daow r then you see one of the loppes that you made were you saw the tie gone up you put you'r (crossings out, with 'bit' added) under this lop and put until it looks allright (presuming you have git a mirror).

S142: Simon

A letter from Simon's mother said:

Simon is 13 years of age and finds great difficulty with reading. I would be most grateful if you would arrange for tests to be carried out as I feel that dyslexia may be his problem.

When I met her personally she said she wished that she had asked earlier.

I kept thinking, I'll wait; I won't make a nuisance of myself... They said he was lazy and didn't try... You can tell him something and a minute later he'll say, "What did you say?" or will have forgotten a message.

Simon read 28 words correctly from the Schonell R_1 test ('reading age' 7 years 10 months) and spelled 18 words correctly from the Schonell S_1 test ('spelling age' 6 years 10 months). Use of both Terman–Merrill and Wechsler tests showed that he was not slow. Yet he made an error in repeating *four* digits (3147 for 3417) and failed both trials at five digits. Surprisingly his performance at Digits Reversed was considerably better, with one success at five digits reversed. (I do not understand this anomalous result, to which the Summary Chart shows virtually no parallels.)

Asked to repeat his 4 x table he said 'Two fours are eight; three fours are twelve; four fours are fifteen; five fours are nineteen; six fours... I can't remember, twenty-seven... thirty-one; eight fours are thirty-one; nine fours are thirty-five; ten fours... I've gone wrong'.

This an extract from one of his school books:

Ju Des The Scarcat ptrad Jesus... necs Day The tumeston was roald a way and The gads was not a slep and Jesus went to The Foloas

His mother reported that he had regularly put 'b' and 'd' the wrong way round and that sometimes his '6' and '9' were 'back to front', though he did not now confuse 'p' and 'q' any more. (This evidence is scored as 'zero' on the Summary Chart since it is based on a report and is not first-hand.) She also said that he could not tell the time until he was aged ten and a half and that in giving the days of the week he would omit Monday even up to age ten. Her own father, so she told me, had been a very poor speller; and in fact I afterwards saw Simon's two brothers (S16 and S88) both of whom were undoubtedly dyslexic.

In my report I wrote as follows:

> Unlike most dyslexic children he was remarkably successful over digits reversed and unlike some dyslexic children he did not need concrete aids to help him with calculation. Despite these two counter-indicators, however, there seems to me to be a whole group of positive signs – b–d reversals (normally outgrown by children of average ability when they are about 8), special difficulty with digits forwards, losing his place both in reciting the 4 x table and months of the year (with reported similar difficulty over days of the week), difficulty over left and right, and in repeating polysyllables, and reported difficulty over telling the time. His spelling has the 'bizarre' character often associated with dyslexia, e.g. ptrad for betrayed, Foloas for followers, and, as with many dyslexic children, there is uncertainty over boundaries between words. Finally, it seems very likely that other members of the family are, or have been, affected, and this I regard as a particularly strong piece of evidence for a specific handicap.

It is worth recording that, unlike the two cases cited so far, Simon was of near-average ability rather than outstandingly bright. This no doubt meant that it was relatively more difficult for him to devise compensatory strategies. It was possible, however, to arrange for him to receive dyslexia-centred teaching, and two years later he was found to have a 'reading age' of 10 years 4 months (gain two and a half years) and a 'spelling age' of 8 years 4 months (gain one and a half years). A report from his teacher reads:

> He is keen to improve his reading and writing and has been encouraged by the comments of his teachers in school about his progress. He reads quite fluently and, where his interest is engaged, with pleasure... He can use a telephone directory and a dictionary. He has practised writing cheques and filling up forms... His written work has improved, though his handwriting is jerky. But he is using words more freely, asks questions more confidently and converses readily. He used to be very diffident but has become more willing to talk as time has passed .... He has grown in confidence generally.

S208: Joanna

Joanna's mother wrote to me as follows:

> I have a daughter of 17 who wishes to enter a Teacher Training College but she is having difficulty in being accepted, partly due to being dyslexic.

Joanna is apparently (sic) typical of many dyslexics in that she was always a bright child, though at Junior School she now tells us that the teachers told her she was alternatively stupid or lazy... When (she) went on to a senior school she was put in the 'B' stream in a Secondary Modern School and her reports showed average and above average results...She has learned to live with her dyslexia and has overcome things like remembering which is left or right by wearing her watch and a ring on her left hand.

So far (she) has sat for and obtained 6 CSE's including Mathematics, English, and Needlework at Grade 1. (At 'O' level she has Mathematics Grade 1, Domestic Science Grade 3 and English Grade 9.) At present she is studying Physics 'O' level and Mathematics and Needlework at 'A' level to be taken this summer.

Joanna is quite determined to be a teacher, no matter how long it takes her to get into College. She is not only a hard worker but also a perfectionist and from first being told she was stupid apparently her attitude has been I'll show them that I am not stupid.

We feel we badly need advice from someone who not only understands studying, but who also has a real knowledge of dyslexia as well. My husband is particularly concerned as he is also dyslexic and therefore knows the problems Joanna is encountering. We wondered if it would be possible to have Joanna assessed...

When she came for assessment Joanna read 79 words out of 100 correctly from the Schonell R_1 word-recognition test (the 'ceiling' is age 15 and this score gives a 'reading age' of nearly 13), and she spelled 57 words correctly from the Schonell S_1 spelling test which gave her a 'spelling age' of just over 10 years 6 months. Her errors included 'liquicd' for *liquid*, 'assiced' for *assist*, 'amoc' (crossed out), 'acomplished' for *accomplished*, and 'primalily' for *preliminary*. Her mother said that there was a large amount of 'mirror writing' in her school books and that Joanna had been told, 'It is stupid'. I copied the following from her geography book.

MAꟼ Oꟻ THE AЯƎA
CROSƨROAD
MATLOƆꓘ
CARBOИIꟻƎROUƧ LIMEƧTOИƎ

She obtained a score of 23 on the Advanced Matrices intelligence test (where average for a university student is set at 21) and she passed 3 items out of 4 at the second highest level of Superior Adult on the Terman–Merrill test.

On the Left–Right test she pointed to her own right hand correctly, but she made mistakes over 'Touch my right hand with your right hand', 'Point to my left eye with your right hand', and 'Touch my right hand with your left hand', and responded correctly to 'Point to my left ear with your left hand' only after detecting an initial error. She said,

'I've got to turn myself round' (though in fact she did not do so overtly). These responses were a clear 'plus'.

She failed to say the word 'preliminary' correctly and her attempt at
'anemone' was 'moneneney'. At the age of 17 the presence of two
errors also gives a 'plus'.

On the Subtraction test she asked me to repeat 'nineteen take away
seven' and commented, 'I thought you said "seven take away nine"'.
She gave the answer '47' to '52 – 9' and said, 'I got the number in my
head but had to think'. Since the error counts as a quarter of a plus and
the request for repetition as a quarter, the whole item is scored as
'zero'.

She reported considerable earlier difficulty over tables, and, after
saying her 7 x correctly up to 'eight sevens are fifty-six', she said 'Nine
sevens'– pause – 'are sixty-four, no, sixty-three, nine' (corrected to
'ten') 'sevens are seventy; eleven sevens are seventy-seven; twelve sevens are' – pause – 'eighty-four. It didn't sound right when I said it'. The
earlier difficulty counts as half a 'plus', and the two corrections count
as a further half, so that there is a full 'plus' even when the two pauses
are not taken into account. She made the further interesting comment:
'I can never get eight eights. I have to say "seven eights" or "nine
eights" and take away but I can say what is eight squared'.

In the case of Months Forwards, she said, 'I've learned them recently', and she in fact went through them with nothing worse than a slight
pause after June. By the scoring rules this response had to count as
'minus', though it still remains astonishing from the point of view of
clinical assessment that a person of her ability should have learned the
months of the year 'recently' at the age of 17.

In the case of Months Reversed she said: 'January – no, that's the
beginning; December, October – no, November, September, October,

November – no'; and, starting again, she said 'December, November,
October, September, June – August, June' – pause – 'July'. This was
clearly a 'plus'.

On the Digits test, when asked to say 8–4–2–3–9 she said '9–3–8;
I've gone wrong' and when asked to say 5–2–1–8–6 she said
'6–8–1–2–5' (which is correct in the reverse order). When asked to say
'3–8–9–1–7–4' she said '3–8–9–1–4–7' and when asked to say
'7–9–6–4–8–3' she said '7–9–4–6–8–3'. This gives her 'highest success'
as 4 and her 'lowest failure' as 5; a tally of 45 counts as 'plus'.

She passed both attempts (and the practice attempt) at three digits
reversed but failed both attempts at four digits reversed. A tally of 34
also counts as 'plus'. It is perhaps worth recording that the four digits
reversed item is given to 9-year-olds in the Terman–Merrill test, while
the five digits reversed item is given to 12-year-olds. Yet on this test
Joanna was passing items at the level of Superior Adult II.

There had been earlier reports of b–d confusion, and this item was therefore scored as 'zero'. The familial incidence item was clearly 'plus', since Joanna was the sister of S177 and the cousin of S172. Although I had no reason to doubt that her father was dyslexic (and the only written communication that I received from him was further confirmation), the score of 'plus' did not depend on this.

The writing of letters the wrong way round is certainly not typical of dyslexic subjects in general; but Joanna was said to have had problems with her eye muscles quite apart from her dyslexia, and it is possible that the two factors in conjunction made her sense of direction even weaker than it otherwise would have been. When her eye-movements were photographed by my colleague, George Pavlidis, they were found to be extremely irregular (Note 5.1).

I was able to confirm that Joanna was very bright and to encourage her in her attempts to train as a teacher. She in fact settled for taking a Nursery Training course rather than a full-scale Teacher Training course, and her mother reported that she had no regrets. Two years later her perseverance received striking recognition in the form of a Duke of Edinburgh award.

I end with extracts from a press cutting sent to me by her mother:

> An invitation to Buckingham Palace arrived last week at the home of__ – the great reward for years of effort to overcome adversity.
>
> At the Palace [Joanna] will be presented with the gold award of the Duke of Edinburgh's scheme – an outstanding achievement for anyone, let alone one fighting the handicap of dyslexia with colour blindness and a further optical defect adding to the problems...
>
> She is now starting nursery nursing at __ College... to use her understanding of the problems to help others... In all modesty [Joanna] can claim that her success has been achieved largely through her own determination.

Chapter 6
The Summary Chart

The following pages contain a summary of the assessment results in respect of 264 subjects, of whom 257 seemed to me to be unambiguously dyslexic and seven to be marginally so. The 257 cases are made up of 223 where there are complete records and 34 where the records are incomplete (see p.26).

The following abbreviations are used:

Int.   = intelligence grade
R_1 = number of words read correctly on Schonell R_1 test
S_1 = number of words spelled correctly on Schonell S_1 test
DF   = Digits Forwards
DR   = Digits Reversed
L–R   = Left–Right
Pol   = Polysyllables
Sub   = Subtraction
Tab   = Tables
MF   = Months Forwards
MR   = Months Reversed
b–d   = presence of b–d confusion
Famil. = presence of dyslexic tendencies in other members of the family ('nk'='not known')

For details of procedures used see Appendix I. Where a line is placed under the score in the R_1, S_1, DF and DR columns, this indicates that the result is within normal limits for a non-dyslexic person. An asterisk indicates incomplete data; where a result is given in brackets this indicates that the testing had already been done at the time of the assessment. An (m) before the subject's number indicates that he was matched for age and intelligence with a member of the control group (see Chapter 7).

In the 'limits' column, Arabic numerals indicate the highest two subtest scores on the WISC (or, in one case, on the WAIS); Arabic numerals preceded by the letters AM indicate the score on the Raven Advanced

Matrices, and Roman numerals indicate the mental age level of the highest two passes on the Terman–Merrill test (AA, SA I, SA II and SA III are the conventional abbreviations for Average Adult and the three grades of Superior Adult). Where an IQ figure is given in brackets this represents a 'composite IQ' (see Chapter 2) obtained elsewhere, the grade-letter for intelligence level being adjusted to one grade higher.

Chapters 8–23 will contain further information about the subjects whose particulars are given in the Summary Chart. My intention in these chapters is to examine in turn some of the different areas where dyslexic-type weaknesses show themselves and to indicate what are the typically dyslexic ways of responding. Not every subject behaves in exactly the same way, but time and time again the same 'picture' emerges: that of unexpected difficulty in a variety of tasks (unexpected, that is, in view of the intelligence and the opportunities that have been available to him), the resultant frustration, in some cases the compensatory strategies (with varying degrees of success) and the relief when the pattern of the handicap is explained.

The evidence contained in the Summary Chart is an integral part of my argument. If, for example, I had simply indicated that subject x mistook left for right on a particular occasion or that at the age of 11 subject Y made errors in reciting the months of the year, then, in the absence of further information, these would be descriptions of isolated occurrences which might not necessarily have any special significance. If, however, there is the additional information that the person who made a mistake in reciting the months of the year was a boy of above-average ability who had had every opportunity to learn them, there is perhaps something a little puzzling, even though an unsympathetic critic might still feel justified in saying, 'He hasn't learned them: so what?' But suppose, further, that the boy is a very poor speller, that he has had difficulty over his tables, that he has a father and first cousin who are also poor spellers and that he still sometimes puts 'b' and 'd' the wrong way round. Even here, these might simply be particular things which this particular child happened to find difficult, though if I were the critic I think that at this stage I should be starting to wriggle somewhat. If it is then shown that large numbers of other people, quite unlike this boy in respect of age, social background, type of schooling etc. display many of the same difficulties, it becomes all but impossible to view such difficulties in isolation.

What I am saying, in effect, is that the phenomena discussed in the following chapters make sense only if considered in conjunction with the information given in the Summary Chart. It is not just *any* person who made a mistake, say, over left and right: it is case number such-and-such who also displayed the other 'dyslexia-positive' indicators which have been systematically recorded.

The central purpose of the Summary Chart is thus to supply a context in the light of which the responses described in Chapters 8–23 can be interpreted.

It has a secondary purpose, however, namely that of serving as a source of data for statistical description and inference. Although quantification has not been my main aim in this book, it by no means follows that all statistical calculation is irrelevant. There is in the first place plenty of scope in the Summary Chart for so-called 'descriptive' statistics, for example statements as to how many of my subjects were left-handed or had dyslexic relatives; indeed the reader will be able to supply his own descriptive statistics from the data if he so wishes. In addition I decided to use a small number of somewhat more elaborate statistical techniques for purposes of comparison. In particular I wished to compare the performance on the dyslexia test of some of my dyslexic subjects with that of controls matched as far as possible for age and intelligence. My reasoning was that if the two groups behaved no differently then there was no justification for speaking of a 'dyslexia' test, since it was failing to pick out distinctively dyslexic subjects; in so naming it I could rightly have been accused of begging the question. The evidence presented in Chapter 7 shows that there were in fact considerable differences between the two groups, and the method of scoring the dyslexia test makes possible a provisional and preliminary attempt to submit these differences to quantification.

Much more, of course, remains to be done. Further comparison of dyslexic and control subjects could well lead to a more sensitive method of scoring. Suitable 'weighting' of the different items in the dyslexia test according to the extent that they differentiated the two groups would almost certainly lead to a more accurate 'index' of dyslexia, while factorial analysis or a related statistical technique could conceivably contribute towards a more accurate classification of the information-processing tasks required in the dyslexia test. Had these procedures been included, however, I would have been writing a different kind of book (Note 6.1).

Despite the number of questions which remain unanswered, I think it can be claimed that the information in the Summary Chart 'sets the stage' for further quantification. The criteria for scoring responses as 'plus', 'zero' and 'minus' have been determined on the basis of what makes sense clinically, and the resultant symbols lend themselves easily to statistical treatment.

Summary chart

Case no.	Sex	Age (years)	Hand	Eye	Int.	Limits	R_1	S_1	DF	DR	L–R	Pol	Sub	Tab	MF	MR	b–d	Famil. Index
1	M	7;5	L	L	W	14,13	8	2	55	3*	+	+	+	+	+	+	+	0 7.5
(m)2	M	7;5	R	R	X	18,16	27	26	44	33	+	+	+	+	+	+	+	+ 9
3	M	7;6	M	L	X	16,15	0	3	56	33	+	−	+	+	+	+	0	nk 5.5
(m)4	M	7;7	R	R	Z	19,16	26	22	45	23	+	−	+	+	+	+	+	0 8.5
5	M	7;9	R	L	W	17,14	12	15	45	33	+	+	+	+	+	+	+	0 8.5
(m)6	M	7;9	M	R	X	18,17	21	15	56	33	+	+	+	+	+	+	0	+ 7.5
(m)7	M	7;11	R	R	Z	18,17	32	5	55	22	+	−	+	+	+	+	+	+ 8
(18,16) (Expected scores on the R_1 and S_1 tests for 7-year-olds: 20 to 30)																		
(m)8	F	8;0	R	R	U	10,11	8	15	56	33	+	+	+	+	+	+	+	nk 7
(m)9	M	8;0	M	L	X	16,15	12	20	56	34	+	+	+	+	+	+	+	nk 7
(m)10	M	8;1	R	L	Z	20,17	31	24	65	33	0	−	+	+	+	+	+	nk 5.5
(m)11	M	8;2	M	R	U	12,11	7	1	45	34	+	−	+	+	+	+	+	nk 6
(m)12	M	8;4	R	R	X	17,16	24	24	55	33	+	−	+	+	+	+	+	+ 7
(m)13	M	8;4	R	R	X	xii,xi	22	18	67	43	0	−	+	+	+	+	+	nk 6
(m)14	M	8;5	R	R	Y	17,17	41	22	65	34	0	−	+	+	+	+	+	+ 6.5
(m)15	M	8;6	M	R	W	xi,xi	40	29	45	44	−	0	+	+	+	+	0	nk 5
(m)16	M	8;6	R	R	X	17,16	38	41	45	33	+	−	−	−	+	+	−	+ 6
(m)17	M	8;6	R	R	X	17,15	24	16	75	34	0	0	−	−	+	+	+	+ 5
(m)18	M	8;6	R	R	X	17,17	8	16	55	45	0	0	0	+	+	+	+	+ 6.5
(m)19	M	8;7	M	R	W	17,14	40	30	55	43	+	0	−	+	+	+	+	+ 5
20	M	8;7	R	R	X	xiv,xiv	26	18	45	33	+	−	+	+	−	+	+	0 7.5
(m)21	F	8;7	M	R	X	xiii,xii	36	22	53	53	+	−	0	+	−	−	−	0 2.5
(m)22	M	8;8	R	R	W	xi,xi	29	23	65	44	+	−	+	+	−	+	0	nk 6.5
(m)23	M	8;9	L	L	Y	20,16	28	21	67	34	+	−	+	+	+	+	+	+ 7

Summary chart (contd)

Case no.	Sex	Age (years)	Hand	Eye	Int.	Limits	R_1	S_1	DF	DR	L–R	Pol	Sub	Tab	MF	MR	b–d	Famil.	Index
(m)24	M	8;10	R	R	W	15,11	25	15	34	33	+	0	+	+	+	+	0	+	8
(m)25	M	8;10	R	R	X	17,16	17	14	45	33	0	+	+	+	+	+	+	0	8
26	F	8;10	R	R	V	xii,x	12	12	67	23	+	+	+	+	+	+	+	nk	8

(Expected scores on the R_1 and S_1 tests for 8-year-olds: 30 to 40)

Case no.	Sex	Age (years)	Hand	Eye	Int.	Limits	R_1	S_1	DF	DR	L–R	Pol	Sub	Tab	MF	MR	b–d	Famil.	Index
27	M	9;0	R	R	X	16,16	50	24	67	33	–	–	–	+	+	+	0	nk	4.5
(m)28	F	9;1	R	R	V	13,11	47	27	55	43	0	–	0	+	0	+	+	+	6.5
29	M	9;1	R	R	X	xiii,xiii	31	25	45	44	0	–	–	+	+	+	+	nk	5.5
30	M	9;1	R	R	Z	20,17	39	30	66	56	–	0	–	+	0	–	+	nk	3
(m)31	M	9;2	R	R	W	14,13	37	24	65	43	–	–	0	+	–	+	+	nk	4.5
32	F	9;2	L	L	V	xii,xi	37	39	56	33	+	0	+	+	–	+	–	nk	5.5
(m)33	M	9;2	L	M	X	xiv,xiii	44	36	45	33	+	0	–	+	–	0	–	nk	5
34	M	9;2	R	L	Z	SAII,SAI	43	25	88	34	–	+	+	+	–	0	–	+	5.5
(m)35	M	9;4	R	M	X	15,15	19	22	66	34	–	–	+	+	0	+	0	nk	5
(m)36	M	9;4	R	R	W	14,14	15	17	56	33	–	–	–	+	0	+	+	0	7.5
37	M	9;5	R	R	W	(IQ 103)	31	21	67	34	+	–	0	+	+	+	0	nk	6
38	F	9;5	L	L	V	15,11	13	22	45	23	+	0	+	+	+	+	0	0	8.5
(m)39	M	9;5	R	R	W	(15,14)	16	17	56	33	+	–	+	+	+	+	0	+	7.5
(m)40	M	9;6	M	L	W	17,13	35	28	34	23	+	+	+	+	+	+	0	0	9.5
41	M	9;7	R	R	Y	19,17	34	25	55	33	+	0	–	+	+	+	+	nk	6.5
(m)42	F	9;7	R	L	V	15,13	26	22	55	33	–	–	0	+	+	+	0	0	4.5
43	M	9;7	R	L	Y	15,15	34	28	65	34	+	–	+	+	+	+	0	0	7
44	M	9;7	R	L	Y	19,19	26	19	55	33	+	+	0	+	+	+	–	nk	6.5
(m)45	M	9;8	R	L	W	xiii,xiii	54	23	2	23	+	–	+	+	+	+	–	0	6.5
46	M	9;8	R	R	X	18,14	31	25	87	34	+	–	+	+	–	+	+	0	6.5

Summary chart (contd)

Case no.	Sex	Age (years)	Hand	Eye	Int.	Limits	R_1	S_1	DF	DR	L-R	Pol	Sub	Tab	MF	MR	b-d	Famil.	Index
47	M	9;8	R	R	Z	20,19	52	36	65	33	+	−	+	+	+	+	−	nk	6
48	M	9;9	M	R	Z	SAI,SAI	39	25	45	33	+	−	+	+	−	0	+	nk	5.5
(m)49	M	9;9	R	L	W	13,12	22	19	34	33	+	−	−	+	+	+	+	nk	8
(m)50	M	9;10	R	R	X	xiv,xiv	47	27	56	45	+	−	0	+	+	+	−	nk	4.5
(m)51	M	9;10	L	R	Y	19,19	46	26	55	44	+	+	−	+	−	−	+	+	5
(m)52	M	9;11	M	L	X	18,17	30	25	54	33	+	+	+	+	+	+	−	nk	8
53	M	9;11	R	R	X	16,16	45	34	56	33	+	0	−	+	0	+	0	nk	5.5
54	M	9;11	R	L	W	15,13	33	34	56	23	+	0	+	+	−	+	+	0	7
55	M	9;11	R	R	U	12,12	30	18	45	23	0	−	+	+	+	+	−	+	7.5

(Expected scores on the R_1 and S_1 tests for 9-year-olds: 40 to 50)

Case no.	Sex	Age (years)	Hand	Eye	Int.	Limits	R_1	S_1	DF	DR	L-R	Pol	Sub	Tab	MF	MR	b-d	Famil.	Index
(m)56	M	10;0	R	R	X	xiii,xiii	39	34	45	34	0	+	−	+	+	+	−	0	7
(m)57	M	10;1	M	L	U	xi,xi	43	40	44	33	0	0	0	+	+	+	+	nk	7.5
(m)58	M	10;1	R	R	V	16,12	10	16	45	23	+	+	+	+	+	+	−	nk	8
(m)59	M	10;1	R	M	Y	17,17	48	26	45	33	+	+	+	+	+	+	+	nk	9
(m)60	M	10;2	M	R	U	12,11	18	13	45	34	+	0	+	+	+	+	0	0	9
61	M	10;3	R	R	Y	SAI,AA	70	56	67	34	+	−	+	+	−	−	+	+	5.5
(m)62	M	10;3	R	R	W	xiv,xiii	54	42	56	34	+	0	0	+	+	+	0	nk	8.5
63	F	10;3	R	R	Z	SAI,AA	56	42	43	33	+	0	0	+	−	+	0	nk	6
(m)64	M	10;4	R	R	Y	19,17	26	19	67	43	+	+	+	+	+	−	+	nk	7.5
(m)65	M	10;6	R	L	W	xii,xii	25	27	65	33	+	0	0	+	+	+	0	nk	8
(m)66	M	10;7	R	R	X	AA,xiv	39	33	67	34	+	+	+	−	+	+	0	nk	6
(m)67	M	10;7	R	R	Y	17,17	47	37	65	44	+	+	0	+	−	+	+	nk	6
(m)68	M	10;7	M	L	X	xiv,xiii	41	35	56	33	+	0	−	+	+	+	0	+	9
(m)69	M	10;7	M	L	W	15,13	40	31	65	33	+	−	−	0	−	+	+	0	6

Summary chart (contd)

Case no.	Sex	Age (years)	Hand	Eye	Int.	Limits	R₁	S₁	DF	DR	L-R	Pol	Sub	Tab	MF	MR	b-d	Famil.	Index
(m)70	M	10;7	R	R	X	14,14	30	10	67	54	+	+	0	+	+	+	-	0	6
(m)71	M	10;8	R	R	W	14,13	46	26	67	34	+	0	-	+	-	-	-	nk	3.5
(m)72	M	10;8	R	R	X	AA,xiv	33	29	55	45	+	+	0	+	+	+	+	+	8.5
(m)73	M	10;8	M	L	W	13,12	41	35	56	33	+	0	-	+	+	+	-	nk	6.5
74	F	10;9	R	R	Z	SAI,SAI	76	42	55	34	0	0	0	+	-	+	-	+	6.5
(m)75	M	10;9	R	L	X	17,16	75	30	55	33	+	0	0	+	0	+	+	nk	7
(m)76	F	10;9	R	R	X	16,14	40	29	45	34	+	+	-	+	0	0	0	nk	7
(m)77	M	10;9	R	M	X	xiv,xiv	52	29	95	44	0	+	0	+	0	+	0	nk	6
(m)78	M	10;9	R	R	V	13,14	29	12	55	44	+	+	+	+	+	+	0	nk	7.5
(m)79	M	10;9	L	R	W	xiii,xiii	45	33	56	33	+	+	0	-	+	+	-	0	6.5
(m)80	M	10;10	R	R	Y	20,16	52	48	56	43	+	0	0	+	+	+	-	nk	7.5
(m)81	M	10;10	R	L	X	SAI,xiv	35	28	67	43	+	-	0	+	-	+	-	+	4.5
(m)82	F	10;11	R	L	W	14,13	30	26	55	54	+	+	-	+	-	-	+	+	7
(m)83	M	10;11	R	L	X	19,18	17	13	45	23	+	0	+	+	+	+	+	nk	8.5
84	M	10;11	M	L	Z	SAI,SAI	40	45	67	33	-	+	-	+	+	+	0	0	6

(Expected scores on the R₁ and S₁ tests for 10-year-olds: 50 to 60)

Case no.	Sex	Age (years)	Hand	Eye	Int.	Limits	R₁	S₁	DF	DR	L-R	Pol	Sub	Tab	MF	MR	b-d	Famil.	Index
(m)85	F	11;0	R	L	V	14,13	41	41	55	34	+	0	0	+	-	-	0	nk	5.5
(m)86	M	11;0	R	R	W	(IQ 104)	54	27	55	34	+	0	0	+	-	+	-	nk	6
(m)87	M	11;0	R	L	X	AA,xiv	41	27	45	33	0	0	+	+	-	+	0	nk	6.5
(m)88	M	11;0	R	R	U	15,10	24	17	66	33	+	0	+	+	+	+	-	+	7.5
89	M	11;1	R	R	Z	20,18	78	55	65	43	+	0	-	+	+	0	0	nk	7
(m)90	M	11;2	M	R	Y	SAIII,SAII	76	54	56	34	+	0	0	+	-	+	+	0	7
(m)91	M	11;2	R	R	W	AA,xiv	33	29	45	33	+	+	+	+	+	+	0	nk	8.5
(m)92	M	11;2	M	L	W	13,14	52	16	56	33	+	0	-	+	0	+	0	+	7.5

Summary chart (contd)

Case no.	Sex	Age (years)	Hand	Eye	Int.	Limits	R_1	S_1	DF	DR	L–R	Pol	Sub	Tab	MF	MR	b–d	Famil.	Index
(m)93	M	11;2	M	L	V	xiii,xiii	30	26	45	33	+	+	0	+	0	–	+	nk	7
(m)94	M	11;3	R	R	Y	SAI,SAI	37	28	45	53	–	0	+	+	–	+	0	0	6.5
95	M	11;3	R	R	Y	AA,xiv	60	21	65	33	+	0	+	+	–	0	+	nk	7
(m)96	M	11;3	M	L	X	16,16	32	22	55	34	0	0	+	+	–	+	+	0	7.5
(m)97	M	11;4	R	R	X	16,15	60	53	67	53	0	+	–	0	–	–	–	+	4
(m)98	F	11;4	R	R	V	14,12	42	29	34	33	0	+	0	+	0	+	+	nk	7.5
(m)99	M	11;4	R	R	W	AA,xiv	67	42	67	44	–	+	+	+	+	+	0	nk	6.5
100	M	11;4	R	R	X	(IQ 120)	67	45	56	33	+	0	+	+	0	+	0	nk	7.5
(m)101	M	11;4	R	L	U	xiii,xii	50	35	45	33	+	0	0	+	0	+	0	nk	6
(m)102	M	11;5	R	R	X	SAI,AA	37	23	45	33	+	–	0	+	0	–	–	nk	6
(m)103	F	11;5	R	R	U	xiii,xiii	27	24	55	23	+	+	0	+	–	+	+	+	8.5
(m)104	M	11;5	R	R	V	13,13	39	31	45	43	+	+	+	+	+	+	0	+	9.5
(m)105	M	11;5	M	R	X	15,15	31	34	45	34	–	+	+	+	0	+	0	nk	6.5
(m)106	M	11;5	R	R	X	15,14	60	44	55	34	0	0	+	+	+	+	0	+	7.5
(m)107	M	11;6	R	R	W	18,15	37	25	55	33	–	0	0	+	+	+	0	nk	6.5
(m)108	M	11;8	R	M	Y	SAI,SAI	42	21	65	33	+	0	0	+	+	+	+	nk	8.5
109	M	11;8	R	R	Z	SAI,SAII	75	63	67	55	+	–	–	+	–	–	–	nk	2.5
(m)110	F	11;9	R	R	X	AM 17	45	32	66	33	+	+	0	+	–	0	0	+	6
(m)111	F	11;10	M	L	W	(IQs 97 & '110–120')	26	20	45	23	+	+	+	+	–	0	+	0	8
112	M	11;10	M	R	Z	SAII,SAII	65	69	78	65	+	+	–	+	–	0	+	0	5
113	M	11;10	R	R	X	SAI,AA	65	28	56	33	+	+	+	+	+	+	+	0	9.5
114	M	11;11	M	M	Y	SAIII,SAI	48	33	55	43	+	0	0	0	+	+	0	0	7
115	M	11;11	L	R	X	19,15	55	36	65	33	0	–	+	0	–	+	0	nk	5.5
(m)116	F	11;11	R	L	V	xiv,xiii	72	34	45	33	+	–	–	+	+	0	+	+	7.5
(m)117	F	11;11	R	R	V	(IQ 'bright normal')	55	41	45	45	–	–	+	+	+	+	0	+	6.5

(Expected scores on the R_1 and S_1 tests for 11-year-olds: 60 to 70)

Summary chart (contd)

Case no.	Sex	Age (years)	Hand	Eye	Int.	Limits	R₁	S₁	DF	DR	L-R	Pol	Sub	Tab	MF	MR	b-d	Famil.	Index
118	M	12;0	R	R	Z	SAIII,SAI	76	38	66	33	-	+	0	+	+	0	0	nk	5.5
119	M	12;0	R	R	Z	SAIII,SAI	74	48	78	34	+	0	-	-	-	-	0	0	3.5
(m)120	M	12;1	R	R	W	15,14	38	33	55	34	-	0	0	+	+	+	0	+	7.5
(m)121	M	12;1	R	L	X	SAI,SAI	56	42	55	44	-	0	0	+	+	+	+	nk	6.5
(m)122	M	12;2	R	L	W	AA,xiv	61	38	67	45	0	+	-	+	-	0	0	+	4.5
123	M	12;3	R	R	Z	SAII,SAII	78	52	78	33	-	0	-	-	-	-	0	0	3
(m)124	M	12;5	R	R	V	(IQ 99)	10	12	67	34	+	0	0	+	+	+	-	nk	6.5
(m)125	M	12;5	R	L	X	SAII,SAI	60	54	56	55	+	+	-	+	+	+	+	nk	6
(m)126	M	12;7	R	R	Z	SAIII,SAIII	82	52	77	44	0	-	-	0	-	+	+	nk	2
(m)127	M	12;7	R	R	Z	SAIII,SAII	82	56	45	33	+	0	0	+	-	+	+	nk	7
(m)128	M	12;7	R	R	X	20,17	26	18	67	53	+	+	-	0	+	+	0	0	6.5
(m)129	M	12;8	R	L	X	SAI,SAI	60	41	66	55	+	-	-	0	-	0	0	+	3.5
(m)130	M	12;10	L	L	X	(IQ122,117)	(36)	(26)	76	34	+	-	+	+	+	+	0	0	7
(m)131	F	12;11	M	L	U	10,10	37	36	55	44	0	0	-	+	-	+	+	nk	4.5
132	M	12;11	R	L	X	SAII,SAI	56	29	67	43	+	0	0	+	+	+	+	nk	7
133	M	12;11	R	R	Z	SAII,SAII	57	43	67	34	+	+	+	+	+	+	0	nk	8.5

(Expected scores on the R₁ and S₁ tests for 12-year-olds: 70 to 80)

134	M	13;0	R	R	V	16,13	50	46	56	33	+	+	-	+	-	-	-	nk	5
135	M	13;0	M	R	Y	SAIII,SAIII	69	52	55	34	+	+	0	+	-	+	-	nk	6.5
(m)136	F	13;1	R	R	W	SAI,AA	35	33	56	53	0	+	0	+	-	0	-	nk	5.5
137	M	13;1	R	R	Z	SAIII,SAIII	89	71	56	34	+	0	-	+	-	+	-	nk	5.5
138	M	13;2	R	L	X	SAI,AA	62	61	78	64	-	-	+	+	-	0	+	0	5

Summary chart (contd)

Case no	Sex	Age (years)	Hand	Eye	Int.	Limits	R₁	S₁	DF	DR	L–R	Pol	Sub	Tab	MF	MR	b–d	Famil.	Index
139	F	13;3	R	L	Y	SAIII,SAIII	83	57	56	43	0	–	–	+	–	–	+	nk	4.5
(m)140	M	13;4	R	R	W	SAI,SAI	24	21	65	33	–	+	+	+	+	+	–	+	8
141	M	13;4	R	R	X	SAIII,SAI	54	28	76	33	+	0	0	+	+	+	0	0	7
(m)142	M	13;5	R	R	U	xiii,xiii	28	18	44	55	+	0	0	+	–	+	0	+	6
143	F	13;6	M	R	X	17,14	62	61	65	23	+	+	+	+	–	+	+	nk	7
144	M	13;7	R	R	Z	SAIII,SAIII	70	66	56	43	–	+	0	+	–	–	–	nk	4.5
(m)145	F	13;8	R	M	W	SAI,AA	75	35	77	55	+	0	+	+	–	0	+	0	5.5
(m)146	M	13;9	R	L	V	SAI,AA	59	37	45	44	–	0	0	+	+	+	+	nk	7
(m)147	M	13;9	R	R	V	SAI,AA	69	46	77	34	+	+	+	+	+	+	–	0	7.5
148	M	13;9	M	R	Z	SAIII,SAII	85	67	55	34	+	+	0	+	–	0	–	–	7
(m)149	M	13;10	R	R	V	13,12	53	40	66	33	0	0	+	+	+	+	–	nk	6

(Expected scores on the R₁ and S₁ tests for 13-year-olds: 80 to 90)

Case no	Sex	Age (years)	Hand	Eye	Int.	Limits	R₁	S₁	DF	DR	L–R	Pol	Sub	Tab	MF	MR	b–d	Famil.	Index
(m)150	F	14;0	R	L	W	15,13	62	41	55	34	0	0	+	+	+	+	+	nk	8
(m)151	M	14;1	R	R	W	SAII,SAI	71	46	77	33	0	0	+	+	0	+	+	0	7
152	M	14;1	R	R	V	SAI,AA	49	35	45	34	0	+	0	+	+	–	–	nk	6
153	M	14;1	L	L	X	SAI,SAI	75	62	66	23	+	0	+	+	+	+	–	nk	6.5
154	M	14;2	R	R	X	AM 18	74	45	56	33	+	0	+	+	+	–	–	nk	7.5
(m)155	M	14;2	R	R	Z	SAIII,SAII	78	62	67	44	–	–	–	+	–	+	+	nk	4
(m)156	F	14;3	R	R	U	AA,xiv	59	44	76	33	–	+	+	+	–	+	–	0	5.5
(m)157	M	14;3	R	L	V	15,13	54	23	67	43	+	0	+	+	–	+	+	0	7
158	M	14;4	R	M	Z	SAIII,SAII	75	48	45	33	+	+	+	+	+	+	0	0	9
(m)159	M	14;4	R	R	X	AM 19	75	58	56	33	0	0	+	–	+	+	0	0	7.5
(m)160	M	14;5	R	R	U	SAI,AA	61	45	55	43	+	+	+	+	+	+	0	nk	7
161	M	14;5	M	R	Z	SAII,SAII	82	54	78	23	+	–	+	+	+	+	–	nk	6

Summary chart (contd)

Case no.	Sex	Age (years)	Hand	Eye	Int.	Limits	R_1	S_1	DF	DR	L–R	Pol	Sub	Tab	MF	MR	b–d	Famil.	Index
(m)162	M	14;8	M	R	X	SAIII,SAII	47	25	55	33	+	+	+	+	+	+	0	nk	7.5
163	M	14;9	R	R	U	xiv,xiv	46	39	45	33	+	+	−	+	+	+	0	nk	7.5
164	M	14;10	R	R	V	12,11	49	25	55	34	−	0	+	+	+	+	+	nk	7.5

(Expected scores on the R_1 and S_1 tests for 14-year-olds: 90 to 100)

Case no.	Sex	Age (years)	Hand	Eye	Int.	Limits	R_1	S_1	DF	DR	L–R	Pol	Sub	Tab	MF	MR	b–d	Famil.	Index
165	F	15;0	R	R	V	AA,AA	53	40	55	43	+	+	0	+	+	+	0	0	8.5
(m)166	M	15;0	R	R	V	SAI,AA	63	37	78	33	+	+	0	+	−	+	−	nk	4.5
167	M	15;0	R	M	V	AA,AA	30	28	67	43	+	+	−	+	+	+	0	nk	7.5
168	M	15;1	R	R	Z	(IQ 132)	92	80	56	23	+	−	+	+	−	+	0	0	7
169	M	15;1	M	L	Y	SAIII,SAIII	72	51	50	34	+	−	0	+	−	+	0	0	6.5
170	F	15;2	R	L	U	SAI,AA	43	24	55	34	+	+	−	+	−	+	+	nk	7
(m)171	M	15;2	R	R	Y	SAIII,SAII	64	46	67	43	0	+	0	0	+	+	0	nk	7
172	M	15;2	M	R	Y	SAIII,SAII	90	77	78	55	0	−	−	0	−	−	−	+	2
173	M	15;3	M	R	Z	(IQ 141)	86	74	66	55	+	−	−	0	+	+	−	nk	4.5
174	M	15;3	R	R	Y	SAIII,SAIII	76	42	89	55	−	+	+	−	−	+	0	nk	4
(m)175	F	15;3	R	L	W	SAI,AA	88	80	55	34	+	+	+	+	−	+	−	nk	5
(m)176	M	15;3	R	L	W	SAII,SAII	53	33	67	34	0	0	0	+	−	+	−	nk	6
177	M	15;4	R	R	Z	SAIII,SAII	55	47	65	44	+	+	+	+	−	−	+	+	7
178	M	15;5	R	R	V	AA,AA	65	46	65	33	+	−	+	+	−	−	−	+	7
179	M	15;7	L	L	V	SAI,SAI	75	30	78	53	+	+	+	+	+	+	−	0	7.5
(m)180	M	15;8	R	R	W	17,14	48	36	55	44	0	+	−	+	−	+	−	0	6
181	F	15;8	R	L	Y	SAI,SAI	53	36	56	33	+	−	+	+	−	+	−	0	6.5
(m)182	M	15;8	R	R	X	AM 19	81	55	65	44	0	+	+	+	+	+	−	nk	7.5
(m)183	M	15;8	R	R	X	SAIII,SAII	93	64	99	44	+	−	−	+	+	+	−	nk	5
(m)184	M	15;9	R	R	X	SAIII,SAII	87	70	55	43	0	+	−	+	−	−	−	nk	4.5

Summary chart (contd)

Case no.	Sex	Age (years)	Hand	Eye	Int.	Limits	R_1	S_1	DF	DR	L-R	Pol	Sub	Tab	MF	MR	b-d	Famil.	Index
185	M	15;9	R	R	Y	AM 28	85	62	77	53	-	+	+	+	-	+	+	0	6.5
186	M	15;11	R	L	Y	SAIII,SAII	90	54	76	64	-	+	0	+	-	-	-	nk	3.5
187	F	15;11	R	L	W	SAIII,SAI	85	71	75	65	+	+	+	+	-	-	-	nk	5
188	M	15;11	R	R	Y	SAIII,SAII	87	72	56	44	-	+	-	+	+	0	-	nk	5.5
189	M	15;11	M	R	Y	SAIII,SAII	79	44	55	33	-	-	-	+	-	+	-	+	5
190	M	15;11	R	R	V	SAII,AA	(58)	(50)	67	55	-	+	0	+	+	+	-	nk	5.5

(Expected scores on the R_1 and S_1 tests for 15-year-olds: over 90)

Case no.	Sex	Age (years)	Hand	Eye	Int.	Limits	R_1	S_1	DF	DR	L-R	Pol	Sub	Tab	MF	MR	b-d	Famil.	Index
(m)191	M	16;0	R	L	W	17,16 (WAIS)	73	58	77	45	0	+	0	+	-	+	-	nk	5
192	M	16;0	L	L	W	(IQ 108)	64	59	67	33	+	-	0	+	-	-	0	0	5
(m)193	M	16;1	R	R	X	SAIII,SAII	58	33	67	33	+	0	+	+	-	-	0	0	6
(m)194	F	16;1	R	R	Y	AM 23	95	85	56	34	+	+	-	+	-	+	-	nk	6
195	M	16;2	M	R	Z	AM 31	75	57	56	64	+	+	-	0	-	-	+	nk	5
196	M	16;3	R	R	X	SAIII,SAII	86	54	67	43	0	+	0	+	-	-	0	nk	5
197	F	16;5	R	R	Y	SAIII,SAII	75	75	56	43	+	+	+	+	-	-	0	nk	6
198	F	16;6	R	R	W	SAII,SAII	76	65	56	43	+	0	+	+	-	-	0	nk	6
199	F	16;9	M	R	W	SAII,SAII	74	77	56	33	0	+	-	+	-	-	0	0	6
200	M	16;9	R	R	Z	AM 31	79	60	78	33	+	+	-	+	-	+	-	nk	5
201	M	16;11	R	R	Y	SAII,SAIII	60	15	56	33	+	+	0	+	+	0	-	nk	7
202	M	16;11	L	L	W	SAI,SAI	42	22	67	43	+	+	0	+	+	-	+	0	8

(Expected scores on the R_1 and S_1 tests for 16-year-olds: over 90)

Case no.	Sex	Age (years)	Hand	Eye	Int.	Limits	R_1	S_1	DF	DR	L-R	Pol	Sub	Tab	MF	MR	b-d	Famil.	Index
203	M	17;0	R	R	Y	AM 25	92	86	56	43	+	+	0	+	-	+	-	nk	6
204	M	17;2	R	R	W	SAII,SAII	80	53	45	44	+	+	+	+	-	+	-	+	8
205	F	17;3	R	R	W	SAII,SAII	82	73	67	33	+	0	+	+	-	-	-	nk	5

Summary chart (contd)

Case no.	Sex	Age (years)	Hand	Eye	Int.	Limits	R_1	S_1	DF	DR	L-R	Pol	Sub	Tab	MF	MR	b-d	Famil.	Index
206	M	17;4	R	R	V	SAII,SAI	81	43	55	34	+	+	+	+	+	+	0	0	9
(m)207	M	17;4	R	R	X	SAIII,SAII	78	58	56	43	-	+	0	+	-	+	0	0	6.5
(m)208	F	17;4	M	M	Y	AM 23	79	57	45	34	+	+	0	+	-	+	0	+	8
(m)209	F	17;5	R	M	Z	SAIII,SAIII	89	76	55	34	+	+	+	+	-	-	-	nk	6
(m)210	M	17;11	L	L	Z	AM 30	92	60	67	64	-	-	0	-	+	-	+	nk	4.5

(Expected scores on the R_1 and S_1 tests for 17-year-olds: over 90)

(m)211	M	18;0	R	R	Z	SAIII,SAIII	92	67	78	43	+	-	+	+	-	+	0	0	6
212	F	18;1	R	R	Y	AM 25	94	87	75	34	+	-	-	-	-	-	-	nk	3
213	F	18;2	R	R	Y	AM 24	96	80	55	43	+	-	0	+	-	+	+	0	7
214	M	18;2	R	L	U	AA,AA	75	39	56	34	+	+	+	+	+	+	0	+	9.5
215	M	18;4	R	L	Y	SAIII,SAIII	92	85	76	44	0	+	-	0	-	-	-	nk	4
216	F	18;5	R	L	Z	AM 31	98	89	67	34	+	0	-	-	-	-	-	nk	3.5
217	M	18;6	R	R	Y	AM 22	94	86	65	55	-	+	-	+	-	-	-	nk	4
(m)218	F	18;11	R	L	X	SAIII,SAII	90	88	78	55	0	+	0	-	+	-	0	0	4.5
219	M	19;0	R	R	X	AM 18	98	88	67	43	+	-	+	+	-	0	-	+	6.5
220	M	19;2	R	R	Z	SAIII,SAIII	93	75	55	44	+	0	-	+	-	-	-	0	5.5
221	M	20;1	R	M	Y	AM 22	92	23	67	45	0	-	-	0	-	-	-	+	4
222	M	20;9	R	L	Z	AM 30	92	77	67	43	-	0	-	0	-	-	-	nk	3
223	M	23;5	R	M	Y	AM 30	93	78	76	55	0	0	-	-	-	-	-	nk	3

(Expected scores on the R_1 and S_1 tests for 18-year-olds: over 90)

Summary chart (contd)

Incomplete records

Case no.	Sex	Age (years)	Hand	Eye	Int.	Limits	R_1	S_1	DF	DR	L-R	Pol	Sub	Tab	MF	MR	b-d	Famil.	Index
224	F	8;5	R	R	V	xi,x	9	1	55	33	*	0	+	*	+	+	+		5.5+
225	M	8;6	R	R	W	xii,xi	10	13	67	33	+	+	+	+	*	*	+	nk	5+
226	M	8;10	L	R	W	(14,13)	13	9	45	23	+	+	+	+	*	*	+	nk	7+
227	M	9;1	M	R	U	11,10	25	23	45	43	+	0	+	+	0	*	0	nk	7+
228	M	9;5	R	L	X	xiii,xii	*	*	65	33	+	0	+	+	+	+	+	nk	7
229	M	9;5	R	*	U	15,14	12	13	67	34	-	+	+	*	0	+	+	+	7+
230	M	9;10	R	L	W	xiii,xii	39	(34)	55	43	+	0	+	+	*	*	-	0	6.5+
231	F	9;11	R	R	V	xi,x	34	25	55	23	+	+	+	+	+	*	0	nk	5+
232	M	9;11	R	R	X	18,14	37	34	78	33	-	-	+	+	*	*	+	0	5.5+
233	M	10;0	R	L	W	xiii,xiii	34	(14)	55	33	-	+	-	*	-	+	+	0	5.5+
234	M	10;7	R	L	W	13,13	27	23	55	34	0	0	+	+	+	+	+	0	5.5+
235	M	10;8	M	M	U	15,13	24	22	45	*3	+	+	-	+	-	*	-	0	9.5
236	F	10;10	R	R	X	SAI,AA	42	29	56	34	-	+	+	+	+	0	+	0	3.5+
237	M	11;2	R	R	Y	20,20	69	*	65	33	+	+	-	+	-	+	+	0	8
238	M	11;3	R	R	Y	SAI,AA	65	46	78	53	0	-	-	*	-	0	+	+	4+
239	M	11;11	R	R	Y	SAII,SAI	57	*	88	43	-	+	0	+	0	+	+	0	6
240	M	12;1	R	R	*	*	30	25	45	33	+	+	0	+	-	-	+	nk	6.5
241	M	12;2	R	R	Z	SAIII,SAII	64	41	55	33	+	+	+	+	*	*	0	0	7+
242	F	12;9	R	L	X	SAIII,SAI	64	32	55	34	+	0	-	+	-	*	0	0	6.5+
243	M	13;4	R	R	X	SAII,SAI	67	58	65	43	0	†	-	+	-	-	-	nk	3.5+
244	M	13;9	*	*	W	SAI,SAI	68	45	55	33	0	0	-	+	+	+	0	0	7
245	M	13;9	*	*	U	AA,xiv	39	23	56	44	*	*	-	+	0	+	+	0	5+
246	F	14;3	R	R	Z	AM 31	86	67	89	67	+	-	-	*	*	*	+	+	3+
247	M	15;2	*	*	Z	SAIII,SAIII	79	62	78	74	+	-	-	0	+	+	0	nk	5
248	F	15;2	M	M	X	AM 20	70	*	45	33	+	+	0	+	+	*	-	+	7.5+

† This item was omitted because the subject had a severe stammer

Summary chart (contd)

Case no.	Sex	Age (years)	Hand	Eye	Int.	Limits	R₁	S₁	DF	DR	L–R	Pol	Sub	Tab	MF	MR	b–d	Famil.	Index
249	M	15;5	R	R	V	SAIII,SAII	79	63	67	34	+	+	+	+	*	*	–	0	6.5+
250	F	15;8	M	R	X	SAI,AA	61	51	78	43	0	0	+	+	*	*	–	nk	4+
251	M	15;10	M	R	Y	AM 25	84	68	2–	65	–	0	0	–	–	–	–	0	1.5
252	F	16;9	L	L	Z	AM 26	92	92	76	43	+	–	0	*	–	–	0	0	4.5+
253	M	17;5	*	*	Y	SAIII,SAII	78	80	67	44	+	+	–	0	+	–	–	nk	4.5
254	M	18;0	M	R	C	SAIII,SAII	96	*	65	55	+	–	0	+	–	–	–	nk	5.5
255	M	19;2	R	R	A	AM 28	83	65	77	44	+	+	+	–	–	*	0	nk	4.5+
256	M	25	M	R	A	AM 31	*	*	77	73	–	0	*	+	–	–	0	nk	3+
257	M	38;8	R	R	A	SAIII,SAIII	82	56	75	44	+	+	+	+	*	*	0	nk	6.5+

Marginal Cases

Case no.	Sex	Age (years)	Hand	Eye	Int.	Limits	R₁	S₁	DF	DR	L–R	Pol	Sub	Tab	MF	MR	b–d	Famil.	Index
258	F	8;1	R	L	Y	xii,xiii	32	24	67	55	+	–	+	+	–	0	–	0	4
259	F	9;3	R	R	Z	20,20	60	42	67	23	+	–	–	*	–	–	–	+	3+
260	M	9;6	R	L	Y	18,16	29	32	65	45	0	–	–	0	–	0	–	+	2.5
261	F	12;7	R	L	Y	SAI,SAII	21	74	77	45	0	0	–	0	–	–	–	nk	2
262	M	13;9	R	R	U	xiii,xiv	68	68	65	34	–	0	*	+	–	–	0	0	4+
263	F	15;6	M	R	W	SAI,SAII	84	80	78	43	+	–	0	+	–	–	–	–	3.5
264	M	18;0	R	R	V	SAI,SAI	85	66	86	54	–	–	–	+	–	–	–	0	3.5

Chapter 7
Control Data

As was pointed out in Chapter 3, the items in the dyslexia test were chosen because it seemed that dyslexic subjects were having unusual difficulty with them. For many years, however, I was, in a sense, working in the dark. I believed that the test was tapping something relevant and important, but I was in no position to convince the sceptical that this was so and I was not without my own moments of doubt. For example, I knew that some dyslexic subjects had difficulty in saying the word 'preliminary', but it was possible that many other persons who were not dyslexic would also have had difficulty. Similarly, even though some of my older subjects could not say the months of the year in reverse order, was it not still possible that many non-dyslexic persons would also have stumbled or hesitated? With some regularity, too, I seemed to be meeting people who were perfectly adequate spellers but who reported that they sometimes hesitated or made mistakes over 'right' and 'left'. Finally I could not help remembering press reports of literacy surveys in schools: x% of children could not do simple addition; y% could not give the date of Christmas day etc. This led me to wonder whether even those tests about which I felt most confidence – for example, saying the months of the year – were more difficult for, say, the average 11-year-old than I had supposed.

Now it was clearly not the case that dyslexic subjects *always* made these mistakes while non-dyslexic subjects *never* made them. It was still possible, however, that dyslexic subjects were more vulnerable on such tasks – that there was a greater *risk* of their making mistakes. The obvious thing, therefore, was to give the dyslexia test to children of the same ages, if possible matched for intelligence, and check whether the adequate spellers performed any differently from the dyslexic subjects. If they did not, then the words 'dyslexia test' were a misnomer and the attempt to pick out children who had distinctively 'dyslexic'-type difficulties by means of it was a failure. In contrast, if there were more 'pluses' among the dyslexic subjects one could say, not indeed that the value of the concept of dyslexia was from that moment fully established, but at least that the classification into 'dyslexic' and 'non-dyslexic' had thus far resisted refutation (Note 7.1).

It could still be objected that reading and spelling failure – however caused – engenders lack of confidence and that lack of confidence engenders uncertainty when a complete stranger fires questions about 'left' and 'right' or makes unexpected requests such as 'Can you say the months of the year?' If this were so, however, one would expect similar lack of confidence to affect the subject's responses to intelligence test items, and one would then have to explain why lack of confidence affected performance on some items and not on others. To meet this objection, therefore, it was necessary to compare the performance on the dyslexia test of the dyslexic subjects with that of a control group matched as far as possible for intelligence level. Full-scale assessment of control subjects has not so far been possible for reasons of time, but although more remains to be done, a start has been made in that a brief intelligence test, a spelling test, and seven items from the dyslexia test, namely Digits Reversed, Left–Right, Polysyllables, Subtraction, Tables, Months Forwards and Months Reversed, have been given to pupils who were adequate spellers (Note 7.2).

For convenience the control subjects have been divided into three age groups, 7–8, 9–12, and 13–18. The 7- and 8-year-olds were given the Standard Progressive matrices (Note 7.3), as were the 13- to 18-year-olds, while the 9- to 12-year-olds were given the Similarities and Picture Completion items from the WISC (Note 7.4). I then devised a rough-and-ready procedure for converting their scores into the grade labels which I had used for my dyslexic subjects (Note 7.5). The result was the following table of equivalents:

Grade	Raven Matrices Score			WISC Scaled Score
	Age 7	Age 8	Ages 13–18	Ages 9–12
Z	31+	38+	57+	32+
Y	28–30	34–37	55–56	29–31
X	25–27	30–33	53–54	26–28
W	22–24	26–29	51–52	23–25
V	19–21	21–25	47–50	20–22
U	15–18	16–20	43–46	16–19

Any subject was excluded from the control group if his spelling age on the Schonell S₁ test was less than 80% of the bottom of the scale for his age level (e.g. 7-year-olds with a score of 16, 8-year-olds with a score of 24, 9-year-olds with a score of 32, and so on (Note 7.6)). Any subject whose first language was not English was also excluded.

This procedure gave a 'pool' of potential control subjects, of whom 132 were selected on the grounds that each could be 'paired' for intelligence grade with a dyslexic subject of the same age (Note 7.7).

Appendix III gives the relevant particulars for each control subject, that is, sex, age, intelligence grade, S_1 score and performance on the seven items of the dyslexia test mentioned above. As a result, it is possible to indicate the number of 'pluses' obtained both by the control subjects and by the dyslexic subjects on the same seven items (Note 7.8).

Table 7.1 gives further details.

Table 7.1 Particulars of dyslexic and control subjects at three different age-levels			
		Dyslexic subjects	Control subjects
1. Ages 7–8			
No. of subjects		21	21
Mean age (years and months)		8;4	8;4
No. in each intelligence grade	Z	3	3
	Y	2	2
	X	10	10
	W	4	4
	V	0	0
	U	2	2
Mean score on S_1 spelling test		19.95	38.19
s.d.		8.29	10.74
2. Ages 9–12			
No. of subjects		80	80
Mean age (years and months)		10;10	10;10
No. in each intelligence grade	Z	3	3
	Y	9	9
	X	26	26
	W	22	22
	V	13	13
	U	7	7
Mean score on S_1 spelling test		29.3	61.3
s.d.		10.99	13.47
3. Ages 13–18			
No. of subjects		31	31
Mean age (years and months)		15;4	14;10
No. in each intelligence grade	Z	4	4
	Y	3	3
	X	8	8
	W	8	8
	V	3	3
	U	3	3
Mean score on S_1 spelling test		49.81	88.16
s.d.		18.39	6.71

Table 7.2 shows the mean (or 'average') number of 'pluses' for dyslexic and control subjects in each of the three age-groups.

Table 7.2 Number of 'pluses' for dyslexic and control subjects in each of the different age-groups

	Dyslexic subjects	Control subjects	Confidence level
Ages 7–8 (n=21)			
Mean no. of pluses	4.95	3.40	*p* <0.00I
Standard deviation	1.00	1.46	
Ages 9–12 (n = 80)			
Mean no. of pluses	5.14	2.24	*p* <0.001
Standard deviation	1.20	1.37	
Ages 13–18 (n=31)			
Mean no. of pluses	4.87	2.05	*p* <0.001
Standard deviation	0.95	1.21	

Table 7.3 Percentages of dyslexic and control subjects who scored 'pluses' on each of the seven dyslexia-test items

	Dyslexic subjects	Control subjects
Age 7–8		
Digits Reversed	10	0
Left–Right	86	79
Polysyllables	24	21
Subtraction	86	62
Tables	90	71
Months Forwards	90	38
Months Reversed	95	71
Ages 9–12		
Digits Reversed	80	48
Left–Right	78	42
Polysyllables	56	24
Subtraction	58	19
Tables	96	51
Months Forwards	60	13
Months Reversed	86	28
Ages 13–18		
Digits Reversed	94	52
Left–Right	65	53
Polysyllables	66	21
Subtraction	63	10
Tables	85	53
Months Forwards	35	3
Months Reversed	79	13

Table 7.3 shows the percentages of dyslexic and control subjects who scored 'pluses' on each of the seven dyslexia test items. (For convenience 'zeros' have been assigned half to 'plus' and half to 'minus'.)

The figures given in Table 7.2 confirm that at all three age-levels the dyslexic subjects were scoring significantly more 'pluses' than the controls (Note 7.9) Those given in Table 7.3 confirm that all seven items were contributing to the discrimination. It is possible that those of higher intelligence grades, both among the dyslexic and the control subjects, score proportionately fewer 'pluses', but this is a matter for further investigation.

The data in this chapter are incomplete. For reasons of time, it was possible to obtain control data in respect of only seven items in the dyslexia test and, even though the procedures have eliminated the possibility of mental handicap, the attempt to 'match for intelligence' has involved assumptions about the comparability of different intelligence tests which may not be fully accurate. The results, however, are so decisive that one must conclude that this particular attempt to 'knock down' the dyslexia concept has been unsuccessful. 'Plus' scores on items purporting to be indicators of dyslexia were found to be far more common among those believed to be dyslexic than among controls; had this not been so the claim that these items are indicators of dyslexia would have become very difficult to defend.

Postscript

Since 1978 I have carried out over 250 further assessments (Note 7.10). Data in respect of 48 dyslexic adults are given in Chapter 31. With regard to the other cases – those aged 18 and under – a full Summary Chart seemed unnecessary, as it would merely be giving the reader 'more of the same'. However, I have data in respect of 122 subjects, judged to be dyslexic not by clinical 'feel', which was what I used in the earlier cases, but by scores on spelling and intelligence tests (Note 7.11). Table 7.4 shows the percentage of 'pluses' of this group in a form similar to that of Table 7.3. (For convenience, 'zeros' have been assigned half to 'plus' and half to 'minus'.)

Table 7.4 Percentages of dyslexic subjects (1978–1991) who scored 'pluses' on each of the seven dyslexia-test items

	Age 7–8 (%)	Age 9–12 (%)	Age 13–18 (%)
Digits Reversed	36	85	85
Left–Right	86	90	89
Polysyllables	57	69	66
Subtraction	93	79	48
Tables	93	100	94
Months Forwards	96	64	36
Months Reversed	100	82	49

Many of the percentages in the two studies have remained very similar. In particular Months Forwards has percentage figures in the first study of 90, 60 and 35 at the three age ranges, compared, respectively, with 96, 64 and 36 in the second study. Tables has a high percentage – never less than 85% – in both studies, while the percentages for Months Reversed are consistent at the two younger age-groups (95 as against 100 and 86 against 82), though there is somewhat less consistency in the Left–Right and Polysyllables items. (The low percentages for the 7- and 8-year-olds on these two items are, of course, an artefact of the scoring system; see Note 7.8.) In general it seems fair to conclude that the assessment procedure described in Chapter 2 has produced broadly consistent results in the two studies.

Chapter 8
Reading Difficulties

If the central thesis of this book is correct, the difficulties experienced by dyslexic subjects over reading should be regarded as manifestations of a wider problem, namely a limitation in the ability to process symbolic material. The presence of such a limitation, however, does not preclude some success at reading. Indeed, as will be shown in Chapters 19 and 31, there is reason to believe that, in society as it exists at present, difficulties over reading are appreciably more likely to be overcome than difficulties over spelling, and far more likely to be overcome than difficulty in remembering digits.

The extent to which my subjects had made progress in reading at the time of the assessment varied considerably and was no doubt in part a function of the amount and quality of the help which they had received. As an initial step, I judged that it would be helpful to note how many subjects had reading ages of less than 80% of the bottom point of the range for their chronological age (Note 8.1). There were in fact 101 of the 223 subjects who satisfied this criterion (Note 8.2).

When the remaining 122 records were examined, however, there was clear evidence that large numbers of the subjects had experienced problems over reading earlier in their lives. In exactly half of the cases (61) there was independent evidence of a history of reading difficulty, either from the letters of referral or from reports by the subject or his parents made during the assessment. When the scores for the remaining 61 were examined, it was found that 29 of them were below the bottom of the range for their age (Note 8.1), 24 were within the range, and 8 were above it (Note 8.3). In this context it seemed justified to take into account the subjects' intelligence ratings. The frequencies were as follows:

Table 8.1 Intelligence and reading age frequencies

Category	Below the range	Within the range	Above the range
Z	8	7	4
Y	3	10	3
X	8	6	0
W	8	0	0
V	1	1	1
U	1	0	0
Total	29	24	8

As was made clear in Chapter 2, intelligence test grades are not easy to interpret; indeed one has no right to expect that intelligence level and reading level, as judged by standard tests, will be highly correlated (Note 8.4). It is significant, however, that seven out of the eight 'above the range' subjects were in the two highest intelligence grades. Moreover even at the level of category X there was no-one who was above the range for his age, and in category W there was no-one who was even on a level with it.

In very few cases was there significant evidence of the *absence* of a reading problem. S203 and S213 were said not to have been late readers, and it was reported that S183, S185, S204 and S223 did not now have a reading problem (though this does not establish that there was no problem at an earlier age). The most convincing negative case among the 223 subjects was S74, who was stated by her parents to have been a fluent reader at the age of 6. Even in her case, however, it is possible that high intelligence had enabled compensation to take place at an earlier age than usual (Note 8.5).

In general, it seems correct to say that in the very great majority of cases where the dyslexic pattern of difficulties is found the subject's performance at reading is affected, but that there are occasional cases where reading difficulty does not appear to have been a major problem.

It is also regularly reported that dyslexic subjects still tend to read slowly even when they have achieved some degree of proficiency. This indeed is what one would expect in view of their slowness at naming digits which are exposed for a brief presentation time (see Chapter 17); for what they are worth I have some incidental observations which support this view. Thus S252, despite a score of 93 on the R_1 test, said to me, 'Mum was always trying to speed my reading up', and when I asked if this worked she said, 'It didn't – I couldn't do it'. S137, who scored 89 on the R_1 test, said 'Most people would read two lines on the board when I'd done only half a line', while S141 said 'If it's a long word on the board I have to have three looks at it'. A letter from the parents of S221, who by the age of 27 had become a successful business man, mentioned that 'it still takes him longer than others to keep up with the figures'. Similarly S257 reported that if he was handed a balance sheet he would either ask his subordinate to summarise it or 'hedge' by saying that he would look at it later.

In addition, it is widely agreed among those who have worked with dyslexic pupils that reading aloud continues to be difficult even when they are reasonably proficient at reading to themselves. Although I did not investigate this particular problem systematically, it received specific mention in quite a number of cases and I suspect that it is widespread. Thus S159 said 'I don't like reading aloud though I'm not a shy person', while S240 said, rather cryptically, 'In reading, it sounds OK by myself, but when I say it to the teacher I get words wrong'. S209 said that she did not like reading aloud; S91 said, 'I can read to myself but when I read aloud I make a lot of mistakes', while, according to her father, S218 had 'never liked reading aloud'. Even the highly successful business man, S257, reported that he was totally taken aback when, as part of a ceremonial, he was without warning called upon to read the rules of the guild to which he had just been elected as president. There seems no doubt that if a dyslexic person is asked to read aloud this often puts him under considerable strain.

One possibility, of course, is that when he reads to himself he reads inaccurately, but because there is no check by means of the spoken word he 'gets away with it' and his inaccuracies are not detected. It should also be remembered, however, that 'finding the right word' is itself a source of difficulty (Note 8.6) and that when a situation requires word-finding, understanding and appropriate intonation all at the same time the 'load' may be so heavy that at least one of the three is affected. It is interesting in this connection that S169 said, 'When I read aloud in class I didn't hear a word of it; the others did'.

Even when dyslexic subjects read to themselves they appear to have difficulty in 'holding in mind' any large quantity of material. For example, in a discussion of examination questions, S166 said, 'I can read it but I can't understand it if it's a long question – I've forgotton by the time I've read it'. Similarly S186 said, 'Long questions are more difficult. They take time to read, especially questions about quotations'. S169 said that any form of reading took him a long time, and he added, 'I read it once, and I read it again to understand it'. In view of the evidence in Chapter 18 it seems likely that a dyslexic person can more readily 'process for meaning' when material is presented auditorily, even though verbatim recall is difficult. When visual material has to be turned into words, however, the spoken representation has not only to be copied but to be *found;* it is this which causes 'processing for meaning' to be less efficient.

Very occasionally I have met subjects who rely in reading on the visual shape of the word rather than on memory for letters. This strategy is well documented in the case of S95. In her initial letter to me his mother wrote: 'His remedial teacher... believes that he reads almost entirely by remembering the shape of the words... I can endorse this myself'. I myself noted that after a particular error on the R_1 test he said, 'I can see the shape of the other word – I realise it's not the shape it should be. They call me "awkward (Brian)" if I don't remember'. There is in fact good reason to believe that in visual matching tasks where no symbols are involved dyslexic subjects are as quick as controls matched for age and intelligence (Note 8.7), and in a sense, therefore, this subject had chosen a procedure at which he was strong. Unfortunately in most reading tasks the combination of shapes is so complex that it is impossible to remember a sufficient amount of detail for accurate recognition, let alone reproduce it correctly in spelling. To be able to symbolise is a way of reducing complexity. Any of us, of course, if we are unsure of the spelling of a word, may try out what it 'looks like' before committing ourselves. This is in effect to ask not 'Are the symbols correct?', but 'Is the shape correct?'. As a fall-back, this is a possible strategy, but even for those who are weak at responding to symbols it is far from being an efficient one.

With regard to methods of teaching reading, the evidence in my files is by no means conclusive, but neither the ITA ('initial teaching alphabet') nor the method of 'look-and-say' comes out with any credit. Admittedly it is impossible to be sure in a particular case whether other methods would have made things better, or worse, or no different, nor can one say how many potentially dyslexic subjects might have come for assessment had not ITA been of help to them. The comments made, however, were alike in being unfavourable. For example, the mother of S7, who was an experienced Primary School teacher, explained that at the age of 5 John had been introduced to ITA. She continued:

> Not only could he not relate and remember the symbols; he developed an overwhelming sense of complete blanketing failure... We indicated our concern at his school and our story was listened to with care and concern. They didn't think it was anything to do with ITA and suggested I learn the ITA script, and help him at home. From January until his 6th birthday in July I spent a deliberately relaxed and happy hour each evening with (John) in which he drew and I wrote in ITA underneath this he copied. We did some reading together. By the July and after one year and one term at school no progress had been made at all with ITA... Mental stress and state even worse.

His R_1 score when I tested him was in fact 32 (the range for age 7 being 20–30). Like his sister, S74, therefore, he had scored above the age-norm, but there is no reason for doubting his mother's view that he had made progress in spite of, not because of, the use of ITA.

Critical references to ITA were also made in the case of S8, S76 and S160, while 'look-and-say' was adversely criticised by the parents of S76, S112, S136, S159 and S164. In the last-mentioned case the report was of 'four years of failure'.

In the light of the above evidence the following conclusions about the reading performance of dyslexic subjects appear to be justified:

1. Dyslexia is not primarily a reading difficulty: many dyslexic subjects learn to read with a fair degree of success.
2. In almost all cases, however, there is a history of early difficulty in *learning* to read.
3. Most dyslexic subjects remain slow readers.
4. Reading aloud continues to present problems.
5. In a few cases they rely on trying to identify the visual shape of the word instead of thinking of the letters as symbols.
6. Neither ITA nor the look-and-say method of teaching are likely to be successful.

This last conclusion is, of course, a negative one and gives no positive guidance as to how dyslexic subjects can best be helped. If one considers reading in isolation from other language skills, however, it is scarcely possible to avoid being negative; before one can come up with positive suggestions, it is necessary to examine in some detail the spelling errors and other types of confusion which dyslexic subjects regularly display.

Chapter 9
Spelling Difficulties

I begin by quoting a letter written to me by a boy aged 11:

Dear Prassr Mails
     Will you plesas see me my name is — and I am 11 years old.
     My techere sase that my I.Q. is norml put I fandit difeclt to rout a can read Falley wall naw But not is wuk as my Frans and I have been going to reading sclooy for to years.
     Mummey came to her you tuk in Bolton Be For Chustomas and we wandr iF I am diclacktic X if you code see me phaps you cude say if this is so ples
PS pleses see me cowikley becars I have my 11 plus soon

I have in fact managed to collect large quantities of spelling by my subjects. In almost all cases they were given the Schonell S$_1$ test, and in addition I regularly made a point of asking for samples of written work to be brought. This meant that it was possible for me to examine school exercise books and occasionally letters home and other spontaneous pieces of writing. In some cases I was able to retain the originals or have them photocopied, while in other cases I made a record in my own writing of mistakes which seemed to me of special interest. One of the things which impressed me ever since the early stages of the research was what I have called elsewhere (Note 9.1) the 'bizarre' character of dyslexic spelling. I have come to realise, as I shall indicate at the end of this chapter, that such spelling is not in fact *limited* to dyslexic subjects but is characteristic of anyone who is 'out of his depth' in the sense that he needs to spell words that are too hard or sophisticated for him (for example a culturally deprived child, a slow child, or, indeed, a bright 6-year-old child attempting to spell words in a spelling test that are set at the 11 year level). It remains true, however, that bizarre spelling is a common characteristic of younger dyslexic subjects, as I shall try to show by means of the examples which follow; indeed this makes sense, since because of the discrepancy between their intelligence level and their spelling performance they are, of all people, among the most likely to be 'out of their depth'.

I shall begin this chapter by indicating some of the differences between bizarre spelling and what, by way of contrast, may be termed 'plausible' spelling. To make this comparison I shall offer a scheme for characterising and classifying bizarre errors. I shall then give examples of single words or short phrases, written by my subjects, which exemplify the different types of error; these will be followed by longer passages (similar to the one quoted at the start of this chapter) so as to show what bizarre spelling is like in context.

If we look at some children's results on the S_1 spelling test, we are likely to find such errors as 'discription' for *description*, 'asist' for *assist*, and 'wellfair' for *welfare*. In contrast, we may also find 'aviod' for *avoid*, 'instistuns' for *instance*, and 'lquied' for *liquid*. It seems plain to me from inspection that the last three are odd or bizarre spellings, in contrast with the first three which are wrong but plausible.

How, then, are the two groups of spellings different? Perhaps the most helpful general formula is to say that plausible spelling involves a relatively more sophisticated knowledge of sound–letter correspondences (that is, the ways in which the sounds which we say are represented by different letters or combinations of letters in the English alphabetical system). A misspelling is plausible if it might be spelled in that way but in fact is not (where the word 'might' implies conformity with some sort of rule or principle which makes such a spelling possible). In contrast, in the case of bizarre spelling, many of the 'rules' or 'principles' (if they merit the term) are highly idiosyncratic, and the knowledge of sound–letter correspondences is much less sophisticated. Indeed, one continually notices the number of things which the speller has *failed* to pick up, for example that words are divided into syllables and that each syllable must contain at least one vowel. This is not to suggest that the ordinary speller knows these things explicitly in the sense of being able to verbalise what the rules or principles are, but once he has reached a certain level of sophistication he implicitly follows such rules and can tell that there is something wrong if they are broken.

The difference is no doubt one of degree. Even in bizarre spelling one can recognise attempts within certain limits to make use of sound–letter correspondences, and there is thus a limited degree of plausibility, while in plausible spelling there are errors which could be avoided if the speller had some highly sophisticated knowledge, for example if he was aware of the Latin derivation of the word 'description'. It therefore seems to me incorrect to say that there are hard and fast dividing lines between the bizarre and the plausible. It is rather that there is a gradual grasping (whether implicit or explicit) of the way in which the English spelling system works, and the more bizarre-looking spellings arise if the person has not acquired a knowledge of certain rules or principles yet attempts spellings which require such knowledge.

The expression 'bizarre-*looking*' is important. It is, of course, the fluent reader who notices that bizarre spelling is bizarre, and it is he who is likely, both when he reads and when he checks spelling, to identify the word as a whole rather than depend on sounding out individual letters. Indeed, it is safe to assume that to many young dyslexic subjects there is no distinction between what is bizarre and what is not since they lack a knowledge of the phonic rules which would enable them to carry out the appropriate monitoring.

In view of the total evidence cited in this book, it seems to me quite impossible to go along with those who say that all the spelling problems of the allegedly dyslexic child would disappear if the teaching methods used in the early stages were adequate. The basic dyslexic handicap, however, is not such as to *preclude* the learning of adequate spelling (Note 9.2); I do not doubt that bizarre spelling can progressively be eliminated as the pupil's knowledge of the English spelling system becomes more sophisticated. The direction of causality I believe to be as follows: as a result of a constitutional limitation the dyslexic child does not learn characteristics of the English spelling system which in a normal environment the non-dyslexic child simply 'picks up'. Suitable specialist teaching can compensate for this and thus, in a sense, absence of such teaching is a causal factor in producing the poor spelling; but it has an effect only if superimposed on the initial constitutional limitation (Note 9.3).

What is it, then, about bizarre spelling which makes it bizarre? In an attempt to answer this question, I undertook the difficult task of attempting a re-classification of spelling errors. I say 're-classification' because various attempts in this direction have been made already (Note 9.4), and I think it is fair to say that different classifications are suitable for different purposes.

One of my difficulties was that when a word is misspelled there may be several different things wrong with it. Thus when S80 spelled *non-existent* as 'nonxextant' one could say that the x-sound had been duplicated, that the combination of letters 'xex' is impossible, and that the word, if pronounced as he wrote it, would have contained the wrong number of syllables. In some cases, therefore, I have indicated alternative error-categories to which the word might equally or near-equally belong. In this particular case 'nonxextant' is in fact classified as a 'false match for order', but I indicate that it could also be classified as an 'impossible trigram', as a misrepresentation of the number of syllables, or as the 'duplicating of a sound' (for a description of these categories, see below). Indeed there are a number of occasions where the 'omission of a sound' and an 'impossible trigram' go together: if a sounding vowel is left out an 'impossible trigram' regularly results.

A second difficulty is that in classifying one is not merely giving a factual report: in putting two misspellings into the same category, one is implying the same theoretical explanation, and this is a matter where one may be in error. In some cases, indeed, one needs to know the context in which the mistake was made. Thus, to cite an example given by my wife (Note 9.5), if an attempt to spell *write* comes out as 'witer', one may misclassify this error if one considers only its visual appearance – correct letters in the wrong order – and overlooks the fact that the child originally wrote w-i-t-e- and later added the 'r'. In other cases a particular theoretical approach may encourage a classification of a particular kind. For example someone in the tradition of S. T. Orton might take the view that the writing of 'was' for *saw* should be classified along with b–d confusion as a special kind of 'reversal', whereas my own classification places it along with 'forgein' for *foreign* – an attempt to rely on memory for the recall of the correct letters coupled with the inability to remember or deduce their order (Note 9.6).

One of the things which this classification achieves is to call attention to the fact that there are certain things which the dyslexic child in the early stages of learning to spell does not pick up, for example that the letters on the page are representations of what we say and that certain combinations of letters, for example 'lqu', cannot arise. It is this failure to 'pick things up' which makes sense of the first four of my categories (see 1–4 below). Another six (5–10) are accounted for in terms of weak immediate memory for verbal material and 'losing the place', while a further two (11 and 12) can be seen as attempts to compensate. The final category (13) is that of b–d confusion, to which I return in Chapter 12.

Any spelling that can be fitted into one of these 13 categories can be regarded as to some extent bizarre, in contrast with spellings such as 'discription' for *description*, cited earlier, which are mistakes but have nothing bizarre about them.

Moreover, by classifying spelling errors in this way one is calling attention to dyslexic weaknesses *which can be put right by teaching*. Let us suppose, for example, that a pupil writes down a combination of letters which, if pronounced according to the normal rules of sound–letter correspondence, would give the wrong number of syllables. From the teaching point of view one can treat this as evidence that he is unaware of how written words can be divided into syllables – an important feature of English spelling which can then be shown to him.

Finally, an incidental advantage from the classification is that one can check whether certain types of misspelling are more common in dyslexic than in control subjects. This may well turn out not to be the case, but if one simply goes by the number of words correctly spelled all possibility of comparison is lost.

For convenience of reference each category has been given an abbreviation of two or three letters or thereabouts. I begin with a description of the first four.

1. The impossible trigram

The first category is what I call 'the impossible trigram' (IT). This involves a combination of three letters which are impossible in normal English spelling because they would represent something unpronounceable, for example starting to spell *liquid* with the letters 'lqu'. As I see the situation, the normal reader picks up, even if not explicitly or consciously, the fact that certain combinations of letters cannot go together; he picks up certain 'rules' of spelling much as the fluent speaker picks up the 'rules' of grammar. Thus it will be plain to most readers of this book that 'sha', 'tep', 'spr' and 'tho' are possible combinations of letters in English words, whereas 'spk', 'wll', 'qww', and 'hja' are not. My suggestion is that a knowledge of sequential probabilities is something which normal spellers simply 'pick up' in the process of learning to spell; for the dyslexic person, however, because of his limitations of immediate memory, there is too much going on, and this kind of knowledge is therefore 'squeezed out'. The result is that he cannot appropriately monitor what he has written and does not therefore recognise that it comprises an impossible combination of letters.

2. Misrepresentation of the sound

The second category is what I call 'misrepresentation of the sound' (MoS). Although there are exceptions, most dyslexic children come to recognise that sounds can be represented by letters, and this is shown in their spelling. There may, however, be difficulty in making the representation accurate, particularly in the case of sounds or vocal movements which are similar; when this happens the word as spelled may contain one or more 'wrong' letters in place of the correct ones, for example 'cet' for *get* (S8) or 'bugger' for *buzzer* (S142)(Note 9.7). In addition, the difficulty in accurate matching prevents them from monitoring what they have written or appreciating where they have gone wrong.

There is a complication here in that some teachers have supposed – somewhat uncritically in my opinion – that such errors can be described as 'auditory'. I do not dispute that hearing loss can be associated with dyslexic manifestations (compare Chapter 20), nor that as a result of hearing loss there are people who, for instance, fail to distinguish 'p' and 'b' or hard 'c' (or 'k') and 'g'. In my experience, however, a child who has written 'pat' when asked to spell the word *bat* can often recognise perfectly well that 'pat' and 'bat' are different when the two words are spoken; I suspect that often the error is not auditory at all but one of memory. It is well established that auditory confusability hinders recall (Note 9.8), and it therefore makes sense that dyslexic subjects, whose recall is weak anyway, should not be wholly secure in knowing which to use of two auditorily confusable letters; this is quite different from being unable, as a result of some weakness in the auditory system, to discriminate that two sounds are different. Moreover, the position is sometimes made more complicated by the fact that the same letter is pronounced slightly differently according to which other letters are near it, for example the letter s in 'sister' has the effect of making the sound represented by the t almost a d-sound. In this case it would be very rash to say that a person who wrote 'sissder' for *sister*, as did my first dyslexic pupil (Note 9.9), *cannot hear* the difference between 't' and 'd'. Similarly, as my wife has pointed out (Note 9.10), the Welsh for 'skirt' is 'sgert', and a child in a Welsh area who, when asked to spell the English word, writes 'sgert' may be confused between the two languages but does not necessarily have a specifically auditory deficiency. In general I suspect – though I am not sure – that most of the errors in this category made by my subjects are memory errors resulting from auditory confusability; this certainly coheres with the idea that dyslexia involves some kind of limitation of immediate memory.

3. Wrong boundaries

The third category of error is that which I call 'wrong boundaries' (WB) between words. The error can take two forms: either a single word is written with a space between the parts as when S74 put 'a nother' for *another*, or separate words are written together without a space, as when, among my early subjects, a young man of 14 (who later went to university) instead of writing *chest of drawers* wrote 'chesetofbrours'. It seems that most of us learn to deal with boundaries between words without much difficulty, but, to judge from their spelling errors, this is one of the things which may become 'squeezed out' in the case of dyslexic subjects.

4. Wrong syllabification

The fourth category is that which I call 'wrong syllabification' (WS). In this case the written word comprises a collection of letters which, if pronounced according to normal English sound–letter correspondence, would result in a word with the wrong number of syllables. Thus if *avoid* were written as 'aviod' and these letters were then pronounced accordingly, the sound would be approximately 'avvi–od', which, unlike 'avoid' contains three syllables and not two; similarly 'instistuns' for *instance* (S97) would contain three syllables instead of the requisite two. These WS errors seem to me to be evidence that the subject has not picked up some of the more sophisticated kinds of sound–letter correspondence. Thus in the case of 'aviod', he is displaying lack of awareness that 'oi' is a digraph, i.e. represents a single sound (or almost so), whereas 'i' followed by 'o' involves two separate syllables. Dyslexic subjects can, of course, be taught to divide words into syllables, and indeed this is an important part of their training, but it is a skill which they sometimes do not acquire unless they are explicitly shown how to do so.

We can also think of dyslexics as being impaired in the area of immediate memory (Note 9.11); and the next six error-types seem to me to be a direct consequence of this impairment.

5. Inconsistent spelling

The fifth error-type may be termed 'inconsistent spelling' (IS). This description is used when the same word is spelled differently within a few lines. I believe that in the majority of cases subjects do not notice the inconsistency and that the reason for this, once again, is because too much is going on. If the present situation is problematic one is in no position to take account of what has gone before (Note 9.12).

6. Wrong letter doubled

The sixth category is 'wrong letter doubled' (WLD), for example 'eeg' for *egg* (S24) or 'sppeling' for *spelling* (S107). I suspect that what is involved here is a knowledge that *something* must be doubled but that the person does not remember or deduce which letter it is. I have come on only a relatively small number of such errors, but I believe they merit being placed in a separate category.

7. Mistaken recall of order

The seventh category is 'mistaken recall of order' (MRO). I am thinking here of situations where the subject draws largely on his memory that certain letters are needed but does not know and cannot deduce the order in which they should occur. Thus he may know that the word *how* contains the letters h, o and w, but may write it as 'who'. I was told that the brother of S221 (who was also dyslexic) once wrote to his parents, 'Dear Mum and Dad, Who are you?' This was not, I am sure, an expression of existential bewilderment!

It should be noted, in view of the special limitations of dyslexics, that reliance on memory is an inefficient strategy. Indeed it is widely agreed that they would be better advised to pay careful attention to the order of letters in the spoken word – and the number of syllables – and then deduce what the order of the written letters *has* to be if there is to be sound–letter correspondence.

My classification of the controversial 'was' for *saw* as an MRO is deliberate. Undoubtedly this mistake is found, though according to my records it is rarer than one might suppose in view of the frequency with which it is cited in theoretical papers. Orton speaks of it as a 'kinetic reversal' – in contrast with the 'static' reversals, 'b' for 'd' and 'p' for 'q' – and he suggests that in these cases the person is somehow going through the letters of the word in the wrong order. It seems to me more likely, however, that the mistake arises because the speller possesses a limited knowledge of how words are made up: he is aware that three-letter words often have a vowel in the middle and consonants on the outside and this knowledge prevents him from writing 'wsa' or 'asw', but, this point apart, the exact inversion of the order of the letters is of no special significance. Similarly he may write 'on' for *no* simply because he is muddled about order, and it may be coincidental that 'on' and 'no' are mirror-images of each other. Despite my respect for Orton I find it difficult to agree with him over this particular aspect of his theory; indeed, interesting though mirror phenomena are, I am not convinced that they are related to dyslexic phenomena at all, and I find it puzzling that the neurological explanations suggested by Orton to account for dyslexic-type mistakes (non-elision of the mirror-image engrams, or traces, in the two halves of the brain) should generate mirror-images in the case of 'static' reversals (e.g. 'b' for 'd') but inverted order of letters (e.g. 'was' for 'saw') in 'kinetic' reversals. A classification in accordance with Orton's ideas would presumably involve the grouping of 'was' for *saw* along with b–d errors, but according to the present classification it involves successful recall of the letters themselves but failure to remember or deduce their correct order.

It follows from the above discussion that the same end-product, namely correct letters in the wrong order, may conceivably occur for different reasons. Even if one does not accept Orton's view of the matter, this point still raises difficulties of classification. Thus, when I came on 'thrid' for *third*, it seemed to me quite likely that the subject was not in fact drawing on his memory but was attempting a phonic representation in which letters and sounds had got 'out of step'; if this was what happened the correct classification of this misspelling is ' false match for order' (FMO, see below). One would have needed to be present at the time of writing, and possibly even to have questioned the subject. However, the 'reliance on memory' explanation seems to me plausible in most cases; and I have therefore, with hesitation, classified as MRO ('mistaken recall of order') those misspellings where all or most of the correct letters are present, albeit in the wrong order.

Moreover even if my explanation is wrong, it is, I think, still justified to record these errors as a single group, since the fact that people can sometimes produce the right letters for spelling a word and yet be unable to put them in the right order, whatever its explanation, remains a puzzling and challenging phenomenon.

8. False match for order

The category of 'false match for order' (FMO) is similar to that of 'mistaken recall of order' (MRO) in that in both cases errors of ordering occur. I believe, however, that they occur for different reasons. False match for order is, I suggest, a 'loss of place' phenomenon and in that respect is comparable with the omission and duplication of sounding letters (OmS and DupS; see below). A typical example of the FMO error is 'aklumpist' for *accomplished* (S249) where there is a mismatch between the 'l' of the written word and the l-sound of the spoken word, the written 'l' occurring too early. Such mistakes seem to me to indicate difficulties similar to those which occur when dyslexic subjects become 'tied up' in saying polysyllabic words (see Chapter 13). They are somehow 'out of step' as a result of having reached later components of the word sub-vocally before the earlier components have been committed to writing. It is, I believe, a case of what psychologists call 'retroactive interference' (in other words later material hinders the correct reproduction of earlier material), and I suspect that the influence of such interference is particularly great when the components of the spoken word are similar either in sound or in the way in which they are articulated. Thus it is the presence of the labials, l, m, n and r which make it difficult for some people to say the word 'preliminary', and this difficulty is no doubt reflected in their misspellings (examples of which I have set out separately). There are also parallels, I believe, with the 'where-have-I-got-to?' response which regularly occurs when dyslexic subjects attempt to say their tables (see Chapter 16).

The concept of 'ordering', however, and the related concept of 'sequencing' both seem to me to raise problems. In particular there are grounds for thinking that it is not *any* kind of ordering task which the dyslexic subject finds difficult, but only tasks which involve the ordering of symbolic material (Note 9.13). Thus a dyslexic subject might well assemble the components of a lock or other mechanism in extra quick time, even though he would almost certainly take longer if reading a book of instructions was necessary. I am reluctant, therefore, to attribute these FMO errors to a failure at ordering *simpliciter*; they seem to me rather to be a manifestation of weak immediate memory when auditorily confusable symbolic material is present.

9. Omission of one or more sounding letters
10. Duplication of one or more sounding letters

Categories (9) and (10) – the omission of one or more sounding letters (OmS) and the duplication of one or more sounding letters (DupS) – can be considered together. An example of the first is 'Agsea' for *Anglesey* (S52) while an example of the second is 'Cheshshire' for *Cheshire* (S117). Any of us may make such errors when we are being 'careless', but I suspect that dyslexic subjects are particularly prone to them because there is too much to hold in mind. Like FMO ('false match for order') they exemplify the phenomenon of 'losing the place'. Thus the subject may suppose that he is further forward than in fact he is, in which case he leaves something out, or he may suppose that he is further back than he is, in which case he repeats the same letter or combination of letters twice. The parallels with the 'Where-have-I-got-to?' response which one regularly finds when dyslexic subjects attempt to recite their tables (see Chapter 16) has already been mentioned. It is perhaps worth adding that those who edit texts which contain corrupt passages – for example, writings in classical Greek or Latin – have sometimes found it helpful to restore the sense of a passage by postulating the occurrence of one or other of these errors. To fail to write the same combination of letters twice over when this is needed (e.g. 'rember' for *remember*) is referred to as 'haplography' (literally 'single writing'), while repetition of a combination of letters which should have occurred only once (e.g. 'animimals' for *animals*) is referred to as 'dittography' (literally 'writing twice over'). As has already been suggested, we all make 'dyslexic'-type errors from time to time, and one would not expect mediaeval scribes who copied classical texts to have been in any way exceptional in this respect (Note 9.14).

11. Phonetic attempt misfired
12. Intrusive vowel

The next two types of error seem to me to arise as a result of attempts by dyslexic subjects to compensate. Because they cannot easily reproduce the correct letters simply by 'remembering' them, they try to use such phonic knowledge as they possess even though it is inadequate for their needs. Category (11), then, is the 'phonetic attempt misfired' (PAM). One can recognise the spellings as phonetic (that is, with letters matching sounds) but the result is incongruous since other necessary conditions for correct spelling are not satisfied. Thus 'whiv' for *with* counts as a case of PAM since the 'w' and 'i' sounds are exactly represented and the 'th' sound approximately so. But the attempt to put the three sounds together has misfired, partly because of the confusion between 'w' and 'wh', partly because of confusion between 'th' and 'v', and partly through ignorance of the relatively sophisticated 'rule' that no word ends in a 'v'.

This particular error could in fact be classified as a misrepresentation of sound (MoS), since it is arguable that there are differences in sound between 'w' and 'wh' (though many people ignore them) and between 'th' and 'v' One could even classify it as an impossible trigram (IT), since at the end of a word 'hiv' is not possible even though it is found at the beginning and in the middle. As was indicated above, however, the categories which I have proposed are not intended to be mutually exclusive.

Possibly PAM is in any case something of a 'ragbag' category, since attempts at phonetic spelling can go wrong for a variety of reasons. Nevertheless it is convenient to group together those misspellings where some kind of phonetic representation has been attempted but which are incongruous because a more sophisticated knowledge of the English spelling system is lacking. Certainly most of the PAM errors can readily be seen to be bizarre.

Category (12) could almost count as a sub-group within category (11). It comprises mistakes where there is an intrusive vowel (IntV), for example the spelling of *swallows* as 'sowollos' which I found among the written work of my first dyslexic pupil (Note 9.15). As can be seen, this is in a sense an attempt at phonetic representation which has gone wrong, and indeed it could also count as a case of wrong syllabification (WS) since the intrusive vowel necessarily specifies an extra syllable which is not present in the spoken word. It nevertheless seems convenient to put such mistakes in a category of their own in view of their likely origin. What I suspect has happened, though I have no firm evidence, is that the subject tries to use a phonetic approach and in so doing says the word extra slowly and carefully. Now if one tries to do this in the case of the word 'swallows' one has to say something like 'ser-woll-owes', and it is therefore perfectly logical to try to represent this extra syllable in what one writes.

13. b–d substitution

My final category, which I style BD, is that of substitution 'b' for 'd' and vice versa whether in upper or lower case letters. This confusion seems to me sufficiently problematic to be discussed separately (see Chapter 12). If it occurs in conjunction with errors belonging in the other categories the bizarre effect is intensified. 'Chesetofbrours' is a good example.

I now pass to actual examples of spelling errors. I have so many of these that I have had to be selective, and I think the most helpful procedure is to start by citing misspellings of single words or groups of words in each of the 13 categories (with possible overlaps and alternative classifications indicated where appropriate). After that I shall present full sentences and longer pieces of writing where many different errors are combined.

In a few cases it is possible that the spelling error had been made appreciably earlier than the time of the assessment. This sometimes happened when parents produced school exercise books of an earlier period. For the most part, however, it is safe to assume that it occurred shortly before assessment. The subjects' ages, which I have included after giving their Summary Chart numbers (see Chapter 6), are thus an approximate guide as to the age at which the mistake occurred.

There are many points about the misspellings which readers will notice for themselves. Of these, I should like to mention three. In the first place, even short words of two or three letters are not always exempt from error; secondly, the logical nature of most of the spellings seems to me to be an indicator of the amount of effort which went into producing them; thirdly, the continuous sentences which follow the single words are often highly sophisticated. This last point underlines the plight of those who have intellectually powerful ideas but who, because of the medium through which they have to operate, namely the written word, are severely handicapped in communicating these ideas to others.

To make the data as complete as possible I have included quite a large number of misspellings in most categories. I doubt if any valid conclusions can be drawn about relative frequencies of types of error, since there was no safeguard against bias in my selection of what seemed interesting; but it is important to emphasise that bizarre spellings are not just occasional curiosities but are regularly found in the written work of large numbers of dyslexic subjects.

Some examples of dyslexic spelling are given in Table 9.1.

Table 9.1 Examples of dyslexic spelling

Target word(s)	Written as	Subject	Age	Other ways of classifying
1. Impossible trigrams (IT)				
quite happy	qwwht hape	10	8	PAM
swallowed	swlowd	14	8	OmS
through	freuu	14	8	PAM
walks	wrrks	24	8	PAM
park	prkr	24	8	PAM
further	frtr	24	8	PAM
people	pilplla	36	9	FMO
made	mde	36	9	PAM
Scotland	Sctland	36	9	OmS

Table 9.1 (contd)

Target word(s)	Written as	Subject	Age	Other ways of classifying
domestic	dmestkig	232	9	OmS
geography	geogrphy	56	10	PAM
hymn	hmy	63	10	PAM
mechanical	micknkle	63	10	OmS
accordance	acordns	63	10	PAM
barley	brliy	64	10	–
combined harvester	conbiy hrts	64	10	MoS
crystal	crestl	72	10	MoS
tidal	tiddl	83	10	PAM
swirling	swrling	83	10	PAM
going	gowing	88	11	-
with	whthe	94	11	PAM
water	watrt	96	11	FMO
usually	uslle	96	11	PAM
started	strted	96	11	PAM
obedient	obetnt	101	11	OmS
marjoram	mreygoron	107	11	PAM
production	prodkshon	108	11	OmS
milk	mlke	112	11	PAM
conquered	cquerd	113	11	OmS
happening	hpaning	113	11	OmS
edge	egn	110	11	PAM
pretend	prtend	110	11	PAM
persuaded	pswaded	110	11	–
wanted	wnntied	110	11	–
different	diffnt	110	11	OmS
successful	succusffl	126	12	PAM, WLD
worry	whre	128	12	PAM
first	frst	136	13	PAM
ground	grwd	140	13	PAM
similarities	smilaartis	145	13	OmS
detergent	dturgent	149	13	–
nothing	nthing	149	13	–
unpopular	uppular	246	14	OmS, PAM
heard	hrad	196	14	PAM
Ephesus	Efusfst	196	14	FMO, PAM
write	wrte	210	17	PAM
fought	forght	213	18	PAM

2. Misrepresentation of the sound (MoS)

job	jop	8	8	–
bell	pell	8	8	–
live	lif	8	8	–
get	cet	8	8	–

Target word(s)	Written as	Subject	Age	Other ways of classifying
Table 9.1 (contd)				
Christendom	chisingdum	23	8	–
during	geuring	34	9	–
needle	megl	72	10	–
paddled	pagelid	103	11	–
exploring	egsbloring	123	12	–
first	firsk	128	12	–
buzzer	bugger	142	13	–
fitted	fidid	152	14	–
nitrogen	nigeragan	163	14	–
hub cap	ubcab	171	15	WB
continued	contnderd	177	15	–
negotiations	nocosiatios	253	17	–

3. Wrong boundaries (WB)

Target word(s)	Written as	Subject	Age	Other ways of classifying
together	to gefer	14	8	–
indeed	in ded	20	8	–
a castle	acasul	34	9	–
forget	for get	57	10	–
eiderdown	I dodown	69	10	–
another	a nother	74	10	–
get ready	getready	74	10	–
cattle market	catellmacet	87	11	–
employer	in ploner	103	11	MoS
in the foreground	intefregound	111	11	OmS
a tennis court	atenis chort	113	11	–
woken	woa kern	100	11	–
chopper	choa per	100	11	–
a type	atipe	135	13	–
no-one	nowon	153	14	–
together	to gether	160	14	–

4. Wrong syllabification (WS)

Target word(s)	Written as	Subject	Age	Other ways of classifying
kittens	kins	36	9	–
oxygen	oschun	72	10	–
watched	wastast	94	11	–
instance	instistuns	97	11	–
sneaked	snecet	113	11	–
next	necese	120	12	–
explanation	explaintion	143	13	–
method	meathered	146	13	–
leaped	leepded	150	14	–
edge	egeg	158	14	–
down	dwonon	160	14	–
assist	asiced	207	17	–
believe	bleav	212	18	–

Target word(s)	Written as	Subject	Age	Other ways of classifying
Table 9.1 (contd)				
5. Inconsistent spelling (IS)				
Aragon	Arergin Aergon	53	9	–
because	becuss becuce	63	10	–
calculation	calcilation calculation calcilation caculation	100	11	–
Joseph	Josheph Joeph	127	12	–
would	whord whored	136	13	–
echoed	ecode ecoad	138	13	–
fire	fier ferar	145	13	–
(The actual sentence was 'fier to make ferar plasyes')				
dinner	dinner diner	151	14	–
(The actual sentence was 'It is dinner time he goes and has diner')				
suddenly	sunndy sunndly	162	14	–
ladies (lady)	laides laydey	191	16	–
Ephesus	Efusfst afess, efese	196	16	–
6. Wrong letter doubled (WLD)				
egg	gee	24	8	FMO
spelling	sppeling	107	11	–
freeze	frezze	162	14	–
7. Mistaken recall of order (MRO)				
else	esle	6	7	FMO
are	aer	23	8	–
snow	sonw	25	8	FMO
each	aech	27	9	–
two	tow	32	9	–
after	afrte	28	9	IT
fuel	fule	31	9	–
window	windwo	33	9	DupS
went	wnet	33	9	FMO
cavalry	cavaryl	33	9	FMO
metal	meatl	47	9	PAM
park	pakr	52	9	–
two	tow	52	9	–
to	ot	57	10	FMO
in	ni	58	10	FMO
to	ot	64	10	FMO
who	how (with crossings out)	65	10	–
army	amry	69	10	FMO
died	deid	69	10	–
drawing	darwing	70	10	FMO

Table 9.1 (contd)

Target word(s)	Written as	Subject	Age	Other ways of classifying
edge	egde	71	10	–
how	who	73	10	–
third	thrid	83	10	FMO
argument	agrument	84	10	FMO
reading	raeding	111	11	–
acid	aicd	237	11	FMO
garden	graden	85	11	–
night	nigth	103	11	–
four	fuor	107	11	FMO
draw	darw	110	11	FMO
Florence	florenec	110	11	DupS
search	sreach	117	11	FMO
bridge	bigder	117	11	FMO
goes	gose	241	12	Possibly PAM
question	qusetion	241	12	IT DupS
goes	geos	126	12	WS PAM
cloud	could	126	12	FMO
golden	gloden	126	12	FMO
basin	baisn	126	12	–
built	biult	127	12	WS
your	yoru	128	12	WS
two	tow	132	12	–
colour	coulor	139	13	–
hair	hiar	143	13	–
nasturtium	nasturtuim	165	15	–
quietly	quitely	171	15	WS
believe	belevie	171	15	WS
soldiers	soilders	178	15	–
tired	tierd	178	15	–
fields	feilds	183	15	–
how	who	189	15	–
poem	peom	192	16	–
avoid	aviod	192	16	WS
arguing	agruing	192	16	FMO
would	woudl	202	16	–
David	Daivd	202	16	WS, IT
of	fo	202	16	–
else	eles	206	17	WS
field	feild	209	17	–
piles	plies	209	17	–
diary	dairy	210	17	–
dairy	diary	216	18	–
again	agian	216	18	WS
prologue	prolouge	223	23	–

Table 9.1 (contd)				
Target word(s)	Written as	Subject	Age	Other ways of classifying

I found 'saw' for *was* in the case of S82 and 'was' for *saw* in the case of S73 and S227; in the case of S21 her mother reported that she had written 'was' for *saw* in the past.

I also came on the following errors which I believe should be classified alongside the above, since they come very near to being 'the correct letters in the wrong order': 'sied' for *said* (S20), 'tsaion' for *station* (S51), 'hoow' for *who* (S64), 'unfarirly' for *unfairly* (S94), 'geuse' for guess (S160), and 'Jeuses' for Jesus (S246).

8. False match for order (FMO)				
remembered	remberded	228	9	–
farmer	framer	52	9	–
sister	sitosr	52	9	–
country	cronty	52	9	–
Tower Bridge	torw brigde	57	10	–
readily	rediyl	62	10	–
mileage	milgeag	70	10	–
ferrous sulphate	efrors sulphate	72	10	WS
percolate	pecrlous	79	10	–
non-existent	nonxextant	80	10	IT, WS, DupS
terrible	terrilb	82	10	–
screamed	creemded	82	10	DupS, WS
Jerusalem	jlosolam	84	10	–
themselves	them sleves	85	11	WB
against	agents	94	11	–
writing	wtihing	96	11	–
people	pelpe	96	11	–
domestic	desimce	98	11	–
especially	epesley	99	11	–
estimate	estnamat	101	11	–
bicycle	biciksl	108	11	–
because	beacs	113	11	–
pressure	persure	126	12	–
ill	lile, changed to ile	132	12	–
your	uoy	132	12	–
referring	ferering	139	13	–
knew	wnew	162	14	–
ignorance	ogronence	167	15	–
ill	li, changed to il	172	15	–
accomplished	aklumpist	178	15	–
topic	popic	189	15	–
domestic	dismostite	197	16	–
entered	enadt	202	16	–
foreign	frogin	210	17	–
exceptionally	expotinaly	210	17	–

Table 9.1 (contd)

Attempts at 'preliminary':

S74	plrinary
S136	primalery
S148	plimenery
S152	pritiremy
S155	plimiary
S179	plirimonery
S177	premanarly
S185	prelimerlary
S206	preremeanally
S208	primalily

Target word(s)	Written as	Subject	Age	Other ways of classifying
9. Omission of one or more sounding letters (OmS)				
father	fther	26	8	IT
suddenly	suddly	32	9	–
Scotland	Sctland	36	9	IT
amount	amt	52	9	–
didn't	dedt	52	9	–
Anglesey	Agsea	52	9	WS
treason	teson	53	9	WS
protestant	prostent	56	10	–
preparation	prepartion	79	10	PAM
effect	efek	84	10	–
drainage	drange	237	11	–
immediately	imeadialy	90	11	–
protestants	proestats	90	11	FMO, WS
exceptionally	explunaly	90	11	FMO, WS
conquered	concert	110	11	WS
imagination	imaduntion	134	13	MoS
didn't	din't	139	13	–
conclusion	caclason	141	13	–
successful	susseful	143	13	–
deficiency disease	defiences diase	244	13	–
mosquito	mositow	145	13	–
malaria	miara	145	13	WS
atmosphere	aterfere	146	13	–
melancholy	melokoly	150	14	–
occurred	occed	153	14	WS
introduction	introdutan	155	14	–
conversation	convistion	159	14	–
attendance	etedents	165	15	FMO
assist	esete	165	15	–
carbon dioxide	cobondox	165	15	–
decision	dession	168	15	WS
attendance	attendce	169	15	WS

Table 9.1 (contd)

Target word(s)	Written as	Subject	Age	Other ways of classifying
marriage	marge	170	15	WS
criticised	critized	175	15	WS
irresistible	erestabl	177	15	WS
pre-historic	prestorick	178	15	WS
interested	intressed	180	15	WS
attendance	adence	180	15	WS
domestic	demstick	180	15	WS
different	diffet	181	15	WS
inorganic	iorganic	185	15	–
decision	dession	187	15	WS
especially	espally	196	16	WS
irresistible	irresable	197	16	WS
syllabus	slabols	199	16	WS
conditions	condions	200	16	–
happened	happed	200	16	WS
anniversary	anvissary	203	17	FMO
exceptionally	exepthaly	207	17	WS
mechanical	mechinal	208	17	WS
different varieties	diffent varites	209	17	WS
mechanical	mechinal	210	17	WS
excessively	excively	213	18	WS

10. Duplication of one or more sounding letter (DupS)

Target word(s)	Written as	Subject	Age	Other ways of classifying
language	languaguage	23	8	–
damage	damageage	32	9	–
their	theirir	46	9	–
square	sqaurare	47	9	–
damage	damiamge	56	10	–
day dream	day dremeam	79	10	–
Eglwswrw*	Eglwswrwrw	83	10	–
edge	egegar	91	11	–
geography	gagragphy	114	11	–
doesn't	dosesant	99	11	–
Cheshire	Cheshshire	117	11	–
exceptionally	exececep-titonally	148	13	–
tree	trere	167	15	–
talk	tokok	167	15	–
forty	fortyty	169	15	–
won	onene	202	16	–
collapsed	collazaped	204	17	–
signature	signinature	208	17	–
financial	finacical	223	23	OmS, WS

* A Welsh village

Table 9.1 (contd)

Target word(s)	Written as	Subject	Age	Other ways of classifying
11. Phonetic attempt misfired (PAM)				
witch	wij	8	8	–
with	whiv	14	8	–
remain	rmen	20	8	IT
used	yost	23	8	–
squeezing	scweecing	23	8	–
choir	cwioer	27	9	–
beautiful	byotiful	27	9	–
ash tray	ach traie	32	9	–
piano	pinou	33	9	–
skidded	sckided	34	9	–
few	fyoow	37	9	–
changing of the guard	chejing out the gord	37	9	–
they	tha	36	9	–
ropes	roaps	47	9	–
cousin	coisn	47	9	–
goes	goase	47	9	–
assist	asisd	47	9	–
baby	baybiy	47	9	–
other	uvr	49	9	WS
our	aor	49	9	–
rice and curry	ris and kure	49	9	–
owns a pub	ons a pud	49	9	BD
experts	eepcts	61	10	–
blue jeans	bluw jens	71	10	–
squirrel	scwirel	71	10	–
blowed	blod	72	10	–
use	yoos	72	10	–
your	yuwer	73	10	–
Alexandra	Alicsandrur	74	10	–
ruin	roowin	75	10	–
jutted	ghutid	75	10	–
carefully	cerfly	75	10	–
people	pepeole	87	11	–
furnace	fernec	87	11	–
driven	driyvur	88	11	–
reasons	resonse	89	11	–
departure	depacher	89	11	–
equaliser	eckerliser	94	11	MoS
during	joring	94	11	MoS
edge	ejeg	98	11	–
sewage	seuge	99	11	–
relief	releeth	100	11	–
potato	ptatow	103	11	–
Europe	urup	107	11	–

Table 9.1 (contd)

Target word(s)	Written as	Subject	Age	Other ways of classifying
educational	egercashonal	108	11	–
highly	hily	108	11	–
squeezed	scwisd	113	11	–
recognise	receynys	127	12	–
radiation	radeasu	128	12	–
next	nexed	135	13	–
injection	ingecshen	138	13	–
decision	disishen	138	13	–
built	byilt	142	13	–
edge	eg	146	13	–
telegraph wires	telegphe whyers	150	14	IT, OmS
area	ereaia	151	14	–
hesitating	hesertaghting	153	14	–
Elijah	iliger	158	14	–
goes through	gos thoow	169	15	–
immediately	amejitley	174	15	–
baggage	bagidgsh	174	15	IT
examined	igzamind	174	15	–
exhausted	egsorsted	178	15	–
furniture	farnichare	181	15	–
cautious	cuitious	188	15	–
hedge	heag	191	16	–
poaching	potshing	191	16	–
edge	ajd	193	16	–
toes	tows	193	16	–
actual	atchial atchel	204	17	IS
eventually	avenchuly advencherly	204	17	IS
syllabus	scyllbus	210	17	–
12. Intrusive vowel (IntV)				
boil	boyul	27	9	–
millions of miles	melions of miy-yils	108	11	–
twenty	tewenty	241	12	–
exactly	ecacctely	158	14	–
13. b–d confusion (BD)				
daughter	borte	23	8	PAM
down	bwon	25	8	MRO
did	bib	26	8	–
daddy	baddy	26	8	–
because	deakos	28	9	PAM
down	bwnd	227	9	DupS
do not	Boo not	57	10	PAM
celebrated	selladratid	64	10	PAM

Target word(s)	Written as	Subject	Age	Other ways of classifying
odd numbers	obd nudners	72	10	OmS
square numbers	spur nudners	72	10	OmS
bubble	budl	72	10	PAM
be	de	75	10	–
bubble bath	dudl dath	96	11	–
February	fadrey	103	11	OmS
alphabet	alferdet	113	11	PAM
bulb	buld	126	12	–
declared	becalad	146	13	WS; IntV
Deuteronomy, Chapter 6	Beut c 6	246	14	–
exhibition	exadtion	177	15	OmS
Bunsen Burner	Bunsen Durner	185	15	–
job	jod	202	16	–
pudding	Pubbing	213	18	–
Scribes	scrids	213	18	–

Table 9.1 (contd)

I pass now to some continuous passages. These will perhaps give the 'flavour' of dyslexic spelling more than does the presentation of isolated words, and in addition they may be of help in indicating to examiners, prospective employers and others that very strange spelling mistakes are not necessarily evidence of lack of ability.

Among the written work of the 11-year-old S95 I found a letter which contained the following:

> Dear David
> I got yor letre and by the way am itritid in mchrie [interested in machinery]

Quite large numbers of my subjects were in fact itritid in mchrie, and it does not take much imagination to be aware of the frustration which they must have felt at the discrepancy between their knowledge of mechanical matters and their ability to put their ideas down on paper.

Here is a piece of even more sophisticated thinking from – surprisingly enough – another 11-year-old (S113). This passage was taken from one of his school books and was written under the title 'My idea of God'.

> I donot beleave in God one reson is that there is no profe that there is such a being as god and a nather is that if you went up to a person that had not herd ether verson and you thold him the siantific verson and the bible he would by most licley to belive in the siantific explanason more than the bible. I do bleave in Chiscianaty but not in god him self. I do not thing that god could make the woarld in six days I thing that plant life was made by serton atoms cuming to gethe but where did the atoms came from?

Here is part of a story by another 11-year-old (S93):

All the time that he wut the little butfil sat on the brim of is hat gust a buv
the left iea at night full When the Miller Went tiod tied to bede the butfliy
folied it wings and slept by the leg of the mills old cher (Note 9.16).

Here is a passage from a 13-year-old (S142) which clearly shows
both high-level scientific aptitude and difficulty in getting his ideas
down on paper:

We can yus, y us the LMF to caclat the same valys

Here are two passages from a 14-year-old (S157):

I have gust cum from whork I was ran ing rather hard I have just den lowk-
ing throw the lowchel cronicul have seen two Descos avertised. I am thinking of starting a Discho it will hcost me about 60£ dut my dad will make me
the amply fiers and some things els...I whont to de a shef when I leve
shcool. when I go to Dacis [dances] evry theing otside I forget my waris and
proplems and the sam at Discos

He also writes:

I like going for walks with gerls I supos it is Becose of my age you *[crossed
out]* I can for get thing and trudes [troubles] when I am with thems dut
gerls can de trudul sum times. Running is an enegetick hody dut I can think
when I am runing like the Book the long lost runner

Here are two very interesting passages from a 16-year-old (S193),
one a dictation from a concert programme, one a piece of spontaneous
writing:

Parvane Op. 50 by Fauré
Comp. in 1887, a year befor the recweum, but publised after ~~tha~~ that work
fo as op. 50, for smal orchestra and oshonal chorus, Fauré himself dicreted
this delicat peas as "carfully rort but not otherwise important". It is a seling
of a texst by Verlane (meny of whos powems Fauré set: eg the unfogetabel
"Clare Daloona"), a pasterel conversation of not grat petick valyou; usaly the
work is performed without the words. Yet the work is sagnificant in the
same wright as some of the Verlane songs sins it is further proof of Faure
abilaty shard with somemay French artists of his time, to recreat the past,
espeshaly the age the of racoco, without lapsing into ~~on a~~ an epectadly
"peryod" maner of expretion. Not the lest fasanating part of the this littal
peas is th ocestration, with it sensative differenshiation of wood-wind tambr-
ers, althou it may not, infact, be by Fauré himself.

One the most difficult thing to wright is something just of the cuff as you lit-
erat perent have not ~~p~~ read the letter propely.

The thing which most illiterats peopel live perpetual feer of, is by geting into a situation were one has to read or by someone ones slipe of the tong, It get into your soshal circals. Luckerly this seldom hapens becaues as one is always one your tows. You have alway got to be ready to drag your frends ~~of~~ out of the room ~~wh~~ were ~~fom~~ famerly are, ~~U we~~ when the conversation gets to deep into the suject "o" leval.

I may be panting a ~~ver~~ very black picker, but to be quite honest it is not as enerjetick all that becaues it become a seconed sens.

The writing of 'comp' for 'composed' in the first passage is presumably a form of shorthand necessitated by lack of time. The difficulty of having to spell in French as well as English is emphasised by the barely recognisable 'Clare Daloona' for 'Clair de Lune', while the ability to be explicit about how he copes with his literacy problems is striking evidence of the way some dyslexic subjects can describe their difficulties without bitterness.

In general, it is plain from the above passages that dyslexic subjects often have plenty to say but that they may have totally disproportionate difficulty in writing it down.

Chapter 10
Confusion between Left and Right

My main source of evidence for confusions between left and right is the responses given by my subjects to the ten Left–Right (body-parts) items in the dyslexia test. Details of these items are given in Appendix I and methods of scoring in Appendix II. For ease of reference, however, the items are repeated here, along with their code letters. They were as follows:

(a) Show me your right hand
(b) Show me your left ear
(c) Touch your right ear with your left hand
(d) (Putting hands on the table) Which is my right hand?
(e) Touch my left hand with your right hand
(f) Point to my right ear with your left hand
(g) Touch my right hand with your right hand
(h) Point to my left eye with your right hand
(i) Point to my left ear with your left hand
(j) Touch my right hand with your left hand

For convenience I have divided the material in this chapter into two sections. In the first I cite evidence which indicates the existence of a general uncertainty on the part of many of my subjects when they were presented with tasks involving use of the words 'left' and 'right'; in the second I cite some of the many examples of compensatory strategies which they had evolved in order to circumvent their difficulty.

General Uncertainties in Left–Right Tasks

Many of the subjects were fully articulate about their difficulties. For example S139 said, 'I once gave my friend directions. I said the right-hand side when it should have been the left-hand side'. S143 said 'I get muddled up sometimes... On a horse they say go round to the right and I am liable to go to the left'. S241 said, 'There's a game called "Lifeboats". I call out "starboard" when it should be "port". I'm told which side is which at the start of the game but I forget it'. The mother of S110 said in a letter that her daughter 'had to give up dancing class because left and right were too confusing'.

Fortunately it is possible for many subjects to laugh at mistakes of this sort which are seldom disastrous. Thus S181 said to me 'People say, "Which way?" I say "right" when it should be "left" and that will take them into a ditch!'

In some cases, however, mistakes were made without the subjects being aware of the fact. For example, when I asked S1 which hand he wrote with, he said rather scornfully 'My left hand, of course', but at the same time held up his right. Similarly S128 gave the following account of his difficulties: 'I spent a lot of time learning it' [i.e. the difference between left and right]. 'I remembered, "Which hand do I write with?" I learned it securely when I was around 6'. Yet despite his use of the sophisticated word 'securely' he in fact made two errors, one on item (h), one on item (j). S148, whose intelligence rating was Z, said: 'Sometimes I get mixed up, not often. I thought of which hand I write with – it becomes automatic'. Yet even after appreciable pauses he had to correct his responses on items (h) and (i). Asked to show me his right hand S70 showed me his left hand, explaining, 'I was going to put my left up; I wasn't thinking'. (By implication the hand which he in fact put up was his right.)

The following are further examples of uncertainties. S54 was described in my notes as having 'paused and looked down at his hands', while S232, after correctly pointing to my right hand in item (d), said, 'No, this is my right' (showing his left), 'no, this' (showing his right), and for all the remaining items was correct for his own side and incorrect for mine. After completing the series S197 said, 'I don't know if I'm doing it right or wrong.' S160 said 'I kept getting "right turn" and "left turn" mixed up'. When S83 was asked to point to my left eye with his right hand (item (h)) there was a long pause, followed by a sigh (which appeared to indicate how difficult he found the task), after which he said 'This one' and pointed to *his own* right eye. S71 correctly showed me his right hand but instantly added 'It's a guess', while S73 incorrectly showed me his left hand but then gave a laugh and said 'This', showing his right. S65 said simply 'I find I get a bit mixed up', while S108 said 'Sometimes I can; sometimes I forget'. S162 hesitated and finally showed me his left hand, saying as he did so: 'I think I've got it wrong – that's left. I always get muddled up'. S4 stopped to think, and after correctly showing me his right hand said 'Is it right?' S44 incorrectly showed me his left hand, saying as he did so, 'I've forgotten'. S135 said, 'If you walk along and someone says "Put your right hand up" you think "Which one?"' Even the highly intelligent and mature S218 reported that 'she sometimes got confused' in giving directions.

An interesting phenomenon was the existence of errors which were consistent. Here is a record of the behaviour of S6 (which I wrote down while a colleague did the testing). Asked by the tester to show her his right hand he showed his left hand; when asked to show his left ear he pointed to his right ear, and when asked to touch his right ear with his left hand he touched his left ear with his right hand. Asked which was the tester's right hand he pointed to her left hand; and he then correctly touched her left hand with his right hand and pointed to her right ear with his left hand – he then indicated that he thought this was a mistake and changed his policy so that thereafter his own right and left sides were correctly given but those of the tester were consistently incorrect. This degree of consistency must clearly have called for very considerable intellectual power (he was only 7 years old), and the picture is clearly not that of a person who fails to distinguish right and left through being too young or insufficiently intelligent.

Similar 'consistent' errors also occurred in the case of S7, S23, S32, S49, S53, S54, S75, S158, S201 and S240, while S26 gave the 'consistent mirror image' answer to all items except (j) (where she 'correctly' touched my right hand) and S111 gave the 'consistent mirror image' answer to all items except (g) (where she was 'correct' in pointing to my right hand but incorrect in using her left hand in order to do so). It is almost certain that these 'correct' responses by S26 and S111 were in fact mistakes by their own standards – something which they would have changed if they had had the opportunity and been alert enough to do so. In this connection the performance of S41 is of sufficient interest to be quoted in full:

> Tester: 'Show me your right hand' (Subject shows his left hand) 'Are you sure?' (Subject looks puzzled) 'Show me your left ear' (Subject shows his right ear) 'Touch your right ear with your left hand' (Subject touches his left ear with his right hand)... 'Point to my right ear with your left hand' (Subject *correctly* points to tester's right ear, though with his own right hand.) In the notes taken at the time I wrote: 'I think this is a *double* error. He's got his own side wrong; so by getting my side 'wrong' he ends up by getting my side right!'

In passing, it is worth noting how unsatisfactory from the point of view of dyslexia research are those large-scale studies which record simply the *number of correct responses*. If the record had merely shown, for instance, that S6 made two correct responses out of 10, the really interesting aspects of his behaviour would not have been recorded, and he would have been classified among those whose two correct responses out of 10 occurred for quite different reasons. The existence of these 'consistent' errors, then, is additional evidence that the subjects were not simply being 'careless' or 'stupid' since in that case the errors would have been purely random. Inconsistency is easy to achieve; consistency in getting the wrong answer is not.

In another respect, however, it seems likely that there is a greater degree of *in*consistency among dyslexic subjects. Such is their uncertainty that one cannot be sure that they will necessarily give the same answers if the various test items are repeated a second or third time, and I found that in some cases they did not. My normal practice was to give the test items only once, but occasionally I gave them more than once, and the following table shows the inconsistent performances of S89, S127, S134, S137 and S145 on their first and second trials. (R = right, L = left; all questions were of the form, 'Touch my ... with your ... hand'. Correct responses are underlined; a stroke indicates a changed response.)

Table 10.1 Inconsistency in performance										
Correct	*S89*		*S127*		*S134*		*S137*		*S145*	
answer	*1st*	*2nd*	*1st*	*2nd*	*1st*	*2nd*	*1st*	*2nd*	*1st*	*2nd*
(d) R	R		L	R	R		R		L	R
(e) LR	LR	RR	RR	LR	RR	RR/LR	LR	LR	LR	LR
(f) RL	LL	LL	RL	LL	LL/RL	RL	LL	RL	RL	RL
(g) RR	LR/LL	RR	RR	RR	LR	RR	RR	RR	RL	LR
(h) LR	LR	LR	RR	RR	RR	LR	LR	LR	RR	LR
(i) LL	RL	RL	LL	LL	LL	LL	LL	RL/LL	LL	LL
(j) RL	LL		LL	LL	LL	LL	LL/RL	RR/RL	RR	RL

In reply to (i) S134 said 'Left to right, did you say?' but gave the correct answer! In the first trial S137 originally responded LL to (j) but changed to RL; the correct answer to (g) in the second trial was given only after a pause, and in reply to (i) he responded RL but immediately added, 'No, that's wrong' and corrected to LL, while in reply to (j) he corrected from RR to RL.

S60 was consistent in giving the wrong answer on my side (i.e. RR, LL, LR, RR, RL, LL), and when I tested him again after explaining what was needed he made five mistakes out of six on *his own* side (LL, LL, RL, LL, RL, LR).

Sometimes the uncertainty is reflected in unusual comments. Thus S201, when asked which was my right hand, pointed to my left and said, 'That is your really right hand... To me that is... oh, lor!' At this point he seemed to realise something, as he then said: 'If I was sat that way' (turning in his seat) 'that would be your left but to me it's your right'. On the first time through he gave the consistent mirror image of the correct answer (see above); on the second time through, he was correct on all the items, the only 'positive' indications being a hesitation and a request for repetition over item (j). S193 reported an experience which is familiar to many of us when the task is more complicated: 'If suddenly you think, "Which is your right hand?", you can't say'.

There is a further phenomenon which some of my subjects mentioned and which appears to be another exemplification of difficulty over left and right, namely difficulty over laying the table. Thus S119 said, 'I still set the knives and forks wrongly', while S241 said 'I get knife and fork the wrong way and put the plate on the wrong side'. Similar difficulties were reported by their parents in the cases of S75, S141, S171 and S244, and the mother of S90 said, 'He sets the table the wrong way round, and one of his problems is that he can't see it!'.

Compensatory Strategies

A large number of my subjects made use of mnemonics and compensatory strategies. One of the ones most frequently cited was that 'you *write* with your *right* hand'. This was used, so they told me, by S28, S48, S54, S63, S75, S76, S82, S93, S125, S130, S132, S135, S148, S157, S177, S194, S202 and S244. S76 said 'If my teacher says "Put up your right hand" I quickly say "Which hand do I write with?"' Asked to show me his right hand S220 said ' I know because I had my pen in it'.

A number of subjects had learned that their watch was on the left hand. S52 said, 'I wear my left hand with my watch on' (sic). 'If I don't have a watch I'd get mixed up… If I'm swimming and haven't a watch I have to copy off other people'. S237 said 'I know my watch is on my left hand; that makes it easier'. S17 said, 'Normally I wear my watch on the right, so I was thinking which hand I had my watch on… I can recognise it a bit as I have a feeling I have my watch on'. At the start of the Left–Right test S126 immediately looked at his watch, and when tested with his watch off he reported that he 'had to think'; he also said that he was liable to become confused in physical education classes when he had to take his watch off. S181 said, 'I write with my right hand and have my watch on my left hand that's how I used to work it out'. Others who referred to their watches were S112, S114 and S195, the last two reporting that they wore their watches on the right hand.

A few subjects had undergone some minor injury on one side of their bodies. Thus S12 said, 'This arm was hurt in rugby so that's how I know sometimes'. S170 reported that she used both her watch (on her left hand) and a scar on the right of her face. S158 said he knew which was his left hand because of an accident to his little finger. S141, after hesitation, correctly showed me his right hand; when I asked him if he had had any difficulty over right and left he said, 'I only know it as it's the one I kick with. I hurt my left knee – they said "Which?" I couldn't tell, but from then on I knew it was my left knee as it was always hurting'.

Other subjects had their own idiosyncratic methods which they were quite willing to talk about. S119 said that he learned left–right at the age of 10 because of a scar on his right hand; 'I always used to get mixed up'. S146 said, 'I think of the piano in front of me'. S248 said ' I paint one toe red and one toe green... I've got a lump on my finger... I have to think, for example at crossroads'. S234, who came from a Roman Catholic family, had learned that his right hand was the one with which he made the sign of the cross. S208 was reported by her mother as having to mark her gloves 'left' and 'right'. S205, in reply to 'Show me your right hand', said 'The only reason I know is I have a lump on my finger'; S212 said 'My left thumb is double jointed so I go with that', while S217 said, 'I wear that ring on my right hand'. S131 said she knew which was her right 'because there's a freckle on my left hand' (my notes record that in response to items (f) and (g) she 'looks at her right hand and works it out'). S102 reported a technique which he did not make fully clear: in reply to 'Show me your right hand' he said, 'I know it because it's the way I sit'. As far as I could make out the technique involved imagining himself in class and also imagining a boy next to him who presumably was known to be on his right or left. S169 said, 'I had to write "left" and "right" on my bike and on the back of my hands'. S67 said 'I always had to turn left to go to school', and S165 said 'I remember the wall outside my house'. S129 said, 'I learned that my blazer pocket was on the left'.

Another strategy adopted by some subjects was that of asking for the question to be repeated or echoing it themselves under their breath (hence my use of the symbols 'RR' and 'EQ'; see Appendix II). For illus-tration purposes here are some examples. When S165 was given item (e) she said, 'Will you say it again?'; when given item (f) she said 'Your right ear?' as a question, and when given item (j) she said 'Will you say it again?' (I in fact did so, and even then she touched my *left* hand with her left hand when it should have been my *right* hand.) S197 in reply to item (f) said 'Did you ask for right ear?' (Other comments included, 'My sister says they were ages trying to teach me... I still don't know if I'm doing it right or wrong'.) S80 in reply to (c) said semi-aloud, 'My right ear with my left hand?' and responded correctly; in reply to (g) he said, 'Could you say that again please?'; in reply to (h) he said to him-self, 'Your left eye with my right hand?', and in reply to (i) said 'Your left ear with my left hand? ...so it's that one'. S59, in reply to (e) said 'Your left hand with my right?' and in reply to (f) said 'My right with your left?', on both occasions responding correctly; in reply to (j) he touched my *right* hand with his left, but when I queried this he repeat-ed the question to himself and finally gave the correct answer.

Now it is, of course, the case that anyone, whether dyslexic or not, needs such 'prompts' from time to time, and since in our society the request, 'Could you say it again, please?', is socially quite acceptable it is not surprising that dyslexic subjects should have learned to make use of it. If my interpretation is correct, however, one would expect this particular series of test items to generate more 'RR' and 'EQ' responses in dyslexic subjects than in controls. This is an idea which requires further investigation.

For some of my subjects the tasks were made easier because of their ability to verbalise what was required; that is to say, they realised that, since I was sitting opposite them, what was on the left for them would be on the right for me and vice versa. For example S109 shut his eyes and thought hard, saying, 'I've got to remember your left is my right'; S145 said, 'I try to work it out by pretending I'm sitting where you are'; S181 said, ''cos your right hand's opposite – on the other side – to my right'; S67 said, 'It's always the opposite', while S220 said, 'Your watch is on the left; I can judge from that watch which side of you you are on' (sic). In reply to (e) S95 said, 'My left with your right? You twist round; your right hand changes'.

Finally, I should like to mention a strategy which has always seemed to me both strange and interesting. Some of my subjects, when given the instruction 'Show me your right hand' or 'Touch my right hand with your left hand', carried out actual movements of their bodies. For example, to determine their own right hand they would go through the motions of picking up a pen and pretending to write and to determine which was my right hand they would turn or half-turn in their seats. In some cases the movements were so slight as to be barely noticeable, and indeed some subjects reported that it was sufficient to *pretend* to be carrying out such movements or to imagine themselves doing so. S51 explained the position to me as follows: 'I was told I was a left-handed writer... I think I'm writing a letter – if it's "left" I put up the hand I'm pretending to write with'. S39 was less articulate but said, 'I have to hold the pen in my hand' (the implication being that this would give him a clue as to right and left because he knew which hand he wrote with). Asked which was my right hand S46 turned in his seat and then gave the correct answer, while S37 said, 'If I was turning round I'd *know* which hand'. S52 who used the 'watch' strategy, turned round in answer to this question but still pointed to my left. S242 said, 'It took me ages to learn it and even now I have to pretend I'm writing... I pretended I had a pen so it was opposite to you'. S209 explained the position as follows: 'I can't do ballroom dancing. When the teacher says "Stand on your right foot" I have to work out which side I am in relation to the road'. S199 said 'I pretend I'm using a knife and fork'; S147 turned in his seat, while S143 had asked for item (j) to be repeated and as a check began to turn round in her seat. S114, when given item (e), said 'Your right with my left?' (It should in fact have been, 'my left with your right'.) 'Wait a minute, let me see'; he then 'correctly' touched my right with his left. In response to (f) he said, 'Wait a minute – I've got to turn round because you're on the opposite side'. S117, without actually turning round, said 'I had to think myself round first'. In response to 'Point to my right ear with your left hand' (f), S100 made a half-turn in his seat and said 'Point to my left ear with your right hand' (attempting to repeat my words). Asked which was my right hand S83 gave the correct answer and then said, 'I turned round'. (He had not in fact done so, except, presumably, in imagination. But he then demonstrated the point by actually turning round.) S61, after struggles with the earlier items, said in response to (i), 'Is it all right for me to turn round', after which he did the remaining two items correctly. Asked which was her right hand S82 gave the correct answer after a pause, and when asked if she found it difficult, said, 'Yes, I remember which hand I write with; I pick up a pen to see'. S81 also paused, and then explained, 'I had to find my kicking foot... I kick a ball with my right or have to lift my leg' (presumably he had been imagining himself kicking a ball). S59 said, 'I have to do this', making a cub salute (presumably he knew that the hand with which he saluted was his right). S67 said 'I always had to turn left to go to school' (meaning, I think, that he had to *imagine* himself on the way to school and that he knew that the side to which he turned was his left). S177, after explaining that he knew his watch was on his left hand, said 'If someone asked me, I used to think "Oh, this"' (meaning, presumably, that he had to direct his attention towards his watch). S187 made several turns, accompanied by the comment, 'I always have to think'. S183 gave a twitch to his left thumb and said 'My right hand is the other one'. S159 said 'I used to turn round and go like that' (movement) 'but I've got it now'. S168 had said 'I have to think which one I write with' and, when asked which was my right hand, turned in his seat; in reply to item (f) (my right eye with his left hand) he pointed to my left eye with his right hand, then said 'No', turned round to check, saying, 'Let's think', and finally gave the correct answer.

As I have indicated elsewhere (Note 10.1), I believe that a helpful account of this behaviour is to be found in the formula 'Doing is a substitute for naming'. It is because the naming skills of these subjects are relatively weak that a procedure which reduces the amount of naming required is sometimes found to be helpful. The American investigators, Spring and Capps, are, I think, making a similar comment when they say that dyslexic persons 'evidence no dramatic inability to function in an environment of concrete stimuli' (Note 10.2).

I have also suggested (Note 10.3) that these responses are not necessarily the outcome of a difficulty over direction as such. It is not the case, for example, that when dyslexic subjects want to leave a room they sometimes walk away from the door instead of towards it (as Alice found was necessary in Looking-Glass World). It seems rather that it is the *words* 'left' and 'right' which cause the problem. Whether this is a complete explanation I do not know; but it is possible that when dyslexic subjects show uncertainty over direction, whether between left and right, between east and west, between 'b' and 'd', between the correct places on the table for the knife and fork, or in other ways, all these problems are the consequence of a weakness at naming. Similarly it is possible that their uncertainty over times and dates (see Chapter 13) should not be described simply as a 'sequencing' difficulty, since there are some tasks, such as assembling the parts of a radio, which a dyslexic person can perfectly well do in sequence. It is rather that verbal labelling is sometimes an aid to sequencing and therefore when such labelling is inefficient the likelihood of faulty sequencing is increased.

If the criterion for showing 'uncertainty over left and right' is taken to be a 'plus' on the Left–Right test as specified in Appendix II, then 149 out of my 223 subjects (76%) showed uncertainty over left and right. Alternatively, if we take only the 132 dyslexic subjects who were matched with the controls (see Chapter 7) the figure is 87 (65%), compared with 36% of the controls. Although this result is highly significant (Note 10.4), it is clear that one should think in terms of tendencies rather than certainties.

Chapter 11
Confusion between
East and West

The main source of evidence about my subjects' awareness of 'east' and 'west' was an adapted version of the Direction items in the Terman–Merrill intelligence test. Direction I contains five items, of which I quote the first two as examples: (1) 'Which direction would you have to face so that your *left* hand would be towards the *east*?' (answer, South), and (2) 'Suppose you are going *west*, then turn to your *right*; in what direction are you going now?' (answer, North). Direction II involves five similar items, while Direction III involves a series of statements, which the subject is allowed to have in writing in front of him, about the distance and direction of travel; he then has to say both the direction in which he is finally going and the distance from his original starting point when he stops.

Direction I is regarded as suitable for the average 14-year-old, Direction II is set at Average Adult, and Direction III at the top grade of Superior Adult. Most of my evidence is therefore derived from the performance of my older subjects, since many of the younger ones would have found such items too difficult. Occasionally, however, it was possible to give Direction I and Direction II to 9-, 10- and 11-year-olds.

I did not use the tests in precisely the way in which the original authors recommended, but adapted them instead in order to make them as meaningful as possible from the point of view of assessment for dyslexia. According to the instructions the subject is not permitted to use pencil and paper, but when I initially allowed my subjects to do so it was clear that a wealth of interesting material was emerging. I therefore continued with the practice, even though this debarred me from using the results to produce an IQ in the standard sense (compare Chapter 2).

Now it was plain in many cases that my subjects knew the kind of response that was needed, that is, the name of one of the points of the compass, even though they did not necessarily come up with the correct one. In contrast there may be younger or slower subjects who either look blank or perhaps reply '*That* way', pointing in some direction, and occasionally there have been subjects who have said, 'But I don't know which way east is from here'. In these cases one can say that the subject has failed to understand the point of the question.

It follows that the tasks involve at least three components, namely (1) understanding the point, (2) working out left and right, and (3) working out east and west. Typically the dyslexic subject, provided he is of suitable age and ability, is successful at (1) but appreciably handicapped over both (2) and (3).

Here are some examples. In response to (1), where the correct answer is 'south', S204 said 'north'. It was apparent, however, when I talked to him afterwards that he had confused 'east' and 'west', and a little later he said, 'If I'd got east and west the right way round I'd have done better'. Similarly, in response to Direction III, when the correct answer is 'west', S179 said 'east', but when I corrected his diagram, in which east and west were interchanged, he immediately said, 'Then it's west'. When I returned to Direction I, which he had earlier failed, he succeeded over item (1) but said 'south' for 'north' in item (2), turning left with his pencil as he said the word 'right'; when I pointed out his mistake he immediately said, 'The north' .

Now the confusions which my subjects showed over the points of the compass, and particularly those over east and west, reminded me very much of the difficulties over 'left' and 'right': there were mistakes, hesitations, echoing of the question, requests for the question to be repeated and special compensatory strategies (including turning in their seats) which were quite often successful.

The following, for example, drew diagrams in which east and west were interchanged: S94, S95, S126, S137, S170, S202, S219, S228 and S244. There were three subjects (S50, S81, and S167) who drew their diagrams as

                                    N

                    W   S

                            E

In each case they started at 'north' and proceeded in a clockwise manner, presumably because they were familiar with the commonly used order, 'north-south-east-west'. Even S221, who was an undergraduate, showed hesitation over his diagram, and although it was in fact correct he turned to me as he drew it saying 'This is east, isn't it?' S175, in response to the first Direction I item, said, 'Could you say it again? Your right hand?' When I said 'No', she then drew a diagram in which west was on the left and east on the right. Next, however, she crossed out 'east' and 'west' and substituted 'east' on the left and 'west' on the right. She then asked, 'Have I got it right? I think it's "west–east"' (indicating west on the left of the page); and, as if thinking out loud, she then said, 'If my left hand faced the east... don't know'. In response to the second item she echoed the question and said, 'East, no south'. With encouragement from me she drew the points of the compass again and said 'Am I looking on to north like that or to the back of it?' I did not understand this question but I had the impression that somehow she was not thinking of *herself* as being at the centre of the diagram even though this is something which is taken for granted by most subjects of this level of ability. I in fact put my pen vertically on the page and placed the cap as its 'left hand', after which she correctly answered all the items both in Direction I and in Direction II.

There was also the same need for mnemonics. S239 said 'Mum told me "WE" so I remember', while S217 said 'I learned it was "WE" across'. S151 said 'I say "Never Eat Shredded Wheat"' (but he nevertheless confused east and west), while this mnemonic was also used by S135 (see below). There were also cases where the subject turned in his seat: thus S212 did so in the case of Direction I and S127 in the case of Direction III, while in response to Direction II, S158 said 'It's much easier with your body'.

S135 not only turned in his seat but actually stood up and turned around the room, these actions being combined with the Never-Eat-Shredded-Wheat mnemonic. It was one of these occasions where I particularly wish the behaviour could have been videorecorded. As a second best I tried to set down in writing what happened as accurately as I could. The whole procedure took an appreciable time, but each stage was purposeful and intelligent. He started by rising from his seat to face the wall on the right, saying as he did so, 'Suppose that's north... You have north, then east... Never eat shredded wheat; so that's south... my left hand (pause) towards the east... so I would be facing south'. This was in fact the correct answer.

His performance seems to me typical of the dyslexic subject in that it shows the ability to make a step-by-step series of deductions and the ability to combine these deductions with use of the appropriate mnemonic. One is also left with a sense of surprise that such strategies are needed at all, since there seems little doubt that in a similar context a non-dyslexic person of the same ability and background would have come up with the answer instantly. Similar compensatory strategies will be referred to in Chapter 15, where an 'instant' answer to 'nineteen take away seven' was impossible for some of my subjects but where a similarly slow step-by-step process often led to the correct answer. The process does not, of course, involve any memory overload; it is rather that a single, non-overloading procedure needs to be used several times over. It is also worth noting that S135, like most other dyslexic subjects, was perfectly capable of 'supposing' that a particular direction was the north. It is symbols which present difficulty, not concrete objects whether real or imagined.

On some occasions there were subjects who went wrong because of
a left–right error. For example, in reply to the item 'Suppose you are
going *east*, then turn to your *right*, in what direction are you going
now?', S81 went through the motion of turning *left* on his diagram and
'correctly' said 'north'. In response to Direction III S185 drew the following diagram, starting at the point X.

Figure 11.1 Response to Terman–Merrill Direction III

The original wording is 'turned to my left and drove east 2 miles',
whereas he turned to his *right* and drove *west* two miles! He then
turned the paper upside down and started again! S193 said, 'You go
south and then turn to your...' at which he became confused, mud-
dling up north and south; and at this point he, too, turned the paper
upside down.

In reply to the first item of Direction I, S81 started by saying 'That
way' instead of naming a point of the compass. When I asked if he
would like to write anything down, he wrote:

N

W   S

E

and when I asked him to try again he wrote:

S

E   W

N

Here the four points of the compass are correctly placed in terms of
relationship but the normal viewer would complain that they were
upside down! Finally this subject produced the correct diagram, after
which he had no difficulty in giving the correct answer. When given
Direction II he used the same diagram, and then, in reply to 'Suppose
you are going *east*, then turn to your *right*, which direction are you
going now?', he turned left and consistently but wrongly said 'north'.

S179 and S174 also drew the points of the compass correctly in terms of relationships, but with south at the top and east on the left, and S174 tried to solve Direction III by means of a grid, as shown in Figure 11.2.

When I queried this he, too, turned the paper upside down! (The other writing in Figure 11.2 shows the very logical way in which he worked out the answer to the Terman–Merrill 'tree' item; see Chapter 15.)

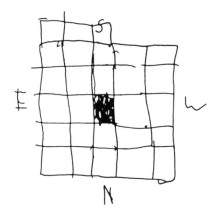

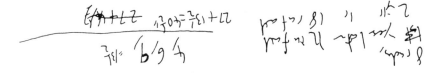

Figure 11.2 Grid to aid calculation of east and west

A further east–west confusion is worth recording, though in fact it did not occur in response to any of his Terman–Merrill Direction tests but in response to a Wechsler test item where the subject has to say what part of a picture is missing. S67 noticed the sun as part of the picture and said: 'If it's rising from the wrong direction – it rises from the west, no, east, and that sun's rising from the west. That's north' (pointing as if the picture were a map). I did not find this statement fully intelligible, but it should be noted that he made the correction from 'west' to 'east' and also (perhaps more interestingly) that he seemed to be under the impression that one could say which were the points of a compass by simply examining the picture. This response is perhaps comparable with that of S175, mentioned above: in both cases there is some ground for supposing not merely that these two subjects were confused over east and west but also that there was something lacking in their understanding of how points of the compass are represented on a two-dimensional surface. Although this lack came to light only in these two cases, it is possible that they are examples of a more general 'uncertainty over spatial relationships' which appears to be part of the dyslexic picture. Factors in the situation which the rest of us take for granted may not have been understood.

Chapter 12
Confusion between 'b' and 'd'

It was plain, even in the early stages of the research, that many of my subjects, including some of the older ones, were confusing 'b' and 'd'. This was clear not only from their performance on the R_1 and S_1 tests but also from an inspection of their school exercise books: they might make a b-sound for a d-sound (or vice versa) in reading and write the letter 'b' for the letter 'd' (or vice versa) in spelling.

There was first-hand evidence of such errors in 75 out of the 223 subjects and reported evidence (which there is no reason to doubt) in a further 71 cases. As an estimate of the incidence of b–d confusion in a dyslexic population this figure (146, or 65%) may be too low, since in the case of some of the older subjects, particularly those unaccompanied by their parents, difficulties at an earlier age would not necessarily have been remembered.

In some cases the confusions were extremely persistent. Of the 47 subjects aged 12 to 14 no less than 14 were scored as 'plus' on this item (that is, they were still making b–d errors at the time of the assessment (Note 12.1), and a further 7 out of the 59 in the age range 15 to 18 were also scored as 'plus'. Only recently I was shown a piece of written work by S126, five years after his original assessment at the age of 12, in which *probably* was written as 'probadly' and *problems* as 'prodlems', both being afterwards corrected (Note 12.2). Such confusions are of course not the norm for older dyslexic subjects, but in view of the apparent easiness of the task by ordinary standards it is remarkable that they occur at all.

It would, I am sure, be a mistake to suppose that dyslexics are the *only* people who confuse 'b' and 'd'. It is a matter of common experience that so-called 'slow learning' children do so and there is evidence from a study by Bottomley that a small number of children with spelling ages under 9 did so even though they were probably not dyslexic (Note 12.3). A great merit of Bottomley's study was that the 50 dyslexic subjects were compared, not with age-matched controls but with younger children of the same spelling age; from this it follows that

any differences in respect of b–d confusion are not simply a manifestation of spelling weakness in general. From the data which Bottomley
provided it has been possible to take the first nine words from the
Schonell S_1 test which begin with 'b' or 'd' and compare the relative
number of confusions by dyslexic and by control subjects. Other types
of spelling error were, of course, discounted. The results were:

Table 12.1 Interchange of 'b' and 'd'		
Word	*Dyslexic subjects*	*Control subjects*
doll	3	2
bell	2	2
by	1	1
brain	1	0
dancing	3	0
damage	1	0
daughter	2	0
domestic	1	0
duties	1	0
TOTAL	15	5

It is interesting that in the case of the control subjects the confusions were limited to words early in the list. It is possible that by the
time these subjects were at a level where they could attempt the later
words any tendency to confuse 'b' and 'd' had been outgrown.
Occasional b–d confusions among non-dyslexic subjects have also been
reported by Pollard (Note 12.4). In general it seems to me likely that
children who show b–d confusion in the early stages do not invariably
present the typical dyslexic picture but that in dyslexic children the
confusion sometimes persists until an older age and that even at a
younger age it is relatively more common.

Now it is usually supposed that mistakes over 'b' and 'd' are basically
errors over direction. I am not myself convinced that the subject's
handedness is a relevant factor, since I found no evidence that the left-
handers or mixed-handers were more prone to b–d confusion than the
right-handers (see Chapter 21). It is still possible, however, that b–d
confusion is 'of a piece' with other typical dyslexic-type errors – confusion over left and right, writing 'ot' for *to*, working from the 'wrong'
end in arithmetical calculation and so on.

Of course 'b' and 'd' are not the only pair of letters which are liable
to confusion. Mistakes over 'p' and 'q' (S4 and S11) and over 'p' and 'b'
(S94) were reported; S13 was said to have written 3 back to front and
S28 to have done the same in the case of 5 and 9. S12 wrote ⌊ for J; S6
was reported to have written 'letters and figures backwards' and similar
expressions were used in the case of S51, S54, S62, S197 and S198. It

was not always clear, however, how recent such mistakes were and it is possible that the parents of non-dyslexic children might sometimes have remembered similar difficulties. S58 'corrected' 'cap' in his S_1 test to 'caq' but this is the only first-hand evidence which I have of p–q confusion in anyone aged 10 or more. There was evidence that S208 wrote 's's (and many other letters) the wrong way round (see p.35), but she appears to be a very exceptional and severe case (Note 12.5), and in none of the 223 records of the Schonell S_1 test is there a single example of an inverted S. Any attempt to explain b–d confusions in terms of mirror-images needs also to explain why p–q confusions do not persist so long and why, after the very early stages, inverted 'S's are relatively rare.

My tentative suggestion is as follows. I do not believe that it is mirror images as such which are the main source of the dyslexic person's difficulty. If objects, pictures, or patterns are mirror-images of each other, all of us may need more time to distinguish between them. Where the dyslexic person has difficulty, because of his weakness at verbal labelling, is with symbols. This means that in the case of symbols which are *also* mirror images one complication may aggravate the other. This makes sense of the fact that some dyslexic children do indeed, if only for a limited period, confuse 'p' and 'q' and write 's's and some numerals the wrong way round; here, however, the uncertainties can be dealt with separately. In contrast, 'b' and 'd' are a unique pair of symbols in that they are both auditorily and visually confusable (Note 12.6). There is therefore a situation where visual processing gives an ambiguous result and where the possibility of an auditory cross-check is reduced. On a 'bad day' any of us may make seemingly 'careless' mistakes (Note 12.7); in the case of a dyslexic person, however, an initial weakness at naming may be compounded by the fact that it is a 'bad day'; if in addition there is absence of cross-check between the visual and the auditory, the probability of error may be disproportionately increased. I do not know if this account of the matter is correct, but some such account is needed if one is to make sense of the relative persistence of b–d confusions in dyslexia when other 'mirror image' confusions have disappeared.

Chapter 13
Confusion over Times and Dates

The confusions described so far – between left and right, between east and west, and between 'b' and 'd' – are alike in that they all involve errors over spatial relationships. To touch a person's right hand instead of his left or to move eastwards on a map instead of westwards is to go to the wrong point in space; similarly to read a 'b' as though it were a 'd' or to write 'b' for 'd' is to be in error about the spatial lay-out of one or both symbols.

In this chapter I shall show that there can be similar uncertainties over times and dates. This, indeed, is not surprising, since successive points in time are sometimes represented by adjacent points in space (Note 13.1), and if spatial representation is in some way faulty it makes sense that temporal representation should be faulty also. However that may be, difficulties connected in various ways with awareness of time were relatively common.

Thus it was reported by his parents that S114 might sometimes say, 'I'll just go down to the shops' even though it was evening and the shops were shut! Still more instructive is the record of my conversation with S130, which went as follows:

Q: 'What day of the week is it?'
A: 'I think it's the 17th.' (It was in fact the 27th.)
Q: 'Yes, but what day of the week?'
A: 'Tuesday. Oh, no, Thursday. I remember, as we came yesterday, so it must be Thursday.'

In the case of S215 I recorded the following remarks: 'It's Wednesday, at least I hope it is; no, it's Tuesday – Thursday, rather. I think at school I used to tell what day it was – we did things in phases, so I remembered what we did on Thursdays – we did art on Thursdays'. It was reported by his mother that S143 could not tell the time until the age of 10 and a half and left out 'Monday' from the days of the week until he was 10. Among others, S57, S149, S154 and S175 were said to have been late in learning to tell the time.

S164 said he did not remember what year it was but knew that he would be 15 next September. I was able to look at the history note book of S214, where I saw on successive parts of the page the dates 1804, 1805, 1806 and 1807, after which 1809 had been changed to 1808 and there were crossings out or corrections for 1810 and 1811. When I asked S10 the date of his birthday he said it was in March but could not give the exact date. He then added: 'But I find Christmas and my birthday move on one day, Saturday this year, Friday last year'. When I asked him the date of Christmas, however, he made no reply.

Uncertainty over dates was specifically mentioned by the parents of S76 and also by the parents of S258 whom – not without some hesitation – I placed in Group II, though I would certainly have placed her in Group I had more supporting signs of this sort been forthcoming. When S171 was asked his date of birth he said, 'Five six – no, hang on; six five nineteen, er –, forty-nine', the correct answer in fact being 6.5.1959. I also had occasion to ask S233 the year of his birth. He replied, 'I've been told it a lot of times'; when I suggested he should work it out (he was 10 and the year was 1972) he said '1862 – no, 1962, – no, 1862'. S204 said that he 'thought' his year of birth was 1957 (which it was) but that he 'couldn't associate dates with events'. Eight years after her initial assessment I was talking to S246, who was taking a degree in embroidery, about the Bayeux tapestry; when I asked if its date was known she said 'About 40 years after the original events in 1666' (instead of 1066).

The recognition by S10 (see above) that his birthday 'moved on one day' each year is particularly interesting. Once again this appears to be a situation where understanding the behaviour of abstract concepts – in this case the use of the days of the week to symbolise the passage of time – is in no way impaired. Similarly it was interesting that some of my older subjects, for example S174, S204, S205 and S218, were successful at the difficult item in the Terman–Merrill test where it is asked how 'beginning' and 'end' are alike. S205 said that they were both 'to do with time' yet when asked to say 'two five nine' in reverse order she said 'nine two five'. Understanding the concept of time is clearly quite different from being able to reproduce symbols in the correct temporal order.

This moment is perhaps a convenient one in which to discuss a related set of difficulties, namely those experienced by my subjects in repeating words such as 'preliminary', 'anemone' and 'statistical'. The evidence from Chapter 7 shows that difficulties over these words were very much more frequent in dyslexic subjects than in controls and, quite apart from evidence derived from the administration of the dyslexia test, it is noteworthy that a number of parents spontaneously mentioned similar difficulties. Thus the speech of S118 at the age of 6 was said by his mother to be full of 'Spoonerisms' (Note 13.2), and among my younger subjects the following mispronunciations were reported: 'proshifency' for *proficiency* (S20), 'Jackercrack' for *Crackerjack* (S25), and 'dikkifult' for *difficult* (S5). Among my older subjects I noted that S188 became 'tied up' in trying to say the word 'susceptible' in the Schonell R_1 word recognition test and that S217 had difficulty in saying the word 'corollary'. S218 reported that she 'got tied up with words' and that 'people laugh at me about it', and her father reported that at a younger age she had said 'tee-sit' for *settee*.

I suspect that auditory confusability can sometimes be an important source of error, and that this may be a more significant causal factor than the length of the word as such. As was pointed out in Chapter 3, there is anecdotal evidence of dyslexic children who say 'par cark' for 'car park' (where length of word cannot be a decisive factor), and, although I have not so far carried out a detailed statistical analysis, I suspect that there have been fewer errors over the longer, six-syllable word 'contemporaneous' than over 'preliminary' which has five syllables and over 'anemone' and 'statistical' which have four. Whether or not this is correct, there is no doubt that dyslexic subjects are more liable than the rest of us to become 'tied up' when asked to repeat certain words, and this appears to be a further example of their weakness at certain tasks involving temporal ordering.

Chapter 14
Recall of Months of the Year

One of the items in the dyslexia test consists of the simple instruction, 'Say the months of the year'. If the subject makes a reasonable attempt at this he is then told, 'Now say them backwards'. The patterns of responding are in many ways like those which occurred with the Left–Right test. In some cases there are actual errors; often there is confusion and at times there is the conscious working out of compensatory strategies. Detailed documentation seems to me worth while, since the task, at least in the case of Months Forwards, is likely to strike a non-dyslexic person as being relatively easy, and indeed the evidence from Chapter 7 shows that 106 out of 132 control subjects scored 'minus' at it, nine of the remaining 26 being under age 9. In contrast only 57 out of the 132 matched dyslexic subjects and only 101 out of my total pool of 223 dyslexic subjects scored 'minus' (Note 14.1).

The following are examples of responses when the subject made actual errors. S188 omitted 'May' and when asked to have a second try omitted it again. S210, who was aged 17 and was in the highest intelligence group (Z), proceeded correctly as far as August and then said, 'October, September, November, December'.

There were also many subjects who named some of the months but failed to name all of them. For example S62 said, 'February, March, June, May, September, August, November, December' – a total of eight months. S25 gave only four months, S43 nine, S52 eight, S62 eleven (but in the wrong order), S124 five, S125 eight (though he claimed to know that there were twelve), S128 ten, S162 five, S164 five and S236 six. Sometimes the same month was repeated more than once, as when S7 said 'November, December, October, November, December, March, April, May, June, July, November, December'. S20 was correct up to September and then said, 'November, December, October, November. No, I can't. I get mixed up'. S38 was correct up to September and then said 'November, December, October, November, December, October, March, April, May, June'. S140 said 'June, where do you start from? June, July, August, September, August, September, August, September,

January. July – oh, I forget – February, August, September – I'm all mud-dled up'.

In addition to the actual errors there were many corrections and signs of uncertainty. S138 said 'January, February, June, no, March, April' and then proceeded correctly. S141 gave the months correctly as far as August, and then said, 'This is where I get stuck – September, November... October I've missed out'. At this point he went back to January and started with his fingers; my notes say that he was 'just about successful'. S159 after responding correctly said, 'Have I missed out August? I usually do'. S158 said, 'Oh, dear! that is hard. April, May, June, July, August, September, December, November – the rightest I've ever said it. It sounded right – normally I get them in an awful muddle'. S157, after a long pause, produced the correct answer but added at the end, 'That's the first time I've done it right'. S173 said, 'January, March, April – or was it February? After that it's May, June, July, August'. Then, slowly, 'October, November, December'. S183 was correct as far as October but then said 'I've missed one out'; he then went through quite correctly but still said 'I've missed one', and after a further cor-rect recitation said, 'Ah! there's twelve that time'. S232 said 'Blimey!', and when after a pause I had prompted with 'January' he said 'February I think it is, March, April, June, July, August, September, October, November, December' (pause), 'April, June, July, August, September, November, December, um – I've finished, haven't I?' S47, after omitting May and October, said, 'I know there's one after November before December'. S99 said 'March, April, June, July, August, September, November, December', and when I said 'Do you know if you have left any out?' he said 'Yes'; when I asked which he said 'March'. One of the most noticeable characteristics of many of the responses was the uncertainty over *order*. Here are some sample com-ments from among the many available. S162 said, 'Oh goodness! where do I start from? Does it matter?' S179 said 'Not in order, no; December, November, June, January, April, March, May – have I said January?'. S44 said 'I've forgotten when it starts', while S59 said 'Where from? Where shall I say them from? I'm always getting muddled'. When I prompted him with January he said, 'February, March, April' (pause), 'May – is it? –, June – I don't know any more'. S26 said, 'Could you tell me the first one?', and when I said 'January' she said, 'January, February, May, July – no, I've left some out; March, April, June, then August... I know it but I can't say the word right... October, the same with this, was the last one I said October? (Yes). Does the next one begin with 'a' – accember?. . . September, October, Devember, how many more? (One) Devember'.

Compensatory strategies and mnemonics are not as easy to find in the case of the months of the year as they are in the case of left/right and east/west. There was one strategy, however, which several subjects used, namely that of counting with their fingers as they said each month so as to ensure that the number of months came to twelve; this was the strategy of S56, S132, S133, S176 and S232. S72 omitted both May and September, saying at the end, 'I know there's not twelve there'. In a number of cases there was the 'epanalepsis' strategy (see Chapter 3). For example it was again S72 who, having said 'June, July', appeared to lose his way and repeated 'June, July' before passing to 'August, October, November, December'. S94 was correct up to April but then started again; he also repeated 'September' when saying the months in reverse order apparently as a way of reorienting himself. S121 was correct as far as 'June, July', albeit with a slight pause and tapping of his fingers after 'March', but he repeated 'June, July' before saying 'August, October, November, December'.

I was particularly fascinated by the strategy adopted by S75, who told me that it was of his own devising. His name was Jason, and he said that he remembered the five months from July onwards because the first letters were given by the letters of 'Jason'. Shortly afterwards I was talking to his teacher, to whom he had proudly said, 'I can do the ones from July onwards', looking, as she aptly put it, like a cat that had got at the cream! More recently still I was at a lecture on teaching methods where the speaker in discussing how to teach the months of the year referred to the 'Jason' months and said afterwards in conversation that this mnemonic was now part of the stock-in-trade of teachers of dyslexic children.

If a person cannot say Months Forwards in the correct order it seems on the face of it inconceivable that he should be correct on Months Reversed; and indeed where Months Forwards was a total failure, or somewhere near it, it was plain that one could score Months Reversed as a 'plus' without putting the subject through the strain of having to attempt a task on which he was sure to fail. It can be seen from the Summary Chart in Chapter 6, however, that very occasionally there was a 'minus' at Months Reversed despite a 'nought' or 'plus' at Months Forwards, or occasionally a 'nought' at Months Reversed despite a 'plus' at Months Forwards. This happened in the case of S30, S34, S90, S93, S116, S118, S122, S151, S219, S237 and S239. The finding is 'genuine' in the sense that the scoring of 'plus', 'nought' and 'minus' conformed with the criteria set out. Since, however, these subjects were more successful at Months Reversed than at Months Forwards one must conclude not that they *could not* have succeeded at the latter but only that they *did not* on this particular occasion. The point is an important one since it underlines the uneven nature of the dyslexic subject's performance and confirms that one should not necessarily think of dyslexic-type difficulties as arising from lack of the appropriate brain mechanisms but from the lower probability of their activation (Note 14.2).

The failures over Months Reversed do not require detailed documentation, but here are four typical 'plus' responses which I quote for

illustration purposes. S46 said 'December, October... I'm sorry, I can't
say any more'; S80 said, 'Oh, crumbs! December, November (pause)
September', while S153 said, 'December, November, August, October,
June...cor!... July, June, April, May... cor!... May, April, March, February,
January'. S203 said simply 'I can't. I get stuck'.

Several of the subjects reported compensatory strategies, the most
common of which was to say a small number of months in forwards
order to themselves and thus 'group' the months for saying in reverse
order. For example S222, an undergraduate, said 'I thought of the
month, then worked in threes, and S155 said, intelligibly if not clearly,
'The ones I know in sequence – you go back to the beginning and get a
few more' (Note 14.3).

At times the subjects' difficulties in saying Months Forwards and
Months Reversed appeared to be similar to those which occurred when
they attempted to say their tables. For example, in the case of Months
Reversed S131 said 'December (pause) November, October, September
(pause), August, July, June, May (pause), April – no, I've gone wrong, I
think... What was the last one?' This response indicates 'loss of place'
in much the same way as do the responses over Tables which will be
reported in Chapter 16.

In view of the number of 'minus' scores, particularly among my
older subjects (Note 14.4), it follows that the months of the year can be
learned, and indeed from the figures in Chapter 7 it is clear that to
dyslexic and non-dyslexic subjects alike they are easier to learn than
tables. It was plain, however, from their comments that several subjects
had not appreciated that after practice correct recitation would become
automatic. Thus S94 said, 'I only learned the months at play group; I
didn't learn them any other time', as though it would be quite natural
for something learned so long ago to have been forgotten. Similarly
S29, after saying 'June, July, August, September, August, September,
June', explained his uncertainty by adding, 'We didn't learn them'.
S208 said 'I've learned these (i.e. the months) recently'. In the
Summary Chart this has to be scored as 'minus', though as a clinical
judgement one can say that the fact that a 17-year-old of above average
ability had only 'recently' learned the months of the year is highly significant. Similarly S143 is recorded as 'minus' for both Months
Forwards and Months Reversed but her mother reported that in fact
she had gone through them with her many times. After successful completion of Months Forwards S181, with almost a sigh of relief, said 'And
that's taken a bit of practice'.

Finally, it is interesting to compare saying the months of the year
with other tasks where nameable items have to be arranged in series. I
seldom asked my subjects to give me the days of the week since in
many cases I had found that they could do so with no difficulty. But
there were occasional reports that this knowledge had not come easily.

Thus S28 was said by her mother to have only recently 'sorted out' the days of the week, while S41 (who was a minister's son) explained that he 'didn't know the order of the days of the week... but Saturday it was bionic man and Dr Who... I got to know it was horrible church on Sunday'. (This was said in front of his father who fortunately had a sense of humour!)

S7 could not say the date of his birthday but knew that it was the start of the summer holidays, while S37 when asked to say the days of the week backwards replied, 'Saturday, Friday, Thursday, Tuesday, Wednesday... I forget'. Such uncertainties, however, were rare and one can be reasonably confident that most dyslexic children of the same age and background as my subjects will show no difficulty in saying the days of the week, at any rate in forwards order.

I found greater uncertainty over knowledge of the four seasons. This again was something which I did not investigate very systematically, but from time to time I came on errors which had a distinctly dyslexic flavour. Thus S83 said 'Winter is first, autumn, summer, winter again'. After S14 had told me that December came in winter I asked if he knew the other seasons, to which he replied, 'Yes, winter, summer, autumn'; and when I asked, 'Do you know any more?' he said, 'Yes, summer'.

Another curious phenomenon which I sometimes found was an uncertainty about the difference between seasons and months and some unwitting slips from one to the other. Thus when asked to say the months of the year S1 said 'January, February, March, April, June, July, August, autumn', while S9 when asked to give the names of some of the months said 'October, November, summer, winter'. Asked if he could say the months of the year S58 said, 'No... Spring, autumn, winter... I've remembered – spring, autumn, winter', and when I asked 'What's the right order?' he said, 'What do you mean?' (Note 14.5).

It seems to me that learning overlay is possible in the case of the days of the week because few children, whether dyslexic or not, can avoid being exposed to them. In that respect they are similar to the lower numbers in the number series. The same names, Thursday, Friday etc., keep appearing, as we say, week after week; this happens 52 times a year, compared with once a year in the case of the months and once a year in the case of the seasons. It is likely, too, that a child needs to know that it is, say, Thursday more often than he needs to know that it is, say, January or spring, particularly if his school has a regular time-table; and even if he learns certain associations – for instance that one plays cricket in summer – the idea of a *sequence* of months or seasons is not necessarily something which will occur to him. It should be noted that length of the series does not appear to be the only relevant factor; otherwise the names of the four seasons would be more readily learned than the names of the seven days of the week.

Chapter 15
Subtraction and Addition

In this chapter the subjects' responses will be classified under three heads, namely (1) those which suggest a basic weakness over calculation in general, (2) those which suggest a specific uncertainty over the direction of the number series, and (3) those which exemplify the use of compensatory strategies. The sources for the data will be the subtraction items in the dyslexia test (see Appendix I), and a number of items from the Terman–Merrill intelligence test which involve subtraction and sometimes addition (Note 15.1).

Weakness over Calculation in General

Just as a dyslexic subject does not easily 'pick up' the details of how words are spelled, so he may also be at risk when required to make seemingly simple calculations with numbers. Thus S42, when asked 9 – 2, replied '8, I mean 7', and when asked 6 – 3 replied '4, no, 3'. In response to 19 – 7 S124 said '2 – I mean 12', while S44 said '13' giving as his explanation, 'I took 9 away from 7, leaves 3' (sic) 'and added 10, makes 13'. (This response indicates not only a weak number sense, since 9 – 7 = 2, not 3, but a confusion over order since he clearly meant 7 from 9, not 9 from 7.) When given 43 – 8 he replied '44... I added 10, and take 8 from 13 leaves 4, then 44'. As I understand the situation he had correctly added 10 to 3 but had both made a mistake over 13 – 8 and forgotten to subtract the 10 afterwards. Once again, as with the answers to the Left–Right items given in Chapter 10, it is the method of working which is of interest rather than the question of whether the end product is right or wrong.

Similar uncertainty is reflected in the response of S113, who, in reply to 6 – 3, correctly said '3' but added: 'I knew that one... I know some of the harder ones but I get most of the easy ones wrong'. When given 9 – 2 S95 said 'Is it 8? No, 7' and when given 6 – 3 he said '3; I think two threes are six'. When S100 was given 9 – 2, there was some long muttering during which he counted forwards from 1 to 7 and finally said '7'; when I asked, 'Are you sure?', he said 'About 50-50'. When S87 was given 19 – 7 he said 'I knew 9 take away 7 is 3 so I made it 13', and when given 43 – 8 he took a piece of paper and said 'I make it 5... I don't know how I did it'; when I asked, 'Can you tell if it is *nearly* right?' he said, 'No', and when I explained that the answer was 35 he said 'So you bring that down there?' (meaning the 3). This response suggests that he was an intelligent boy who was willing to learn certain rules of calculation, such as bringing down a number into a different row, but that he had not picked up a basic knowledge of how the number series behaves. I do not doubt that the properties of the number series can be taught, just as correspondence between letters and sounds can be taught; what is important in the case of the dyslexic subject is that one cannot take for granted that he will acquire such knowledge, as other children acquire it, during the course of ordinary experience at home and school.

It is, of course, possible for parents to be aware of the child's basic lack of understanding. Thus in the case of S60 his father reported that he 'hadn't got the concept of what dividing etc. are', while in the case of S232 his mother said, 'He has little idea of the relationship of one number to another; for example he would have difficulty in saying whether 282 was greater than 268'.

The following record of the behaviour of S104 is evidence of high reasoning power and, indeed, of some verbal fluency in describing this reasoning, which was nevertheless coupled with uncertainty over an elementary number relationship. When first asked 19 – 7 he replied '8', and when asked how he got it he said that he did not know. He then made another attempt and said '13', giving the following explanation: 'I put one on the 19 to make 20, and 7 and 4 make 10 so after that I... when I add 4 to make it... instead of having 4 you knock off one so it comes to 13'. I have been able to reconstruct what I believe to be his argument, which runs as follows: 'Bring both terms to the nearest 10: 19 becomes 20 by adding 1 and 7 becomes 10 by adding 4 (sic). One therefore adds 4 to 20 – 10, which gives 14, and one 'knocks off' the one needed to bring 19 up to 20, thus ending up with 13'. This reasoning is entirely correct, and the only mistake is that 10 is 7+3, not 7+4. What is remarkable is that a boy of this reasoning ability should not have known that 7 + 3 = 10!

In contrast I was defeated by the explanation of S86 as to how he arrived at 11 for 19 – 7. 'I went up to 10; another 10 would make 19, so I did 11'. If there was any logic here I did not discover it. Possibly his 'logic' was the same as that of S162, who in reply to 44 – 7 said '32', which he said was 'mainly a guess and mainly a bit of working out'. S99, in reply to 52 – 9, said explicitly, '42... I think it was in the 40s and then I did a guess' .

Sometimes errors and corrections seemed to have been generated by the memory load which some of the subtraction tasks involved. Thus S63 gave 52 – 9 as 46 and explained afterwards 'I remembered it as 55 and took away 9'. In reply to 43 – 8 S155 said '35, sorry, 34 – no, 35', while S154 said '37' and then said '53, was it? No, 43, take away 8; no, it was 36; no, I was right, 47; no, 37'.

Sometimes the subjects' spontaneous comments indicated the strain under which their handicap placed them. Thus S114, in reply to 9 – 2, said '8 – I mean 7. I make slips in my exam but I check it. When some-one's racing me against the clock I'm fast saying it in my mind but when I get it down I make slips. When I'm being timed I feel I must beat the clock – I came top but didn't get in Set 1'.

Even the relatively mature S201 showed uncertainty when I gave him 6 – 3. He first echoed the word 'three', as if to repeat to himself that this was the number to be taken away, and then said 'No! Minus three'. Without the explanatory concept of dyslexia the failure by a bright 16-year-old to answer this item instantly would be truly astonishing.

There was also an interesting comment from S96 who said that when he had to write 'a thousand and fifty' he had started by putting 1000.

Further evidence of uncertainty over numbers is to be found in the many requests for repetition made by my subjects when some calcula-tion was required. For example, S182, in response to 19 – 7, said '8, no 9. You said 18... You said 19 take away what?'. Both S203 and S58, in response to the same question, said '19, was it?... 12', while in reply to 44 – 7 S96 said 'Was it 40 take away 7?'. S99 echoed the question when given 6 – 3 and S131 did so in the case of both 52 – 9 and 44 – 7, while S93 asked for both 19 – 7 and 44 – 7 to be repeated. S175, in reply to 44 – 7 said 'Thirty, oh, heck! – What was it? 44?', and when I repeated '44 – 7' she said '36... I got lost again'. S185 gave 33 as the answer to 44 – 7 but corrected it to 36; when I asked, 'Are you sure?', he said, 'I think so; what was the number again?' S159 when asked 52 – 9 said 'Forty... ' followed by an s-sound, as if he was about to say 46 or 47, and then said, 'I'm sorry; what was it again?'; when I told him he gave the answer as '44' and, showing signs of crossness with himself, cor-rected this to 34.

In general there can be no doubt that many dyslexic subjects show a basic uncertainty over number which is often strikingly at variance with their ability in other directions, not least their ability to grasp some quite abstruse mathematical ideas.

Uncertainty over Direction of the Number Series

The difficulty, however, is not simply that of remembering symbols as such (including the number symbols in particular) but of remembering the direction in which to move when numbers have to be arranged in order. Uncertainty over left and right is no doubt a contributory factor here; but when an instruction such as 'x take away y' is given orally (with values for x and y supplied) and the subject wonders if the instruction was 'y take away x' it appears that there is a confusion of temporal order in addition. It is, of course, a tiresome complication that in some arithmetical operations it is necessary to go from right to left and in others from left to right; indeed there are some tasks, including parts of long multiplication and, in certain contexts, the presentation of graphical data where there is initially a choice of direction even though it is necessary to be consistent thereafter.

If he has to express, say, the number 'fifty-nine' in figures the non-dyslexic child very quickly learns to put the 5 on the left and the 9 on the right. He also learns that in the case of the 'teens' the order is the other way round (Note 15.2). The dyslexic child, on the other hand, because of his uncertainty over direction, may fail to 'cotton on' to this characteristic of the number system unless he is specially taught, and even then he may become confused or make mistakes. For example S227 was reported to have written 24 for 42, while S232 was said by his mother 'sometimes to tackle sums from the left-hand column'. According to his father S135 used to put '3 × 9 = 72', while S167, when travelling with his parents, had said 'That petrol's reasonable – forty-seven' when in fact the figure on the petrol pump (long years ago, it now seems!) was 74.

S70, during his assessment, needed to write the number 18; to achieve this he wrote an 8 and then added a 1 on the left, saying, 'I don't know which I do first', while S57 said, 'I used to get them all wrong – all double numbers; I sometimes put them the wrong way round'. S4 said the number 'ninety-two' and wrote 29. Sometimes there appears to be a muddle over the actual words 'backwards' and 'forwards' (possibly because there is no 'permanent tag' for backwards and forwards in the number series, since to reach any number one has to go backwards from a higher number and forwards from a lower one). Thus S5, when given 24 – 2, said 'Easy – I went backwards and found out that number – 24, 25, 26, 27'. He then hesitated, as though he had made an error, and said 'Did I go back three?'. It seems that by implication he meant that the correct answer should have been 26, which in his terminology would have been 'back' two. When I asked the leading question, 'Did you go forwards?' he said 'Backwards'.

It is also possible for dyslexic subjects to 'get things the wrong way round' in time as well as in space. For example S140, in response to 9 – 2, said, '9 take away 2... 2 take away 9... I thought you meant take away 9 from 2'; and in reply to 52 – 9 he said, 'Is it 9 take away 52?... 47, I think... 43'. In reply to the same item, S90 said, '47, no, 57' (taking 2 from 9 instead of 9 from 2); S56 asked, 'Is it 8 from 43 or 43 from 8?', while in reply to 9 – 2 S45 said '2 take away 9? 7'. S143, in reply to

19 – 7, paused for a long time and finally said, '16... 9 from 7 and I added 10 on'. I do not follow her logic here but in any case she should have said '7 from 9'. In reply to 52 – 9 she said, '55, no, 45. Take 2 from 9 and add 4 on'. Here, I suspect, she had in fact correctly taken 9 from 2, despite the incorrect verbalisation, and if, like some of the other subjects (see below), she had incorrectly reached 41, the adding of the 4 would explain the 45 (though I am still not clear how she arrived at the 4 in the first place). In reply to 19 – 7 S208 said, 'Can you say it again, please? I thought you said "7 take away 9"'.

For 52 – 9 a common response was '41'. This was given by S107, S112, S127, S133, S138, S144, S150, S160, S162, S174, S177 and S201, while S185 and S212 both said '41' and corrected it to '43'. The most likely explanation seems to be that they took away 10 from 52, correctly reaching 42, but *then moved in the wrong direction*, i.e. downwards to 41 rather than upwards to 43.

I should like at this point to cite two pieces of evidence reported by Griffiths (Note 15.3), both of which illustrate directional errors. In one case a dyslexic boy, aged 13, of above average intelligence, had been shown how to multiply 176 x 6 by the Egyptian 'duplatio' method (which calls only for addition and for multiplication by 2). He correctly set out:

1	176
2	352
4	704

knowing that he had to add 352 and 704 for the correct answer, but in fact he added 253 and 407. Another boy was given the exercises:

Ex. 1	79	Ex. 2	304	Ex. 3	5927
	56		275		7246
	90		493		3193
	+ 85		+ 629		+ 6455

His comments were recorded on tape. For Exercise 1 they were: '80 and 90, 170, 220, 290, 299, 305, 305, 310'; he then, correctly, wrote 310 as the answer. These comments show that he was adding the numbers in the left-hand column first, working upwards and 'correctly' ending at 290; he then worked *down* the right-hand column, adding 9 and 6 to get 305, staying at 305 because of the 0, and correctly ending at 310. In the case of Exercise 2 he said, '1000, 1200, 1500, 1570, 1660, 1680, 1684' (which he repeated twice, presumably as an epanalepsis in order to keep his place), '1689,1692, 1692, 1701'. The reader who follows his logic will see that he started in the left-hand column and went upwards, went down the middle column, and finally went down the right-hand column. It is interesting to note that despite these directional oddities the correct 'place values' for thousands, hundreds, and tens were fully understood. For Exercise 3 the method was too difficult for him to operate. The end product was:

$$
\begin{array}{r}
5927 \\
7246 \\
3193 \\
6455 \\
1\,7\,7 \\
\hline
21228 \\
\hline
\end{array}
$$

He started, as usual, with the left column, which came to 21, wrote down the 2 and added 1 to the next column; since $1 + 9 + 2 + 1 + 4$ comes to 17 he wrote down 1 and added 7 to the third column; thus 7 $+ 2 + 4 + 9 + 5$ gave 27, so he wrote down 2 and carried 7 to the right-hand column which he then wrote as 28. Working from left to right can still give the correct answer if suitable safeguards are observed, as is shown in the case of Exercises 1 and 2; in Exercise 3, however, instead of observing these safeguards, he transferred the 'carrying number' from left to right instead of from right to left and this led him into error.

One must conclude, therefore, that uncertainties over order and over left and right are a regular source of difficulty for dyslexic subjects when they attempt calculation.

Compensatory Strategies

Finally, there were all kinds of compensatory strategies as a result of which the subjects sometimes reached the correct answer, albeit in a laborious – and often highly idiosyncratic – way. Before describing the evidence in detail I should like to make some tentative suggestions as to why these strategies were necessary and what they were designed to achieve. For this purpose it will be helpful to distinguish between arithmetical tasks where the answer can be given instantly and arithmetical tasks which call for counting or deduction. If, for example, the task is $19 - 7$, one can be confident that the great majority of readers of this book will say that they 'just know' that the answer is 12.

Now it seems likely that the range of items which the dyslexic subject 'just knows' is severely limited (Note 15.4). The great majority of my subjects were able to give the answer to $24 - 2$ instantly, but $19 - 7$ presented them with much more difficulty. It is possible, of course, even in the case of $24 - 2$, that some of them did a rapid count, but this was certainly not apparent. In contrast, even those who arrived at the answer 12 for $19 - 7$ often used aids, for example their fingers or marks on paper. The suggestion was made in Chapter 10 that in some contexts, for a dyslexic subject, doing can be a substitute for naming; and I think it likely that the tapping of their fingers or the writing of marks on paper are further examples of such 'doing'. Once the rule has been grasped that one finger-tap or one mark on paper represents each number in the number series, the subject can proceed indefinitely, and there is no need for him to rely on 'just knowing' the answer to any calculation. I suspect – though this is by no means established – that there is some kind of threshold value, perhaps around 4 (Note 15.5), and that when the number to be added or subtracted is less than this – as in 24 – 2 – an 'instant' response is sometimes possible. When larger numbers are involved, however, the units have either to be counted out one by one or else to be grouped as sums of smaller numbers. For example, if the question is 44 – 7, the 7 can conveniently be split into 4 and 3; 44 – 4 is immediately seen to be 40, and 40 – 3 (which may well not be known instantly) can be worked out, with only minimal risk of error, by means of finger-taps. As in in the case of reciting tables (see Chapter 16), the multiples of 10 are in an important sense 'anchor points'.

The main strategies were in fact the use of fingers, the use of marks on paper and the breaking down of larger numbers, in particular 7, 8 and 9, into smaller units so that two short calculations were possible in place of one longer one. The first of these two calculations would normally be chosen so as to bring the subject to the most suitable 'anchor point'.

Among the subjects who noticeably used their fingers as an aid to calculation were S8, S9, S23, S24, S38, S43, S47, S59, S65, S68, S79, S83, S96, S99, S100, S111, S113, S117, S124, S135, S145, S157, S158, S165, S175, S181, S197, S205 and S212, and this list is almost certainly not exhaustive. S12 told me that he used his toes! At the time I had no exact data on the extent to which non-dyslexic subjects use their fingers in similar tasks. However, Ashcraft and Fierman have now produced evidence, based on a study of reaction times, which suggests that most children in an ordinary classroom abandon the strategy of 'counting' at about age 9 (compare Note 25.6). It is therefore noteworthy that some of my subjects were still relying on counting at age 14 and later.

The following are examples of the use of marks on paper as an aid to calculation. S3, when asked to solve 19 – 7, drew a line consisting of 19 dots arranged vertically; he then drew a line under the seventh dot and counted up the remainder. S232 used strokes for the first three items (9 – 2, 6 – 3 and 19 – 7) but not for 24 – 2. S230, when given 19 – 7, wrote as follows:

					1	2	3	4	5	6	7	8	9	10	11	12
1	2	3	4	5	6	7	8	9	10	11	12	13	14	15	16	17	18	19

This enabled him to give the correct answer. S40 used dots on paper even for 6 – 3.

Similar 'concrete aids' were used by some of my subjects when they attempted items from the Terman–Merrill intelligence test. For example, in the third 'cans of water' item (Note 15.6). S95 made nine marks, each about 1 cm long, vertically downwards on the paper, and placed five further marks alongside the bottom five, while S94 drew two rectangles, one with nine bars across, one with five bars across. Figure 15.1 shows the three diagrams used by S175 for all three items.

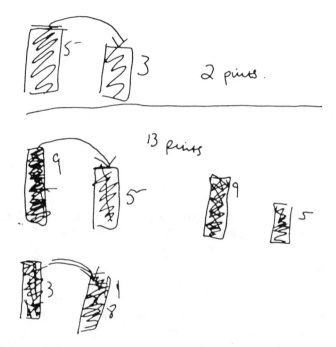

Figure 15.1 'Concrete aids' for numerical calculation

A number of my subjects also needed concrete aids in order to solve the 'boxes' item (Note 15.7). For the fourth 'box' item S158 put a rectangular figure down 21 times, while S162, for the third and fourth items, wrote

1	1
3	4
3	4
3	4
3	4

S109 and S178 spontaneously drew the boxes while S137 produced the drawing shown in Figure 15.2.

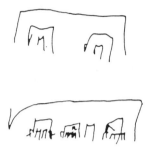

Figure 15.2 Similar 'concrete aids' for the Terman–Merrill 'boxes' item

Many of the subjects were able to be quite articulate about their compensatory strategies, and in most cases it was possible by means of suitable questioning to understand the logic of what they did. S7, when given 19 − 7, explained 'I started to think nineteen, eighteen, seventeen, sixteen counting in my head how many numbers I took away'. In response to the same item S46 echoed the question subvocally, murmured 'no ... nineteen ... twenty-two ... no, not twenty-two ... twelve ... What do you call it?' (He appeared to be searching for the word 'add'.) He then explained: 'Add three on to make it ten, then take away by ten, then' (pause, as if stuck), 'add three to the other one – it makes what do you call it, twelve'. (In other words, he turns the 7 into a 10 by adding 3, so has to turn 'the other one', 19, into 22 by adding three and then subtracts 10 from 22.) S61 said, 'I put down nineteen, take-away sign, and seven; I took seven off nine, counted seven, eight, nine from seven to nine missing out the seven, it made two, and one for nineteen made it twelve'. (In other words he gets the difference between 7 and 9 on a 'one-by-one' basis and then correctly retains the 1 in the tens column.)

S64 said, 'Nineteen – there's ten in. From ten I took seven and added the other nine'. S179 said, 'I put seventeen, and there was two more to nine, so it had to be ten and two'. S249 said, 'It's rather complicated. I added the seven to itself, which is fourteen, and added the remainder to the seven'. S164 said that his method was to 'count up from seven to nineteen and note how many counts', though because of a slip in counting he gave the answer as 'eleven' instead of ' twelve'. It was clear that some of the more sophisticated subjects tried to look for logical procedures which would make calculation easier. This point was made explicit by S193, who, when asked 9 − 2, said, 'Five, yes... no, seven. I was looking for a pattern; I have one or two patterns for taking away'.

In reply to 52 − 9 S84 said, 'What was the question again?'. After calculation he gave the correct answer, and explained that he was 'self-taught': 'Take the two away, this leaves you seven, and see how many are left from seven, so it's forty-three'. (This seems a good example of the ability to use multiples of 10 as 'anchor-points'.) S100 and S111 both did the same sum by working backwards on their fingers, until nine fingers were used up. S100 also said that he could do 6 – 3 because he 'remembered three is half of six'. When I gave him 9 – 2 for the second time he muttered to himself, counting forwards from 1 to 7, finally saying 'seven'; and when I asked him if he was sure he said 'About fifty-fifty'.

In reply to 44 – 7 S169 said 'Thirty-... five; no, thirty-eight, thirty-six, thirty-seven; four, no, four minus seven minus three, so minus three from forty gives thirty-seven'. The reasoning here is not fully clear, but once again it appears to be an attempt to divide 7 into 4 and 3 and make use of 40 as a multiple of 10.

In a number of cases I have seen complex reasoning co-existing with elementary difficulties over calculation. Thus it was plain, in the Terman–Merrill cans-of-water item, that S109 was fully clear as to the kind of solution that was needed, but only after careful working out was he able to discover that 9 + 4 = 13! Similarly S201, when given the Terman–Merrill 'tree' item (Note 15.8), produced some fully coherent arguments, marred only by the fact that he believed the difference between 18 and 27 to be 11 !

When one looks at the attempts of dyslexic subjects to do subtraction and addition, the overall picture is often that of a highly sophisticated person, well capable of quite complex logical reasoning, who is nevertheless severely restricted in his ability to give instant answers, and who therefore has to resort to strategies – often of his own devising – which are time-consuming and may sometimes involve considerable risk of error.

Chapter 16
Reciting Tables

When I started to use recitation of tables as a test for dyslexia it was immediately obvious that almost all my subjects were having difficulties, often very severe ones. The following were some of the characteristics which were particularly noticeable: (1) loss of place, as exemplified by questions such as 'Was it six sevens I was up to?'; (2) consistent errors in which a correct deduction is made from a faulty premise, for example, 'Two eights are fifteen; three eights are twenty-three'; (3) a variety of slips such as changing to the 8 x table during the course of reciting the 7 x or saying 'eight eighties' for 'eight eights'; (4) the adoption of compensatory strategies, for example the use of fingers, the use of epanalepsis (i.e. taking up what one said earlier as a means of getting back 'on course', see Chapter 3), and the saying of the table without the 'preamble' ('one six is…, two sixes are… , etc.).

These things are by no means uncommon in children who are not dyslexic (see Chapter 7), but a distinction should be drawn between those who have not spent much time learning or practising their tables (whether because they are still young, because they were absent from school, or because in their school tables were not taught) and those who still fail despite long and hard efforts.

In dyslexics these tendencies are so widespread that detailed documentation would be monotonous. I shall therefore limit myself to citing a small number of examples from each age level.

Age 7

It appears that at this age the number sense in a dyslexic child can sometimes be extremely confused. When asked to say the 3 x table, S5 said: 'Two threes are four; four threes are five; five threes are six; six threes are seven; seven threes are eight; eight threes are nine; nine threes are ten'. S6 said: 'I know all the answers but I hate saying it'. He said his 3 x correctly up to 'four threes are twelve', and continued, 'Six threes… no, five threes are fifteen… no, fifteen; six threes are eighteen;

nine threes are twenty; three threes are twenty-three – which one am I on now?' When asked to say his five times he said, 'I can give the numbers, five, ten, fifteen, all right'.

Age 8

The picture is not all that different at age 8. When asked to say his 3 ×, S26 responded 'One two is two; two twos are six; three twos are nine; four twos are eleven; five twos are fourteen; six twos are seventeen; seven twos are... no'. S12, when asked to say his 4 ×, was correct up to 'three fours are twelve'; he then said 'Four fours are fifteen and – um – five fours are nineteen and five – six – fours are twenty-three and – um – seven fours are... what did I get up to? Thirty-three, did I?'

S20 said, 'Do I have to say "one three is" as I can't do it like that?' When I said that he need not, he started 'Three, six, nine' etc. and continued correctly up to fifty-one when I stopped him. When required to include the 'preamble' he said, 'One three is three; two threes are six; four threes are... no, I've missed one out; four threes are twelve; five threes are fifteen; six threes are seventeen – eighteen; eight threes are twenty-one, nine threes are twenty-four; seven – um – ten threes are thirty'.

When asked if she could do her tables, S8 said, 'I can do some, but I forget half way through'. Asked to say his 2 ×, S11 said, 'One two is two; two twos are four; three twos are six; seven twos are nine; eight twos are ten; nine twos are thirteen; ten twos are fourteen; eleven twos are fifteen; twelve twos are twenty-four'.

Age 9

At this age I sometimes tried the more difficult 6 × and 7 × tables, but some of my subjects were still unsure over the 3 × and 4 ×.

S43 said his 3 × correctly up to 'five threes are fifteen'; he then said 'Six threes are twenty-one; seven threes are twenty-four; eight threes are twenty-seven; ten threes are thirty; eleven threes are thirty-three. Twelve threes are thirty-six.' On the 4 × he was correct up to 'three fours are twelve', after which he said, 'Five fours are sixteen; seven fours are twenty-one – I'm stuck !'.

The performance of S38 was extremely curious. She said, 'I did tables once – I keep getting them backwards'. She wrote '02' and asked if that was the way to write 'twenty'. When I started her off with 'One two is two' she said, 'Two twos are four' (pause); 'eight and eight is' (long pause) 'seventeen; three and three are six; six and six is twelve; ten and ten is twenty.' When I indicated that she could write down her 3 × table and said 'One three is three' she wrote

20	20	20
30	30	30
40	40	40
50	50	50
60	60	60
70	70	70

S46 said his 7 x correctly up to 'four sevens are twenty-eight'; he then said, 'five sevens are thirty-two; six sevens are thirty-eight, thirty-nine. What am I up to? Was it six sevens? Seven sevens are forty-two – that's wrong. Forty-two, yes, I think it is... forty-nine, fifty-six, sixty-three. What do you call it? I must have got some of them wrong. Seven sevens are forty-two; six sevens must be wrong'. (My notes say, 'Fascinating sub-vocal speech – too fast to take down'.)

Age 10

Even some of the 10-year-olds had difficulty with the 3 x and 4 x. S61 said 'One three is three; two threes are six; three threes are... three threes are twelve, no, three threes are nine; four threes are twelve; five threes are fifteen; four threes – have I just done four threes?... Five threes are eighteen; six threes are twenty-one... which one am I on?'

S58 produced the following strange series (though it is one that is not wholly lacking in logic): 'Two threes are six; six threes are twelve; twelve threes are twenty-two; three twenty-twos are thirty-six'. When I tried him on the 4 x, he said, 'Four twos are four; four fours are eight; eight twos are sixteen; sixteen twos are twenty-six; twenty-six twos is forty-six; forty-six twos is seventy-six – sixty. I mean sixty-six'.

S83 said his 2 x correctly, but without the preamble, as far as thirty-six. He then murmured 'thirty-seven' *sotto voce* before saying 'thirty-eight' and, later, after saying 'forty-two' he murmured 'forty-three' *sotto voce* before saying 'forty-four'. I stopped him at 50, and not surprisingly he did not know how many twos it was. When he was asked to include the preamble he said, 'One two is two – there's two twos in every two; two twos are four; three twos are six; four twos are ten; five twos are two – four, six,... um... twenty – oh, twenty-two, twenty-four, twenty-six... oh, twenty-six, thirty'. (I did not follow his logic over the last part.)

Similar uncertainty was shown by many of those who attempted their 6 x and 7 x . For example, S75 recited his 6 x correctly up to 'three sixes are eighteen'; he then paused and said 'three' as an epanalepsis, and continued 'Four sixes are twenty-four; five sixes are thirty; eight – six eights are thirty-six; seven sixes are forty-two; eight sixes are forty-two; eight sixes are fifty-eight' (pause); 'nine sevens are... um... fifty-one... um... eleven, ten sixes are sixty; eleven sixes are sixty-six; twelve sixes are seventy-two'.

On a few occasions there was the substitution of a similar sounding number for the correct one. Thus S74 said her 6 × table correctly up to 'nine sixes are fifty-four' and then said, 'ten sixties are sixty; eleven sixties are sixty-six; twelve sixties are seventy-two' (Note 16.1).

Age 11

Even some of the 11-year-olds were having difficulty with the 2, 3 and 4 ×. Thus S105, when asked to say his 2 ×, responded 'Once two is two; two twos are four; two, no three twos are six; four twos are' (pause) 'eight; five twos are ten; six twos are twelve; seven twos are fourteen; eight twos are sixteen; seven twos... eight twos are twenty' (long pause); 'ten twos are twenty-two'. S107 said his 4 × correctly up to 'seven fours are twenty-eight' and continued: 'Nine fours are thirty-two, twelve... eleven... have I had nine fours? Nine fours are thirty-two; ten fours are thirty-six; eleven fours are forty; twelve fours are forty-four'.

S91, when asked to say his 3 ×, said: 'One three is three; once threes are four – no, one threes are six; three threes are nine – no, I get all muddled up'. S92 said his 3 × correctly as far as 'four threes are twelve' but continued. 'Five threes are sixteen; seven threes are eighteen; nine threes are twenty-one; eleven threes' (pause)... 'ten threes are thirty-four; ten threes are thirty-seven; eleven threes are forty; twelve threes are forty-three'.

S98 could say her 4 × correctly as far as 48 provided she did not include the preamble. When she was asked to include this she was correct as far as 'seven fours are twenty-eight' and then said 'Where am I up to?' When encouraged to 'have a go', she said, 'Four sixes are twenty-eight; seven sixes are... seven fours are thirty-two; eight fours are thirty-six; nine fours are forty; ten fours are forty-four; eleven fours are forty-four; twelve fours are forty-eight'.

S111 was able to get as far as 'five fours are twenty' using her fingers. She then said, 'Five fours are twenty-four; six fours are thirty; eight fours seven fours... thirty-four; seven, oh!, have we done seven fours? – thirty-eight; eight, er, nine fours are... ' (counts on fingers) 'forty; ten fours are forty-four'.

There were many typically 'dyslexic' responses over the 6, 7 and 8 ×. When asked to say his 6 × table, S95 said, 'One six is six; two sixes are twelve; three sixes... oh, gosh!' (pause); 'I know... no, I don't, eighteen'. He then proceeded correctly as far as 'eight sixes are forty-eight'. He then said, 'What's next? Nine sixes are fifty... oh, gosh, fifty-four. What's next? That's nine sixes; ten sixes are sixty; eleven sixes are sixty-six; twelve sixes are seventy-two – must be seventy-two as I know two sixes are twelve'. His 7 × was correct up to five sevens are thirty-five;... 'I usually say five sevens are thirty-six. What's next? That's *five* sixes; six sevens are forty-two; eight sevens – now, let's see; ah! it's fifty-six; five,

six, seven, eight, so seven eights are fifty-six. Where am I? I've forgotten
where I am. I was on seven – five, six, seven, eight; seven nines are
sixty-three; seven sev ..., no, seven tens are seventy; seven elevens are
seventy-seven and seventy twelves – seven twelves – no wonder I'm getting all confused – are fourteen, so eighty-four using the same system'.

S74 had clearly learned to use the '10 x table' as an aid. He said his
7 x correctly as far as 'seven sevens are forty-nine'. He then said, 'Eight
sevens are fifty-five – I've gone wrong somewhere. I was adding the
seven and I knew the next number wouldn't go on. If it had got to
sixty-five I knew it couldn't go on like that ... If it's seventeen times
nine I put ten nines are ninety and I say, Nine sevens, that's sixty-three;
then I add them together'.

S90, so his mother told me, had pinned his tables up in his bed-
room and eventually learned them, 'but they were very hard work'.
When asked to say his 7 x he was correct as far as 'seven sixes are forty-
two'; he then said, 'Eight sixes are fifty-four ... oh, dear! – gone wrong
... ten sixes are sixty; eleven sixes are sixty-six; twelve sixes are eighty-
four'. It seems that even hard work in learning tables does not guarantee success, at any rate in a context where one has to recite them
aloud.

Age 12

At least three of my 12-year-olds (S120, S124 and S131), out of a total
of 16, were still having difficulty in reciting the 4 x, while of those who
were given the 6, 7 and 8 x only one came out as 'minus'.

S120 said his 4 x correctly up to 'seven fours are twenty-eight', after
which he said, 'Nine fours are thirty-two, no, seven fours are thirty-two;
eight fours are thirty-six; nine fours are forty – no, nine fours ... *ten*
fours are forty; eleven fours are forty-four; twelve fours are forty-eight'.
S124 was correct up to 'three fours are twelve' after which he said,
'Four fours are fifteen, no, twenty; five fours are twenty-four; six fours
are twenty-seven; six fours are twenty-eight; nine fours – no, seven
fours are thirty-two; eight fours are thirty-six; nine fours are – I don't
know; I'm lost'. S131 was correct up to 'four fours are sixteen, after
which she said, 'Five fours are eighteen ... Can I just say the numbers
as it gets me muddled up?'

Here are two typical performances with the 7 and 8 x. S125 said his
7 x correctly up to 'five sevens are thirty-five' and then said, 'Six sevens
are forty-five, no forty-three – forty-two; seven sevens are forty-nine; five
sevens are fifty-six; six sevens are forty – no, fifty-three' (the intonation
of the 'forty' suggesting that a number in the forties would have followed and that he did not simply mean the number forty) 'and then –
what is it now? I've got them muddled. Nine sevens are ... um ... sixty;
ten sevens are sixty-seven'. S133, when attempting his 8 x said, 'One

Reciting Tables   129

eight is eight; two eights are sixteen; three eights are twenty-eight; four eights are thirty-six; five eights are forty; six eights are forty-eight; what am I on? Seven eights are sixty-four; eight eights are ...' (pause) *'eight eights are sixty-four'*, after which he finished without further error. S127 said his 6 × correctly up to 'nine sixes are fifty-four', but then said 'Ten sixties are sixty; eleven sixties are sixty-six; twelve sixties are –, no, twelve sixes are seventy-two'.

Age 13

Even at this age there were still subjects who had difficulty with the 3 × and 4 ×. Thus S147 said his 3 × correctly up to 'three threes are nine', after which he said, 'Four threes are eighteen; five threes are twenty-one; six threes are twenty-four; seven threes are twenty-seven; eight threes are thirty; nine threes are thirty-three; ten threes are thirty-six; eleven threes are fifty-nine; twelve threes are forty-two'. From 'eight threes' onwards he was overtly using his fingers. S143 said her 3 × correctly up to 'eight threes are twenty-four', and then said, 'Five – no, where are we? Nine threes are twenty-seven; ten threes are thirty; six tw ...' (as if she had been about to say 'twelve' but had stopped herself); 'eleven threes are thirty-three; twelve threes are thirty-six'. S142 said his 4 × correctly up to 'three fours are twelve', after which he said, 'Four fours are four ... fifteen; five fours are nineteen; six fours – I can't remember – twenty-seven, thirty-one; eight fours are thirty-one; nine fours are thirty-five; ten fours – I've gone wrong'.

Even omission of the preamble does not guarantee correctness. For example, when I asked S141 if he had had any difficulty over tables he said, 'I had to go through a lot of this. I could say "Two, four, six, eight" but not "once two is two", like that'. I asked if he would like to say his 6 × 'the easy way', to which he responded, 'Six, twelve, eighteen, twenty-four, thirty, thirty-eight, forty-two, fifty, fifty-six ... no, that's not right; can I start again?' On the next attempt he went through correctly to 72, though with a slight pause at 42. I then asked if he would like to try it 'the hard way'. He was correct as far as 'five sixes are thirty' but added 'I'm on six, am I?'. He continued, 'Six sixes are thirty-six; seven sixes are forty-two; eight sixes are forty-eight; nine sixes are fifty-four – sixty; seven sixes are sixty-six; eight, no – where am I on? Eleven sixes are sixty-six; twelve sixes are seventy-two'. It is possible that the substitution of 'seven' for 'eleven' is another example of an error arising from auditory confusability comparable with those already mentioned (Note 16.2).

Age 14

Among my 14-year-olds there was still one subject (S162) who failed at the 2 ×. The following is a record of my discussion with him. I started by asking him to say his 4 x, to which he replied, 'One four is four; two fours are eight; three fours are sixteen or something – I never can remember them'. I then asked him to try his 2 x, to which he responded: 'Two twos are four; three twos – I'm all mixed up – two twos are four; three twos are six; four twos are nine; five twos are eleven; six twos are thirteen; seven twos are fifteen; eight twos are eighteen, I think; nine twos are twenty; ten twos are twenty-two; twelve twos are twenty-three'.

S158 also had difficulty with his 4 x. His responses were: 'One four is four; two fours are eight; three fours are sixteen; five fours are eighteen; five fours are twenty-two; six fours are forty – um – forty-six; seven fours are fifty-two – how could they be? Oh, help! I'm all lost now'. When I gave S152 what I thought would be an easy task, namely that of saying the 4 x without the preamble, his response was: 'Four; eight; twelve; twenty-four; thirty-six; forty-two'.

When I asked S156 if she had had any trouble with her tables she said that they were 'a nightmare'. Her 6 x was correct up to 'five sixes are thirty', after which she said, 'Seven sixes are thirty-six; eight sixes are forty-two; nine sixes are forty-eight; ten sixes are sixty; eleven sixes are sixty-six; twelve sixes are seventy-two.'

When I said to S164, 'Did you have any trouble with tables?' he replied, 'I still have'. On the 6 x his responses were: 'One six is six; two sixes are twelve; two twelves are twenty-four; three twelves are forty-eight'. When I asked him to try the 4 x he said, 'One four is four; two fours are eight; three fours are sixteen; three fours' (sigh) 'no – twenty-two; four fours are forty...' (pause, with intonation implying a number in the forties to follow) ... 'I'm lost again'.

Age 15

S181 had difficulty with her 2 x. With a slight pause after 'two twos are four' she was correct as far as 'seven twos are fourteen'. She then said, 'Oh, I've lost count. Eight twos' (using fingers) 'are fourteen; nine twos are sixteen; ten twos are eighteen; ten twos' (said not as a correction but as if she was saying the next number up) 'are...' (pause for use of fingers) 'twenty'.

S166 said 'I can do it on paper but I can't do it aloud.' He said the 2 x correctly up to 'five twos are ten'; he then said 'Eleven twos are twelve; twelve twos are fourteen.' I then suggested that he should write out his 7 x, and he wrote:

$$
\begin{array}{rcccr}
1 & \times & 7 & = & 7 \\
2 & \times & 7 & = & 14 \\
3 & \times & 7 & = & 21 \\
\cancel{3}4 & \times & 7 & = & 28 \\
8 & \times & 7 & = & 56
\end{array}
$$

$$9 \times 7 = 61$$
$$10 \times 7 = 68$$
$$11 \times 7 = 75$$
$$12 \times 7 = 92$$

Writing down, however, was usually an aid. S177 had got into serious difficulty over his 6 x. When I gave him 'one six is six' he continued, 'Two sixes are twelve; three sixes are thirty-eight. I can't do the rest; what was the last one I said?'. However, when I allowed him to write down the answers, he wrote '44, 50, 56, 62' etc. all 'correctly' at intervals of 6 as far as 98.

S179 said his 4 x correctly up to 'three fours are twelve' and then said, 'Four fours are fifteen; five fours are nineteen; six fours are twenty-three; seven fours are twenty-six; eight fours are thirty; eight fours are thirty-four; nine fours are thirty-eight; ten fours are thirty; eleven fours are thirty-three; twelve fours are thirty ...' (pause, indicating that a number in the thirties was to come) ' ...six – thirty-seven'.

I did not normally ask my subjects to say the 9 x. This was because, more than the 6, 7 and 8 x, it allows for learning overlay. In the early stages of the research I had met subjects who had been told either to 'drop one each time' (the second figure being, successively, 9, 8, 7, 6 etc.) or to check that the two figures in conjunction added up to nine – 1–8, 2–7, 3–6 etc.; and if either strategy has been taught there was the possibility that the dyslexic handicap would be masked. When S170 was asked to say her 9 x, however, she made the typically dyslexic responses of using her fingers and 'skipping' to the wrong table: 'One nine is nine; two nines are eighteen; three nines are' (pause) 'twenty-seven; four sevens are ... four nines are thirty-six; five nines are' (uses fingers) 'forty-five; six nines are fifty-four; seven nines are' (pause, uses fingers) 'sixty-four; eight sevens are seventy-three; nine sevens are eighty-two; ten sevens are seven ... are ninety; eleven nines are ninety-nine; twelve nines are a hundred-and-eight'.

Age 16

This is the first age level at which none of my subjects had difficulty with the 3 x or 4 x. The overall picture, however, though sometimes more sophisticated, is not basically different.

Here are three typical efforts. S191 was correct over his 6 x up to 'six sixes are thirty-six'. He then said, 'Seven sixties are forty-two; eight sixties are forty-eight; nine sixes are fifty-two; ten sixes are sixty; eleven sixes are sixty-six; twelve sixes are fifty-eight – I get lost, I get muddled'. S200 was given 'one seven is seven' to start him off; he then said, 'Two sevens are fourteen; twenty-one; twenty-eight; thirty-five'. This omission of the preamble was his own choosing. When I asked him to put in 'how many sevens' it was, he was correct up to 'three sevens are twenty-one' and then said, 'Seven fours are twenty-eight – no, yes, twenty-eight; five sevens, no, seven sevens are thirty-five; eight sevens are forty-two; nine sevens are forty-nine; ten sevens, um, what am I doing? It can't be. What were ...? I'm a bit confused. I was on ten sevens and got to forty-nine'.

S193 gave an interesting account of his difficulties. 'I never learned my tables but I have a number of numbers which I can do easily; for example, three sevens multiplied by two is forty-two ... they made me learn them but I never did'. When he attempted his 6 x he was correct as far as 'four sixes are twenty-four', after which he said, 'Six sixes are thirty-six; seven sixes are thirty-two; eight sixes are thirty-eight; nine sixes is for–' (as if it was to be a number in the forties) ' ... what was the last one? Fifty-four; six sixes – no, ten sixes are sixty; eleven sixes are sixty-six; twelve sixes are seventy-two'.

Age 17

It is still the same story at this age. In attempting her 6 x, S205 was correct as far as 'eight sixes are forty-eight'. She then said, 'Nine sixes are ...' (laughs) 'I've got to add it up. What am I on ...? Fifty-four; ten sixes are sixty; eleven sixes are – eleven – eight sixes are seventy-two'. ('Are you sure?') 'Oh, sorry! Twelve sixes are seventy-two'.

S209 said her 6 x correctly up to 'six sixes are thirty-six' and then said, 'Seven are forty-two; eight are forty-eight; nine are' (pause) 'fifty-four; ten are sixty; sixty-six, eleven; seventy-two are twelve'. This appears to be an attempt to make the task easier by reducing the time-interval over which the multiplier has to be held in mind.

S204 muttered inaudibly to himself some of the time. When I started him off with 'one seven is seven' he said, 'Two sevens are fourteen – no, twenty, no, fourteen; three sevens are twenty-one; four sevens are twenty-eight' (pause); 'thirty-six; I think; five sevens are thirty-five – that's wrong oh – yes!, forty-nine – good at tables' (said sarcastically); 'forty-nine; fifty-four, I think – fifty-six, I think. What are we up to so far? Next one's forty-two, forty-nine'.

Age 18

Even among my oldest subjects there is no change in the basic pattern, only an increasing degree of sophistication and in some cases use of compensatory strategies.

S213 said to me, 'I don't know my tables even now'. She was correct on her 7 x as far as 'four sevens are twenty-eight'. She then said, 'Five sevens are thirty – heavens!, thirty-five; six sevens are forty-two; seven sevens are forty-nine; eight sevens are' (pause) ... 'seven sevens are forty-nine; eight sevens are fifty-six; nine sevens are' (pause) 'sixty-three; ten sevens are seventy; eleven sevens are seventy-seven; twelve sevens are eighty-' (pause to work out number in the eighties) 'four – no, eighty-five'.

S219 said his 7 × correctly as far as 'four sevens are twenty-eight'. He then said, 'Five sevens are thirty-six – thirty-seven; six sevens are thirty-eight; seven sevens are forty-five' (uses fingers); 'no, five sevens are forty-five; six sevens are fifty-two – I've got to make sure it's right – I've got to check up'. He then recited from 'five sevens are thirty-five' to 'twelve sevens are eighty-four' correctly.

S220 said his 7 × correctly up to 'four sevens are twenty-eight'. He then said, 'Five sevens are' (pause) 'thirty-five; six sevens are' (pause) 'seventy-two – I've just got to add. Six sevens are forty-two; seven sevens are forty-nine; eight sevens are fifty-six. What are nine...? Nine sevens are – seven off ninety which is eighty-three; ten sevens are seventy; eleven sevens are seventy-seven; twelve sevens are eighty-five; thirteen sevens are ninety-two; I'd be worse if I didn't play darts'.

89% of my subjects (199 out of 223) scored 'plus' on the Tables item of the dyslexia test, or 119 out of 132 (90%) if we take only the dyslexic subjects who were matched against controls. In contrast there were 71 'pluses' among the 132 controls (54%)(Note 16.3). Clearly, therefore, difficulties over tables are not found solely in dyslexic subjects, and it seems likely that they occur in anyone who has not had the requisite amount of practice or experience. What is interesting about so many dyslexics is that in spite of all the opportunities available to them the difficulties still persist.

Chapter 17
Recall of Digits

I had noticed at an early stage of the research that many of my subjects appeared to be weak at the recall of auditorily presented digits, whether in the 'forwards' or 'reversed' condition. From the norms given in the Terman–Merrill test, it was plain that a 9-year-old of average ability could be expected to succeed in at least one trial out of three at 'four digits forwards' and a 12-year-old in at least one trial out of three at 'five digits reversed'. Yet even some of my older subjects were making errors over 'three digits reversed' and those who obtained passes at the Superior Adult grades of the Terman–Merrill test were consistently failing at 'five digits reversed' even though this is set far lower down the scale. I also found that subjects who scored well above the average on some of the other sub-tests of the WISC were consistently below average on the Digit Span sub-test. A check on the literature in this area (Note 17.1) fully confirmed that among poor readers of all kinds a distinctive weakness in the area of 'digit span' was extremely common.

It was during the early 1970s that I first decided to make a study of the responses of dyslexic subjects to visually presented digits. The conditions in such an investigation are different from those of auditory presentation not only because a different sense modality, vision, is involved but also because, if one so wishes, the digits can all be presented simultaneously. We are so made – and this is no doubt a point of considerable theoretical interest – that if digits, or other symbols, are presented to us auditorily they have to occur in succession, whereas if they are presented visually they can be either simultaneous or successive.

It was not a standard part of the assessment to present digits visually, but examination of my records showed that I had usable data in respect of 40 out of my 223 subjects, along with two other subjects (S237 and S245) from my 'incomplete records' group (Note 17.2). As I had data on the performance of all my subjects when digits were presented auditorily, it was possible not only to examine the performance of each of these 42 subjects in the visual condition but to compare it with their performance in the auditory condition.

To avoid the dangers of premature grouping, I have presented the data for each subject separately (see Table 17.1). My procedure was to show the subject the tachistoscope (a device for exposing stimulus material for controlled periods of time; Note 17.3), explain what was required, namely that when the presentation was over he should report the numbers which he had seen on the screen, and then expose about 30 cards at varying exposure times. These times were decreased or increased according to the subject's success or otherwise in reproducing the correct digits, larger numbers of readings being taken near the 'limits' of his success. A somewhat complicated method of scoring enabled me to take account not only of whether he had responded with the correct digits but whether he had given them in the correct order (Note 17.4).

Table 17.1 shows the performance of each subject when six digits were exposed. The first column gives the mean (average) exposure time for three presentations of six digits near the range at which he had just started to make incorrect responses. The second column gives the subject's mean score out of a maximum of 6 for the three presentations. In addition, to make possible a comparison between different subjects despite variations in exposure time, I calculated a figure, presented in the third column, which I termed the 'comparison ratio'; this is the subject's hypothetical score at an exposure time of 1000 ms (one second) by extrapolation from the actual score at the specified exposure time. Thus a score of 4.2 at an exposure-time of 2000 ms would give a comparison ratio of 2.1 (Note 17.5). Finally, so as to make comparisons between each subject's performance in the visual condition and in the auditory condition, I have extracted from the Summary Chart (see Chapter 6) the highest series length for which the subject gave a correct response on Digits Forwards and used this, along with the comparison ratio, as a basis for assigning each subject to a 'visual grade' and to an 'auditory grade'. The grade labels are 'high' (H), 'medium' (M), 'low' (L) and 'very low' (VL) (Note 17.6).

One of the most striking points about Table 17.1 is the excessively long time needed by some of the subjects to respond correctly in the visual condition. Some data for adequate spellers have been collected by Pollard (Note 17.7), from which one can infer that the typical non-retarded 9–12-year-old will have a comparison ratio of about 6; although comparisons are not straightforward because of differences in the experimental conditions, the figures obtained by Ellis and Miles (Note 17.8) make it highly improbable that the typical normal speller aged 10–14 would have a comparison ratio of less than this amount. Yet four subjects in the present study needed over 6000 ms (6 s) before they could get somewhere near a correct answer and 24 others needed

Table 17.1 Comparison of subjects' recall of digits in conditions of visual and auditory presentation

Subject no.	Mean exposure time (ms) (visual)	Mean score	Comparison ratio	Maximum no. of digits forwards (auditory)	Visual grade	Auditory grade
3	2500	4.3	1.73	5	VL	L
7	1500	4.67	3.11	5	L	L
12	2000	3.67	1.83	5	VL	L
16	6000	4.67	0.79	4	M	VL
20	3000	5.00	1.67	4	M	VL
21	1833	4.67	2.56	6	L	M
33	7000	5.00	0.71	4	M	VL
34	2000	4.00	2.00	8	L	H
40	2500	5.00	2.00	3	L	VL
49	667	5.33	8.42	3	H	VL
50	2000	3.00	1.50	5	VL	L
53	3000	3.75	1.25	5	VL	L
56	2333	4.33	1.86	4	M	VL
60	8000	3.00	0.38	4	M	VL
62	1600	5.00	3.13	5	L	L
69	3667	5.33	1.45	6	VL	M
74	1467	5.00	3.41	5	L	L
79	1200	5.00	4.17	5	M	L
84	1000	5.33	5.33	6	H	M
86	2000	3.66	1.83	5	VL	L
87	1467	5.33	3.63	4	L	VL
88	4000	4.67	1.17	6	VL	M
90	1200	5.00	4.17	5	M	L
102	2000	5.00	2.50	4	L	VL
104	4667	5.00	0.94	4	VL	VL
107	3000	4.33	1.44	5	VL	L
108	2000	5.33	2.67	6	L	M
112	1833	5.33	2.99	7	L	H
121	3000	4.33	1.44	5	VL	L
136	1500	5.00	3.33	5	L	L
146	1500	5.33	3.55	4	L	VL
149	2000	4.66	2.33	6	L	M
159	1000	5.33	5.33	5	H	L
165	8000	4.33	0.54	5	VL	L
174	1067	4.00	3.75	8	L	H
193	1200	4.67	3.89	6	L	M
197	1233	5.00	4.06	5	M	L
202	1600	4.67	2.92	6	L	M
208	1000	4.67	4.67	4	M	VL
213	933	4.33	4.64	5	M	L
237	1000	5.00	5.00	6	H	M
245	1333	4.00	3.00	5	L	L

1500 ms (1.5 s) or more. Only four subjects had a comparison ratio of 5 or above, and only one subject (S49) produced a result which would have led to a prediction of 'non-dyslexic' had no other information about him been available (Note 17.9). Slowness at processing visually presented symbolic material was thus extremely widespread.

Now it has sometimes been suggested that a distinction should be drawn between the 'visual dyslexic' and the 'auditory dyslexic'. There are, however, various reasons for doubting the validity of this distinction (Note 17.10), and it seemed to me that a possible way of throwing further light on the problem was to compare each subject's performance in the auditory condition with his performance in the visual condition. The idea of two types of dyslexia – one characterised by a predominantly visual weakness and one characterised by a predominantly auditory weakness – would receive strong support if most of the subjects could be classified without ambiguity as belonging to one type or the other: a high score in the visual condition and a low score in the auditory condition would suggest 'auditory dyslexia' while a low score in the visual condition and a high score in the auditory condition would suggest 'visual dyslexia'. Table 17.2 shows no convincing evidence for such a grouping.

Table 17.2 Numbers of subjects in each grade (auditory and visual conditions)					
		Auditory condition			
		High	Medium	Low	Very low
	High	0	1	1	1
	Medium	0	1	3	6
Visual condition	Low	3	5	7	3
	Very low	0	2	8	1

The high scorers in the visual condition were not necessarily the low scorers in the auditory condition, nor vice versa, and indeed 19 of the 42 subjects obtained 'low' or 'very low' scores in both conditions (Note 17.11). This finding does not prove that the distinction between 'visual dyslexia' and 'auditory dyslexia' is valueless but it provides no active support for it. It seems more likely that most dyslexic persons are slow at processing symbolic verbal material irrespective of the sense modality through which the material is presented (Note 17.12).

Chapter 18
Additional Evidence

This chapter contains a number of findings on topics which it was not possible to investigate fully or systematically. Of necessity, therefore, the evidence is somewhat uneven in quality, but many of the results seem to me interesting and suggestive.

Memory for sentences

In a number of cases I was able to give my subjects the sentence memory item which occurs in the Terman–Merrill test (year xi, no. 4). It runs: 'At the summer camp the children get up early in the morning to go swimming'. This turned out to be an interesting test because it was just marginally too long for many of them, even in cases where they had no difficulty in understanding the gist, and it was often helpful to determine how many trials were needed before they were word-perfect.

The results were very clear. On almost all occasions the main points of the sentence were given, but it was very common for one or two words to be left out. Here are a few examples from the many available: S63, S77, S114, S120, S137, S159, S163, S170, S181 and S213 left out 'in the morning'; S176 left out 'early'; S184 ended up 'early to go swimming in the morning', while S121 ended 'get up early and go to the baths'. An unusual reproduction, apparently combining an error based on auditory confusability with an error of ordering, was made by S140, who said, 'The children get up early in the morning to go fishing to the summer camp (Note 18.1). Since this item is regarded in the Terman–Merrill test as suitable for 11-year-olds it is highly significant that some of the errors mentioned above should have occurred in subjects aged 13 and over who, with the exceptions of S163 and S170, were graded W or higher in intelligence rating.

Particularly interesting is the fact that some subjects needed five or more repetitions and were not always word perfect even then. Here is a record of the responses of S93 over seven trials, the original sentence being repeated by me between each trial:

(1) At the summer camp the children in the morning get up early to go swimming.
(2) At the summer camp the children get up early to go swimming.
(3) At the summer camp early in the morning the children go swimming.
(4) At the summer camp the children get up early to go swimming.
(5) At the summer camp the children get up early in the morning to go swimming (correct response).
(6) At the summer camp the children get up early to go swimming.
(7) At the summer camp the children get up early to go swimming.

Here is a further series, this time from S49:

(1) The little boys get up in the morning and go and have a swim.
(2) At the summer camp the boys get up early in the morning to have a swim.
(3) The summer – no, the boys get up in the morning and go and have a swim.
(4) At the summer camp the children get up early in the morning and go for a swim.
(5) At the summer camp the children get up in the morning and go for a swim.

I have similar records for S59, S75, S83 and S99. The conclusion appears to be that a dyslexic subject can be very strong at 'processing for meaning' but is sometimes extremely weak at verbatim recall.

Other memory problems

S139, according to her mother, 'could never learn nursery rhymes. This struck me as odd'. Difficulty in rote learning was also mentioned in the case of S25 and S218. Difficulty in following instructions was regularly mentioned, and the mother of S110 commented on the fact that instructions often needed to be repeated. Several subjects mentioned the need to 'go back' when they became lost (the 'epanalepsis' strategy mentioned in Chapter 3). For example, in connection with learning the alphabet, S206 said, 'If I want to know what comes after H or I, I have to go back to the start'. S34 said, 'I don't like long stories. They stop in the middle of a page – it gets your turn – you have to begin from the top of the page to get it properly... When Mrs __ reads a story I can remember right back but what's just happened I forget'.

When we arrived at the word 'anxious' in the Schonell S_1 test, S209 said, 'That's one of the words Mrs __ went over with me but I can't remember what she said about it'. An admirably succinct statement was given by S63, who simply said, 'I'm a quick forgetter'.

In some cases mathematical calculation was affected. For example S214 said, 'I've never liked mental arithmetic. I'd just work half of it out and I'd have forgotten it before I could work out the rest'. A particularly insightful comment was made by S155, who said, 'If I have to work something out at maths and have to keep something else in my head I use my fingers. You get confused easily when you try to remember something and keep something else in your head'.

Copying from the blackboard

Difficulty in copying from the blackboard was mentioned on many occasions, for example in the cases of S4, S61, S145 and S227. A related difficulty was that reported by S175 who had been studying Macbeth and found it difficult to locate particular passages which she wished to examine.

Learning a foreign language

Difficulty with written French was also commonly reported and for interest a copy of a French dictation by S115 is given below (Figure 18.1). I was told that S147 had been good at oral French but had had severe problems in learning the difference between acute and grave accents. I think it likely that only a very bright dyslexic subject would be able to achieve 'O' level standard in written (as opposed to oral) French, and my experience was that those who had struggled with it were usually very relieved at the thought of giving it up. Possibly languages which are phonically more regular would present less difficulty – a point made to me by S168 who, in connection with the Polysyllables item of the dyslexia test, said, 'I do a lot of this in Spanish. The words are similar and you've got to pick out the differences'.

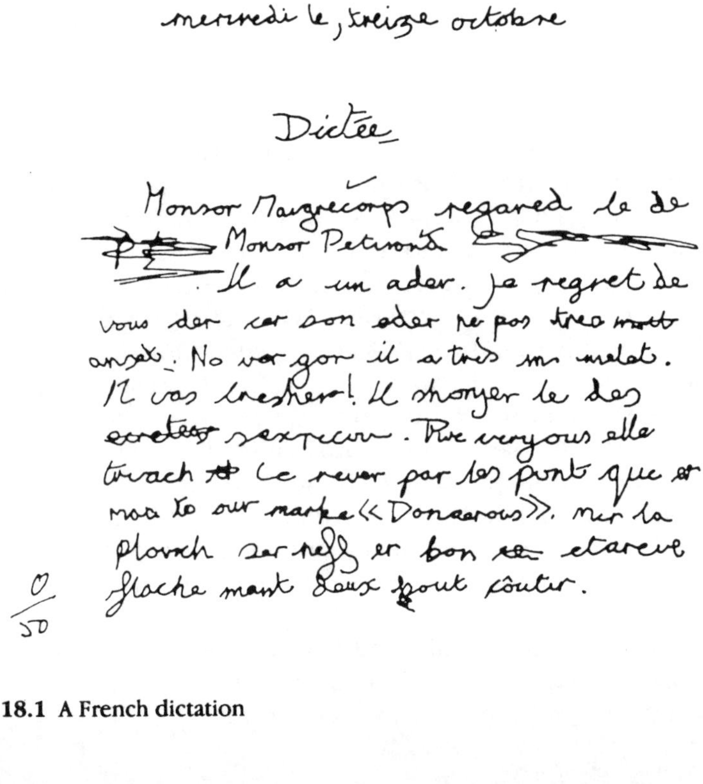

Figure 18.1 A French dictation

Finding rhymes

In some cases I gave my subjects the Terman–Merrill rhymes test. This is an item given to 9-year-olds in which they are asked to say (a) a colour which rhymes with *head*, (b) a number which rhymes with *tree*, (c) an animal that rhymes with *fair*, and (d) a flower that rhymes with *nose*. Those who appeared to be having difficulty were given a supplementary test (see Appendix I): words were presented in pairs (e.g. 'cat/dog' 'cat/fat', etc.) and they were asked to say 'yes' if the words rhymed and 'no' if they did not.

The number of subjects who displayed difficulty over rhymes was not large; but when they did so my impression was – as with so many other dyslexic manifestations – that in some way they had 'missed out'; in other words it was not simply that the items were too hard for them but rather that they were at a loss to know what was needed.

My records give the following data in respect of S1:

Table 18.1 Data for S1

Stimulus	Response
hit/bit	yes
cat/dog	yes
cat/mat	no
bet/set	no
cat/mat	I've said it before; yes
cat/hat	no
cat/hit	no
bat/sat	yes
egg/bacon	yes – no, it should be bacon and egg

With one subject (S49) I went over the items a second time because I had serious doubts as to whether he would be consistent. The following table shows his responses:

Table 18.2 Data for S49

Stimulus	Response (first time)	Response (second time)
cat/dog	no	yes
cat/sat	yes	no
mouse/elephant	yes	yes
mouse/house	yes	yes
fish/dish	yes	no
fish/water	yes	yes
butter/gutter	no	yes
butter/jam	yes	yes
egg/bacon	no, yes	yes

S88 went through the whole list replying 'yes' indiscriminately, and when I asked him, 'What exactly *is* a rhyme?' he replied, 'Something like "Jack and Jill"', without any awareness, so it seemed to me, of the fact that 'Jill' and 'hill' in the next line are similar sounds. S181 gave 'two' as the number that rhymed with 'tree' and 'fish' as the animal that rhymed with 'fair'. She was able to respond correctly to the pairs of items, but when asked about 'egg and bacon' she said, 'I don't know why – I just don't think they do rhyme. They're always together but I don't think they rhyme'. It is hard to see how a person who had really understood the notion of 'rhyming' could say that she did not *think* that two words rhymed, since the matter is surely one for immediate recognition. Similarly S75 in reply to 'mouse-house' said 'No – yes' (changing his mind) and in reply to 'egg–bacon' he said 'yes' and corrected this to 'not really'. The responses of S72 were puzzling and ambiguous. He responded correctly with 'red' as a rhyme for *head*, but when asked for a number that rhymed with *tree* he said, 'Trente – no, that's French', and when I asked if 'trente' rhymed with 'tree' he said, 'No, not really'. He responded 'yes' and 'no' correctly to all the pairs of words, with the exception of 'egg and bacon', to which he said, 'Yes, no', and, when I asked which, he said, 'Yes, they do'. Asked to give two words that rhymed he said 'Sit and bit – no, that doesn't rhyme'. When I asked what a rhyme was he said, 'A word that flows into the other one – they kind of flow – they are similar words'. S179 gave 'red' as the colour that rhymed with *head* but only after a long pause; he gave 'two' as the number that rhymed with *tree*, and failed to give rhymes to either *fair* or *nose*. He said 'yes' and 'no' correctly to all the pairs of words, and when I included 'two and tree' and he said 'no', I pointed out that 'two' could not be right for the earlier item. He then said 'Three – yes, I think so; they've both got "e" at the end'. A subject whom I described in an earlier book (Note 18.2) was able to do the Rhymes test by means of a similar compensatory strategy: if one has not grasped the idea of auditory similarity it is still possible, in the case of older subjects, to spell the two words and note if they end in approximately the same letters.

The existence of a difficulty on the part of poor readers over recognising if words rhyme has also been reported by Bradley and Bryant, whose subjects were required to give the 'odd one out' from a list of words such as *nod, red, fed, bed* (Note 18.3). I find it hard to believe that this difficulty arises from any kind of hearing deficiency of peripheral origin, although by analogy with the acquired aphasias I would not object to calling it an 'auditory agnosia', provided one appreciates that even those dyslexic children who display it may well grow out of it. What is involved, I suspect, is the formation of some kind of linkage or association between words such that the person can classify the cat–sat relationship as similar to the hit–bit relationship. If the language system

is in some way deficient, as in dyslexia, the development of this particular linkage may not come easily, in much the same way, perhaps, as, for
some dyslexic children, the recognition that the letters which we write
represent the sounds which we hear does not come easily. It does not
follow that such failures are permanent or incurable; the position
seems to be that dyslexic children do not invariably 'pick up' various
forms of language skill which in non-dyslexic children can be taken for
granted.

Bell-ringing

Next I should like to call attention to a curiosity which was mentioned
on two occasions (S244 and S246). Both had attempted to learn bell
ringing and both had had to give it up because they could not keep
count! I suspect that this task necessitates holding in mind a verbal
record of the number of previous rings which have occurred; the person therefore has to count at speed, and the difficulty experienced by a
dyslexic subject is presumably a special case of the 'loss of place' phenomenon which has been described in Chapters 13 and 16.

Driving a car

I am sometimes asked if dyslexic persons are in any way at risk in driving a car. The question is presumably raised because of possible confusions over 'left' and 'right'.

There are occasional references to car driving in my records. Thus
S248, who used a lump on her finger as a mnemonic, said, 'I have to
think, for example at crossroads'. S253 said, 'I do have difficulty in
defining left and right; it was terrible when I started learning to drive'.
S205, when asked 'Show me your right hand', said 'The only reason I
know is I have a lump on my finger... One of my faults [in her driving
test] was turning left when he said "right"'. If, however, as seems likely
(Chapter 10), it is the *words* 'left' and 'right' which are a source of confusion for dyslexic subjects rather than the directions as such, there is
no reason to think that a dyslexic driver would be more prone than
other drivers to cut across traffic, since one can tell that another car is
approaching without any knowledge at all of the words 'left' and
'right'. Moreover, if a guide tells a dyslexic person to turn left and he
mistakenly supposes that he is being asked to turn right, he would have
to be a very incompetent driver before he turned right across a stream
of oncoming traffic; if he failed to wait this would be nothing to do
with misunderstanding the instructions.

I know of several dyslexic adults who are very good drivers and of
none who have been involved in any serious accident (see also Chapter
31).

It therefore seems to me entirely sensible that a dyslexic person should learn to drive a car if he believes himself to have the necessary competence. Few, if any, actions in life are totally risk-free, but I do not believe that there is any distinctive risk (certainly not any appreciable one) if a dyslexic person is in charge of a car.

Wetting and soiling

Although wetting and soiling are commonly believed to be signs of stress, the occasions when they were mentioned during my assessments were remarkably few in number. The bed-wetting of S7 has already been mentioned in Chapter 5. In addition I was told that up to age 8 S158 was 'still bed-wetting and full of nervous twitches', that S211 used to wet the bed until age 9, that S169 soiled until the age of 10, and that S207 had until recently had a persistent soiling problem. I did not specifically ask questions in this area, and it is therefore hard to be sure that there were no other cases of wetting or soiling among my subjects, but these were the only cases where the matter was spontaneously mentioned. It is interesting that Sandhya Naidoo (Note 18.4) reports no higher incidence of wetting or soiling among her two dyslexic groups than among her controls. Since it is clear that many dyslexic children are under appreciable stress, it is possible that the commonly accepted idea that wetting and soiling are signs of stress is itself in need of revision.

Chess

I was told on several occasions that my subjects had been successful at chess. S62, who came to me at the age of 10, was said to be able to win against his mother; the skills of S118 were said to have been particularly encouraged at Junior School, and S179 said that he could beat anyone in the school except for two boys. At first glance it might seem that chess involves calculation and that there is a large amount to remember. It is different, however, from a skill such as reciting tables, since (except in blindfold chess) the information about the position of the pieces is available whenever one wishes to be reminded of it. Moreover a dyslexic person has no difficulty in *imagining* such and such to be the case and there is therefore no reason why he should not pass in his imagination to several moves ahead; nor does this involve any 'memory overload' since the different moves can be considered successively and do not have to be held in mind all at once. All that needs to be considered at one instant is the piece and the place to which it is moving; even possible threats from the opponent's pieces can be considered successively. I see no reason, therefore, why dyslexic subjects should not be good at chess, and from the above evidence it is plain that some of them are.

Music

Enough of my subjects were gifted musically to convince me that for a dyslexic person success in this area is entirely possible. If there is a drawback one might expect it to arise from a difficulty in *reading* music, not from any difficulty in appreciating it. In particular, an orchestral score is so full of symbolic material that one would expect a dyslexic person to have considerable difficulty with it (though a conductor, if dyslexic, would presumably be able to rely on his musical knowledge), and one would also expect relative difficulty with piano music, where two staves have to be read simultaneously. On the other hand, since despite early struggles a dyslexic person eventually learns to read a book there seems no reason why he should not also master musical notation in the same way.

The reports which have reached me, though few in number, seem on the whole to bear this out. Thus S72 and S74 had passed Grade Two at the piano, though the latter was reported to have difficulty in reading the bass clef 'even though she knew what was there'. She had also passed Grade Four on the flute. S193 had been successful at the piano, and when I asked him about reading music he said, 'I read it slowly. I'm less ahead than most people would be for the amount of learning I've done. My sight reading is a bad point; I know it all but it's slow. Then eventually my fingers remember'. S147 had been deputy-leader of his school choir and had sung in oratorios, while S241 had apparently had considerable success on the flute (Note 18.5). The only counter-example which I have recorded was that of S112 who according to his mother 'could not make headway with the piano because of his left–right problem', though it was not clear what exactly this problem was.

I think it probable, therefore, that a dyslexic person is as likely as anyone else to be gifted musically, and that although the reading of musical notation may be something of a barrier, once this barrier has been overcome (as in the reading of an alphabetic script) there is no reason why good progress should not be made. It is perhaps a pity that young children sometimes equate 'doing music' with learning the names of the notes on the stave (E G B D F etc.), since any weakness in this area may give them the impression that they will be unsuccessful at music; this may in fact be quite mistaken. The situation is not unlike that when a dyslexic child mistakenly concludes from his difficulties over calculation and tables that he is 'no good at maths' (Note 18.6).

Art and craft

It is likely on general grounds that the spread of talents and interests among dyslexic children is as varied as it is among other children. One must also suppose, however, that those talents which are least affected by the handicap will be the ones which tend to flourish. In particular, art is something at which a dyslexic subject can be successful without having too many dyslexic-type problems to overcome. Some of my subjects were in fact extremely gifted in this area. For example, S171 and S199 were aiming at going to Art School, while S46, S54 and S150, among others, showed me some quite remarkable drawings. S179 gave me a mosaic comprising small dots of many different colours, which had clearly involved many hours of patient work. S123 had made beautiful carvings of a rabbit and a stoat, while S257, despite his lack of success at school in other ways, told me that he had done well at art and woodwork. S120 had pottery and painting as his hobbies, and S112 was reported to have considerable talent for technical drawing.

Creative writing

Many of my subjects showed remarkable powers of literary appreciation and expression. For example, the school books of S192 showed some extremely imaginative writing, and his mother when she first wrote to me said: 'He loves poetry, however, and does appear to understand some difficult poems. When I read his own writing I am always amazed at the depth of feeling especially when I consider the almost total lack of reading experience'. In the school books of S46 I found:

> A yellow frightened moon slid itself behind the dark clouds as an owl hooted murnfully from the black woods. It was cold and strangely quiet here.

Presumably in this case the spelling had been amended. Sometimes, however, the poor spelling can increase the pathos, as in the following line which I found among the school books of S204:

> I feel so much pain in this garbag hiepe called time.

The following was written by S237 about his memory:

> My morey is a Labourinth (crossings out) of passegs with an old sage moveing for on to room to another thats how I rember things when I am not tring.

To conclude, I should like to quote two samples of written work by S128, the first a piece of imaginative prose, the second a humorous poem. This is the first:

> I am a TT rider about to start the race

> I can bearly hear the reving up of the powerful race bikes my mind is dume to everything exept the starters flag the smell of the 5 star 4 stroke petrol

the tention wich was bilding up in me was unberable I just had to go suden-
ly the checked flag droped and I was away among the screming gutsis,
BMWs, BSAs and Nortons to name but a few

This is the second:
> I am a gnu
> Sick of typhoo
> But just between you and me
> I drink beer, sparkling beer
> And so do all the other gnus I knew
>
> But now I've reformed
> I drink typhoo
> Boo-hoo-hoo
> Gnu-gnu-gnu
> Sadly gnu.

One of the paradoxes of dyslexia is that although in a sense it is a 'language disability' it is not the kind of disability which precludes creative
writing.

Chapter 19
Improvement over Time

As was indicated in Chapter 6, the Summary Chart provides a large quantity of material for statistical analysis; although in the present book no attempt has been made to treat the data exhaustively, there is one area, that of improvement over time, where I thought it appropriate to introduce a somewhat higher degree of statistical technicality.

Ideally it would have been helpful to have had longitudinal studies of all the subjects in the sample, so that each individual's changes in performance could be investigated as his age increased. Unfortunately there is only a limited amount of evidence in this area, since relatively few of my subjects came for a second assessment (see the postscript to this chapter). It may still be of interest, however, to compare, not the same subjects at different ages, but how far those of different age-groups perform differently.

The items chosen for study were reading, spelling, Digits Forwards, Digits Reversed, Months Forwards and Months Reversed (Note 19.1). The question at issue is whether – or to what extent – the older subjects were more successful at these items than the younger ones (Note 19.2).

Table 19.1 shows the subjects' reading scores, Table 19.2 their spelling scores, Table 19.3 their Digits Forwards scores, and Table 19.4 their Digits Reversed scores, all in relation to age; Table 19.5 shows the percentage of subjects at each age level scoring 'plus', 'zero' and 'minus' on Months Forwards and Table 19.6 gives the same information in respect of Months Reversed. For ease of inspection the scores in the reading and spelling tests have been grouped in tens and in all six tests the ages have been grouped in years. In the calculations which follow later in the chapter, however, the actual scores have been used and the ages were recorded to the nearest month (Note 19.3).

Inspection shows that the older subjects were considerably more successful at reading than the younger ones, somewhat more successful at spelling, but only marginally more successful in the other four tests.

To express the relationship to age of each of the six tests with greater precision it was decided to make use of the statistic known as the correlation coefficient. This figure (written as 'r') lies between +1 and −1 and indicates the extent to which increase in one variable (for example, reading score) can be predcted from increase in another (for example, age). In what follows age is symbolised by 'a' and scores on reading, spelling, Digits Forwards, Digits Reversed, Months Forwards and Months Reversed (Note 19.4) by the letters 'u', 'v', 'w', 'x', 'y' and 'z' respectively. Calculation gave the following results:

Table 19.1 Reading and age: Table of frequencies

Score on R_1	7	8	9	10	11	12	13	14	15	16	17	18
						Age in years						
90–99	-	-	-	-	-	-	-	-	4	1	2	9
80–89	-	-	-	-	-	2	3	1	7	1	4	-
70–79	-	-	-	3	4	3	2	6	4	6	2	1
60–69	-	-	-	-	7	3	4	2	3	2	-	-
50–59	-	-	3	4	5	3	4	2	5	1	-	-
40–49	-	3	6	10	6	-	-	4	2	1	-	-
30–39	1	3	13	6	8	3	1	-	1	-	-	-
20–29	3	7	3	3	3	1	2	-	-	-	-	-
10–19	1	3	4	3	-	1	-	-	-	-	-	-
0–9	2	3	-	-	-	-	-	-	-	-	-	-
Mean	18.00	24.63	34.93	41.52	49.18	55.56	60.44	63.80	71.19	71.42	85.00	92.11
s.d.	11.61	11.48	11.64	16.07	15.86	21.16	19.35	12.63	17.67	13.86	7.52	6.87

Table 19.2 Spelling and age: Table of frequencies

Score on S_1	7	8	9	10	11	12	13	14	15	16	17	18
						Age in years						
90–99	-	-	-	-	-	-	-	-	-	-	-	-
80–89	-	-	-	-	-	-	-	-	2	1	1	7
70–79	-	-	-	-	-	-	1	-	5	2	2	1
60–69	-	-	-	-	2	-	4	2	2	2	1	1
50–59	-	-	-	1	3	4	2	2	4	4	3	-
40–49	-	1	-	6	5	4	3	6	6	-	1	-
30–39	-	1	6	8	7	4	3	2	5	1	-	1
20–29	2	8	18	8	14	2	2	3	2	1	-	-
10–19	2	8	5	6	2	2	1	-	-	1	-	-
0–9	3	1	-	-	-	-	-	-	-	-	-	-
Mean	12.57	20.05	25.62	30.55	34.09	39.06	46.19	43.47	51.88	55.00	63.75	78.78
s.d.	9.50	8.24	5.79	11.28	13.77	13.36	16.76	12.65	17.17	21.56	13.98	15.41

Table 19.3 Digits Forwards and age: Table of frequencies

No. of digits	7	8	9	10	11	12	13	14	15	16	17	18
						Age in years						
9	-	-	1	1	-	-	-	-	1	-	-	-
8	-	-	2	-	-	-	-	-	1	-	-	-
7	-	1	-	-	1	4	4	3	6	2	-	4
6	-	7	7	10	9	7	3	3	8	4	2	3
5	4	6	12	10	11	4	7	6	10	6	4	3
4	3	5	5	8	11	1	2	3	-	-	2	-
3	-	-	2	-	-	-	-	-	-	-	-	-
Mean	4.57	5.10	5.27	5.20	4.94	5.88	5.56	5.40	6.04	5.67	5.00	6.10
s.d.	0.53	1.05	1.36	1.08	0.93	0.89	1.03	1.06	1.08	0.78	0.76	0.88

Table 19.4 Digits Reversed and age: Table of frequencies

No. of digits	7	8	9	10	11	12	13	14	15	16	17	18
						Age in years						
6	-	-	-	-	1	-	1	-	2	1	1	-
5	-	1	1	2	3	3	3	-	6	-	-	2
4	-	5	5	7	5	5	3	3	9	5	4	5
3	5	12	18	18	22	8	8	10	8	6	3	3
2	2	1	5	2	2	-	1	2	1	-	-	-
Mean	2.71	3.32	3.07	3.31	3.36	3.70	3.69	3.07	4.00	3.67	3.75	3.90
s.d.	0.49	0.67	0.70	0.71	0.86	0.79	1.08	0.59	1.02	0.89	1.04	0.73

Table 19.5 Months Forwards and age: Percentages scoring 'plus', 'zero' and 'minus'

	7	8	9	10	11	12	13	14	15	16	17	18
						Age in years						
Plus	100	89	62	59	33	63	31	67	35	17	25	20
Zero	0	0	14	7	18	0	0	0	0	0	0	0
Minus	0	11	24	34	48	38	69	33	65	83	75	80

Table 19.6 Months Reversed and age: Percentages scoring 'plus', 'zero' and 'minus'

	7	8	9	10	11	12	13	14	15	16	17	18
						Age in years						
Plus	100	95	83	90	67	62	50	93	73	25	62	30
Zero	0	0	10	0	18	13	25	7	4	8	0	10
Minus	0	5	7	10	15	25	25	0	23	67	38	60

$$r_{au} = 0.78 \qquad r_{ax} = 0.30$$
$$r_{av} = 0.73 \qquad r_{ay} = 0.37$$
$$r_{aw} = 0.26 \qquad r_{az} = 0.35$$

These figures indicate in particular the very low extent to which it is possible to predict performance in the Months and Digits tests from the subject's age (Note 19.4).

To determine the degree of 'improvability' in the six different tasks regression lines were fitted to the data described in Tables 19.1 to 19.6 (Note 19.5). These were found to be:

Reading:	$y = -25.05 + 0.52x$
Spelling:	$y = -21.67 + 0.41x$
Months Forwards:	$y = -0.58 + 0.0103x$
Months Reversed:	$y = -0.69 + 0.0078x$
Digits Forwards:	$y = 4.22 + 0.0079x$
Digits Reversed:	$y = 2.35 + 0.0074x$

where y is the score on each test and x the age in months. The slope for reading (given by the formula $\tan^{-1} 0.52$) was found to be 28° and that for spelling 22°; none of the other four slopes was greater than 1°.

Table 19.7 gives the confidence levels for the differences between the slopes of the regression lines, that is, the likelihood that the difference between a particular pair of slopes could have occurred simply as a chance fluctuation.

Table 19.7 Confidence levels for the differences between the slopes of the regression lines

	Reading	Spelling	Digits Forwards	Digits Reversed	Months Forwards
Spelling	†				
Digits Forwards	‡	‡			
Digits Reversed	‡	‡	*		
Months Forwards	‡	‡	NS	NS	
Months Reversed	‡	‡	NS	NS	NS

NS = not significant ($p > 0.05$); * $= p < 0.05$; † $= p < 0.01$; ‡ $= p < 0.001$.

Caution is needed, however, in the matter of interpretation, since the figures were not based on longitudinal studies but relate to different subjects at the different ages; any reference, therefore, to 'improvement over time' is thus a kind of collective statistical improvement rather than the improvement of a particular individual.

Common sense suggests that reading and spelling, because of their social usefulness, are normally given large amounts of practice and that this explains the higher scores of the older subjects. In the case of months of the year the data in Chapter 31 show that some older dyslexics eventually master them, though it is likely that dyslexics in general will take longer to do so than age-matched controls (Note 19.6). Mnemonics are of course possible, for example the 'Jason' mnemonic mentioned in Chapter 14; and in the case of Months Forwards success was in fact achieved by 101 out of the original 223 subjects and by 37 out of the 48 subjects reported on in Chapter 31 (Note 19.7). Moreover, once Months Forwards are known a variety of strategies make it possible to say Months Reversed, for example saying two months forwards at a time to oneself and then inverting them.

The relative lack of improvement over the two Digits tests is less easy to interpret. The idea of a 'capacity limitation' is not excluded, but there is no way of knowing how much might have been achieved as a result of practice. With regard to the other differences, the figures show that progress at spelling in dyslexic subjects falls further behind the norm than progress at reading; this means in effect that they are differentially weaker at spelling relative to controls, over and above their weakness at reading. This is perhaps no surprise, since recognition of the correct word when it is already written is an easier task than creation of the correct letters from nothing, and if one is handicapped an easier task is more likely to be conquered by effort than a harder one. The slightly higher correlation between Digits Reversed and age, in comparison with that between Digits Forwards and age, is not easy to explain; it could be due to sampling error (since the difference is only just within the 5% significance level, see Table 19.7), or it is possible that the compensatory strategy of 'saying them forwards first' was marginally easier to acquire than the compensatory strategy of 'grouping' in the case of Digits Forwards. This latter explanation, however, is speculative, and the factors which lead to improved performance in the two Digits tasks require further systematic investigation.

Postscript

A full re-assessment was possible in the case of 23 of my subjects. The results are set out in Table 19.8.

For each subject the information in the first line has been extracted from the Summary Chart (with the data on handedness, eyedness, and 'limits' excluded); the second line then gives the data at the time of re-assessment, namely age, score on the R_1 test, score on the S_1 test, score on the two Digits tests and the results of the dyslexia test scored in terms of 'plus', 'zero' and 'minus'. A further column gives the time-interval in years and months between the two assessments, the next two columns the gains in 'reading age' and 'spelling age' respectively, and the final two columns the rates of gain in each case, that is, the

Table 19.8 Re-assessment data

Case no.	Sex	Age	Int.	R_1	S_1	DF	DR	L–R	Pol	Sub	Tab	MF	MR	b–d	Famil	Index	Interval (years, months)	Reading age gain (years, months)	Spelling age gain (years, months)	Rate of reading gain	Rate of spelling gain
3	M	7;6	W	0	3	56	33	+	–	+	+	+	+	0	nk	5.5	0;7	2;2	1;6	3.7	2.6
		8;1		22	18	56	33	+	–	+	+	+	+	0	nk	5.5					
6	M	7;9	X	21	15	56	33	+	+	+	+	+	+	0	+	7.5	5;1	4;4	1;7	0.9	0.3
		12;10		64	31	64	43	+	+	–	+	–	+	0	+	7.5					
10	M	8;1	Z	31	24	65	33	+	–	+	+	+	+	+	nk	6	4;5	5;11	4;2	1.3	0.9
		12;6		90	66	87	77	+	–	–	+	0	+	0	nk	4					
13	M	8;4	X	22	18	67	43	+	–	+	+	+	+	+	nk	6	7;4	6;11	6;0	0.9	0.8
		15;8		91	78	78	45	0	–	–	+	–	–	0	nk	3					
18	M	8;6	X	8	16	55	45	0	0	0	+	–	+	+	+	6.5	1;6	2;5	1;4	1.6	0.9
		10;0		32	29	55	43	–	0	–	+	–	–	0	+	5					
19	M	8;7	W	40	30	55	43	+	0	–	+	+	+	+	0	5	2;1	2;1	1;6	1.0	0.7
		10;8		61	45	65	43	+	+	–	+	–	+	0	0	7					
22	M	8;8	W	29	23	65	44	+	–	+	+	+	+	0	+	6.5	6;11	4;11	4;7	0.7	0.7
		15;7		78	77	55	44	+	+	–	+	–	0	0	+	7					
35	M	9;4	X	19	22	66	34	–	–	+	+	0	+	0	nk	5	7;7	5;10	4;0	0.8	0.5
		16;11		77	62	45	34	–	+	–	+	–	+	0	nk	5.5					
39	M	9;5	W	16	17	56	33	+	–	+	+	+	+	0	+	7.5	6;10	3;7	2;8	0.5	0.4
		16;3		52	44	66	34	+	–	–	0	–	–	+	+	5.5					

Table 19.8 (contd)

Case no.	Sex	Age	Int.	R_1	S_1	DF	DR	L-R	Pol	Sub	Tab	MF	MR	b-d	Famil	Index	Interval (years, months)	Reading age gain (years, months)	Spelling age gain (years, months)	Rate of reading gain	Rate of spelling gain
43	M	9;7	Y	34	28	65	34	+	-	+	+	+	+	0	0	7	3;4	2;10	3;0	0.9	0.9
		12;11		62	58	56	45	+	0	-	+	-	+	0	0	5.5					
		16;5		85	79	34	44	+	+	+	+	0	-	0	0	7.5					
48	M	9;9	Z	32	25	45	33	+	-	-	+	-	0	+	nk	5.5	6;9	4;10	4;8	0.7	0.7
		16;6		87	72	76	43	+	0	-	+	-	-	+	nk	5.5					
53	M	9;11	X	45	34	56	33	+	0	-	+	0	+	0	nk	5.5	6;3	4;10	3;11	0.8	0.6
		16;2		93	73	66	43	+	0	-	0	-	0	0	nk	5					
61	M	10;3	Y	70	56	67	34	+	-	+	+	-	-	0	+	5.5	4;1	2;6	3;2	0.6	0.8
		14;4		92	88	56	34	+	-	+	+	-	0	0	+	7					
		16;1		*	*	56	45	+	-	0	+	-	-	0	+	6					
63	F	10;3	Z	56	42	43	33	+	+	0	+	-	-	0	nk	6	4;1	2;7	2;7	0.6	0.6
		14;4		82	68	66	43	-	+	0	+	-	-	0	nk	4					
64	M	10;4	Y	26	19	67	43	+	+	0	+	+	+	+	nk	7.5	6;0	4;1	3;8	0.7	0.6
		16;4		67	56	65	54	0	+	-	+	+	0	0	nk	6.5					
94	M	11;3	Y	37	28	45	53	-	0	+	+	-	+	0	0	6.5	3;4	3;5	2;0	1.0	0.6
		14;7		71	48	55	43	-	0	-	+	-	-	0	0	4.5					
96	M	11;3	X	32	22	55	34	0	0	+	+	-	+	+	0	7.5	3;1	5;7	3;8	1.8	1.2
		14;4		88	59	56	43	+	-	-	+	-	-	0	0	5					

Table 19.8 (contd)

Case no.	Sex	Age	Int.	R_1	S_1	DF	DR	L–R	Pol	Sub	Tab	MF	MR	b–d	Famil	Index	Interval (years, months)	Reading age gain (years, months)	Spelling age gain (years, months)	Rate of reading gain	Rate of spelling gain
110	F	11;9	X	45	32	66	33	+	+	–	+	–	0	0	+	6					
		16;9		80	58	76	23	0	+	–	+	–	0	0	+	6.5	5;0	3;6	2;7	0.7	0.5
118	M	12;0	Z	76	38	66	33	–	+	0	+	+	0	0	nk	5.5					
		19;6		94	72	56	34	–	+	–	+	–	–	0	nk	4.5	7;6	1;10	3;5	0.2	0.5
143	F	13;6	X	62	61	65	23	+	+	+	+	–	–	+	nk	7					
		17;5		81	75	45	43	+	+	–	+	+	–	0	nk	6.5	3;11	1;11	1;5	0.5	0.4
		26;11		*	*	55	32	+	+	+	+	–	0	+	nk	7.5					
190	M	15;11	V	(58)	(50)	67	55	–	+	0	+	+	+	–	nk	5.5					
		19;1		(72)	(64)	78	44	+	+	–	+	–	–	–	0	4.5	3;2	1;5	1;5	0.4	0.4
202	M	16;11	W	42	22	67	43	+	+	0	+	+	–	+	0	8					
		33;1		79	37	66	33	+	+	0	+	–	–	+	0	7	16;2	3;8	1;4	0.2	0.1
258	F	8;1	Y	32	24	67	55	+	–	+	+	–	0	–	0	4					
		14;6		86	75	66	65	+	–	–	0	–	–	–	0	2	6;5	5;5	5;1	0.8	0.8

gains in reading age and spelling age divided by the time-interval between the two assessments (Note 19.8).

Now it is clear from Table 19.8 that almost all the subjects showed considerable gains in both reading and spelling, with reading consistently showing the larger gain. Of the 12 subjects who were first assessed at ages 7, 8 or 9 (S3, S6, S10, S13, S18, S19, S22, S35, S39, S43, S48 and S53), all had gained at least two years in reading age when they were re-assessed and only S6 had a rate of spelling gain of less than 0.4. Of the remaining 10 subjects (exclusive of S258, see below) only S64 had a reading age of under 12 (70 words correct) on re-testing, and six had a reading age of 13 (80 words correct) or over. All of them, however, remained relatively weak spellers, five having spelling ages of under 11 (60 words correct) and only three having spelling ages of over 12 (70 words correct) (Note 19.9).

With regard to performance on the dyslexia test, Table 19.8 shows that out of the 22 subjects (exclusive of S258) 17 had an index of 5 or more 'pluses' on the second testing. Quite independently, therefore, of my first-hand knowledge of their earlier difficulties there would have been grounds for a positive diagnosis in these cases. Even S13, though his index was only 3 on the second occasion, displayed weakness at Digits Reversed and typically dyslexic difficulties over Tables, and in the context of his high intelligence and relatively weak spelling a diagnosis of dyslexia would therefore have seemed extremely likely (Note 19.10). There is therefore stronger reason for saying that this would be true of the other cases.

In devising a scoring system for the dyslexia test I had in fact been influenced by the idea that signs of dyslexia would be present at all ages. If this is the case and the scoring system is adequate, there will be only minimal changes in the dyslexia index (total number of 'pluses') over time. Table 19.9 gives a frequency distribution of these changes between the first and second assessments. It will be noted that although overall there were fewer 'pluses' on the second assessment, five of the 22 subjects actually scored *more* 'pluses'.

If we ignore whether the difference is positive or negative, we find that the mean value of the differences is 1.16, with a standard deviation of 0.81. If it is legitimate, therefore, to generalise on the basis of these 22 cases, it can be concluded that when a dyslexic person comes back for reassessment their dyslexia index is unlikely to change by more than two points. The time-intervals involved were between 7 months and 16 years.

At this point it may be helpful to refer to the case of S258, who at the time of the first assessment left me uncertain as to whether she was genuinely dyslexic (Note 19.11). When I assessed her the second time there were still difficulties over Left–Right and over Tables; her score of 6 on Digits Forwards, though not low enough for a 'plus', was

Table 19.9 Frequency distribution of differences in dyslexia index between first and second assessments

Difference	f	Difference	f
+2	1	–0.5	2
+1.5	1	–1	4
+1	–	–1.5	3
+0.5	3	–2	4
0	3	–2.5	–
		–3	1

on the weak side, and there was the further evidence that when digits were presented visually for 8/10 s her 'comparison ratio' (see Chapter 17) was only 5.0 which again is less than would be expected in a non-dyslexic person of her age and ability. If anything, therefore, I would be more inclined to go for a 'positive' diagnosis of dyslexia than I was at the first assessment, even though the scoring system showed her as having only two 'pluses'. The truth seems to be that from time to time one meets people who are only very slightly or marginally dyslexic (Note 19.12).

It is also worth noting that 20 out of the 23 subjects scored 'plus' on the Tables item, the remaining three (S39, S53 and S258 scoring 'zero'). This means that not a single subject went through the 6 x, 7 x, and 8 x tables without some appreciable degree of stumbling.

One additional piece of evidence is worth mention, namely that six of the subjects on re-assessment did the Raven Advanced Matrices test. Table 19.10 shows the scores and the resultant intelligence grade, with the earlier intelligence grade given in brackets.

Table 19.10 Scores on Advanced Matrices test

Subject no.	Score	Intelligence rating (with earlier rating in brackets)
13	26	Z (X)
35	26	Z (X)
39	21	X (W)
64	22	Y (Y)
118	26	Z (Z)
143	21	X (X)

These figures are interesting in that in all six cases the intelligence rating obtained at the first assessment either remained the same or actually improved. Caution is needed, of course, since (1) only six subjects were involved; (2) from the way in which the grades were determined (see Chapter 2, p. 12) some degree of inexactness is unavoidable; and (3) any attempt to compare later performance on the Advanced Matrices test with earlier performance on the Wechsler or Terman–Merrill tests can only be an approximation. Despite these possible objections, however, the figures seem to me to be worth citing. I have sometimes wondered if, in my anxiety to help and encourage my subjects, I have been guilty, in using the concept of a 'selected IQ' (see Chapter 2), of over-estimating their ability. In the case of an Advanced Matrices score, however, no 'selection' of items is possible; if these six cases are in any way typical it follows that there cannot have been over-estimations on any large scale. In addition the figures suggest that if tests are used (such as the Advanced Matrices) which do not involve the dyslexic subject's areas of special weakness, the actual figure for 'intelligence level' need not decrease; this confirms the idea that in their 'good' areas dyslexic subjects mature at the same rate as anyone else. Further discussion of possible reasons for the success of dyslexics at the Advanced Matrices test will be found in Chapter 31.

The evidence contained in the postscript confirms that dyslexic subjects can improve their performance in all kinds of ways as they grow older, and that even at reading and spelling there can be appreciable gains if the conditions are right. Even so, however, it is clear that traces of the handicap remain; it seems that these are particularly likely to show themselves in difficulty over saying tables and difficulty over remembering digits. It is therefore incorrect simply to describe a dyslexic child as 'behind' at reading or spelling and therefore able, or partially able, to catch up; a less misleading formulation is to say that he is handicapped but can achieve considerable success in learning to compensate (Note 19.13).

Chapter 20
Familial Incidence

On some occasions it was possible to assess more than one member of the same family. This was true in the cases shown in Table 20.1.

In addition, I had at an earlier date assessed the elder brothers of S17, S120, S170 and S229, and the cousin of S116. More recently I had assessed the younger brother of S23 and S61 and the sisters of S39 and S97 (Note 20.2), while a colleague using the same criteria had assessed the sister of S68 and the brother of S221. In all these cases the diagnosis was positive. S172 was the cousin of S177 and S208, and S104 was the cousin of S140. In addition I had ample evidence from discussion over many years that the mother of S219 was dyslexic (Note 20.3). These results, taken in combination, gave me an assured 'positive' family history in 50 out 257 cases (Note 20.4) (see those marked 'plus' in the Summary Chart in Chapter 6).

There were in addition plenty of other cases where it seemed at first sight likely that another member of the family was affected. In accordance with the procedure described in Appendix II such cases were scored as 'zero', my intention being to make a distinction between those cases where I myself had observed difficulties in another member

Table 20.1 Brothers and sisters	
Brothers *Ss:*	*Brother and sister(s)* *Ss:*
2 and 51	6 and 110 (Note 20.1)
14 and 108	7 and 74
16, 88 and 142	12, 82 and 248
22 and 238	18 and 117
24 and 178	34 and 246
55 and 106	72 and 103
92 and 148	129 and 224
189 and 204	122 and 28
	177 and 208

of the family at first hand and those cases where I had to rely on the reports of others. With regard to scoring, however, the real problem arose when it became necessary to decide whether the reported evidence was sufficient to count as a 'zero' or whether it was not. In general I accepted reports of late reading as meriting a 'zero'; for example the sister of S1 was said not to have read until age 9, an uncle of S45 not until he was aged 12, and the father of S38 not until he was aged 14. Except in the case of late reading, however, I required some kind of twofold confirmation before scoring a zero, for example that a particular relative regularly muddled left and right and *in addition* could not remember telephone numbers.

On some occasions one or other of the parents, after listening to my account of their child's difficulties on the reading, spelling or dyslexia tests, reported similar difficulties in themselves; provided more than one such difficulty was mentioned the result was again scored as 'zero'. This was true, for example, in the case of S23 whose father reported that he himself was a poor speller and had never succeeded in learning his tables. (When a younger son came several years later for assessment and was also found to be dyslexic the original 'zero' was changed to 'plus'.)

The category 'nk' (= 'not known') was used (1) when there was insufficient evidence for a 'zero', (2) when no evidence was available either positive or negative, and (3) when the parents reported that they knew of no relatives similarly affected. Thus S125 was scored as 'nk' since the only evidence was that his father was a poor speller, and similarly S62 was scored as 'nk' since it was reported only that he tended to spell phonetically. If I was in doubt I tended to go for 'nk' rather than 'zero', since a critic could argue that in the assessment situation there were social pressures on the parents to 'oblige' by finding dyslexic relatives if at all possible! It may well be that I have overcompensated for this – somewhat speculative – possibility, and I suspect that the number of cases scored as 'zero', namely 72, is probably an underestimate of the number of cases where there were in fact dyslexic relatives.

Nine of the subjects had been adopted, and in these cases familial evidence was virtually impossible to obtain (Note 20.5). In a further 14 cases the subjects were not accompanied by their parents and, not surprisingly, could not answer questions about the family history with any confidence. If these 23 are subtracted from the total of 257, this leaves 234, of whom 122 (50 + 72) almost certainly had a positive family history. If, as is likely, the figure of 72 for the zero category is an underestimate, then in any sample of dyslexic subjects it appears that one should expect familial incidence over 50% of the time.

Does it follow, then, that the familial incidence of dyslexia is something which requires explanation? This question is not as absurd as it seems, for there are clearly plenty of characteristics which occur in more than one member of a family but which in themselves seem to be of no special significance. For example, there could well be two members of the same family who enjoyed swimming, and if this is unimportant and the familial incidence of dyslexia is important, wherein lies the difference?

The answer appears to depend on the relative unlikelihood of certain features occurring in conjunction. If, for example, one takes poor spelling on its own, this is perhaps a somewhat surprising phenomenon in those, like most of my subjects, who had adequate intelligence and the opportunities to learn, and the surprise is therefore the more if two members of the same family are both poor spellers. This, however, could happen from time to time simply as a chance coming together of two relatively infrequent events. If a person is dyslexic, however, it is not just *two* such events which co-occur but many more. Thus although the control data show that such weaknesses can quite well occur from time to time in those with no spelling problem, yet as the number of positive indicators increases the probability of their occurring by chance in two members of the same family rapidly decreases; since there is evidence in some families of three, four, or even more members being affected, the hypothesis of 'random spread' (as there might be random spread of the enjoyment of swimming) has to be rejected. For example, unless there had been some familial factor it seems inconceivable that the mother of S97, along with her son and daughter, and the father of S55 and S106, along with his two sons and their elder brother (assessed before 1972), should all have been dyslexic. In contrast, if several members of a family are gifted at swimming the main causal factors are likely to be good physique and enhanced opportunities.

Now the most obvious explanation of the familial incidence of dyslexia is to postulate a genetic factor. In other words, because of their genetic make-up certain individuals are predisposed to dyslexic-type difficulties. It is important, however, not to accept this hypothesis without considering alternatives.

A suggestion which is sometimes put forward is that one should take into account the unconscious or 'dynamic' factors in the family situation. For example, it could be argued that children sometimes unconsciously identify with a parent or sibling and therefore 'choose' the same things to be weak at. This idea, however, seems to me entirely speculative, and the onus is clearly on those who accept it to present relevant evidence. Moreover, it is hard to see how a child of, say, 8 could know that his father was a relatively weak speller or relatively weak at recall of digits. In addition, even if he knew, it is hard to see why he should imitate these particular facets of his father's behaviour when there was so much else to choose from, and why children in other families should imitate precisely the same facets of *their* parents' behaviour. There is the further difficulty that where one parent is affected and not the other, it would be necessary, if the 'identification' hypothesis were to be made convincing, for independent criteria to be formulated as to why it was this parent with whom the child identified; and where two siblings were affected one would have to assume that they identified themselves not with either parent but with each other. Finally, if one considers a family such as that which I have described elsewhere (Note 20.6), where the members visited the USA and found several second cousins similarly affected, it is hard to see how there could be 'identification' with previously unknown relatives living on the other side of the Atlantic! In general, the 'unconscious identification' hypothesis seems to me to be psychodynamic speculation run wild!

Nor is it convincing to lay the blame on poor teaching, since it would then be necessary to explain why other children, exposed to precisely the same teaching, had learned to read and spell perfectly well.

If, however, it is correct to look for constitutional factors in the causation of dyslexia, then it is also at first sight plausible, in view of the incidence of familial dyslexia, to suppose that these constitutional factors are genetically determined. To be strict, perhaps one should speak of a genetic predisposition rather than of a genetically transmitted agent whose effects are 100% certain, since we know, after all, that dyslexic tendencies can to some extent be counteracted by suitable training, and we do not know the limits of such counteraction. The view that some kind of genetic factor is involved has of course received very considerable support (Note 20.7).

In a number of cases, however, the parents, when carefully questioned, said that they knew of no affected relatives. Although it is hard to establish a 'negative' with complete assurance, since it is always arguable that mild forms of the condition among relatives would have gone undetected, it is unlikely that any large number of these parents were mistaken, and if this is correct it follows that there are at least some cases (the so-called 'sporadic' cases) where dyslexic-type difficulties occur in those whose relatives are all unaffected. In a few cases, too, there was evidence of more gross physical damage – an early history of hearing loss in S8, S37 and S198, a history of convulsions in the case of S83, a suggestion of very slight brain damage in the case of S143, a report that S167 was 'brain damaged and slightly spastic' and a report in the case of S174 (via his mother) that 'Dr — says that in his view there is a physical condition caused by damage at birth which has also caused the dyslexia'. The proportion of such children finding their way to Bangor may well be small since our assessments were known to be educational rather than medical; but the above evidence makes clear that the dyslexic group of difficulties can sometimes be associated with factors of this kind.

In the cases where there is early hearing loss it seems at first sight likely that this is a causal factor. Indeed such a causal connection would be in no way surprising since the earliest language for all children except the deaf is *heard* language, and it makes sense that deprivation of heard language should lead to a stunting of the mechanisms for processing verbal stimuli. It also makes sense that slight physical impairments, perhaps sometimes classifiable as mild cases of spasticity or epilepsy, should result in the typical dyslexic picture even though intelligence level is unaffected. It seems to me that, at least in the present state of knowledge, these subjects, too, should be classified as 'dyslexic' since, as in the sporadic cases, there is no evidence for differences in behaviour pattern or for believing that different teaching methods are needed.

With regard to gender ratio, 208 of my 257 subjects were male and 49 female. This gives a male-to-female ratio of about 4.25:1. The reason for this imbalance is not clear, but since it has been reported in population studies as well as in studies of 'referred' cases (such as the present) it is most implausible to suppose that it is merely a function of the referral system – that parents more often seek help for their sons than for their daughters. There can be no doubt, in my view, that dyslexia is more common in males than in females (Note 20.8).

In brief, the evidence from the present research (1) confirms that dyslexia sometimes runs in families, (2) establishes that it can also occur when no-one else in the family is affected, (3) supports the view that it (or something similar) can occur as a result of a physical deficit such as early deafness, and (4) gives some degree of support to the view that it is more common in males than in females (the actual ratio in this particular enquiry being 4.25:1). From the literature in general it seems virtually certain that familial dyslexia is genetically determined.

Chapter 21
Handedness and Eyedness

It has been supposed in the past that there is some connection between dyslexia and unusual patterns of handedness and eyedness. Various suggestions have been made about the nature of this connection. The simplest view is that there is an enlarged proportion of left-handers in a dyslexic population; a more sophisticated view is that the dyslexic person shows poorly developed dominance, or in other words is neither strongly right-handed nor strongly left-handed, while a third view is that many dyslexic persons are 'cross-lateral', in other words right-handed and left-eyed or left-handed and right-eyed.

Even in the early stages of the research I had felt doubts as to whether handedness and eyedness were as important in dyslexia as these views implied. The first necessity, therefore, was to obtain more data, and it was for this reason that tests of handedness and eyedness were included in the dyslexia test and given to all my subjects. In addition, one of my students, Joanna Watts, gave identical tests to 62 local schoolchildren, aged 8–11, who had been selected on the basis of adequate scores on a spelling test. This procedure gave a control group with whom the dyslexic subjects could be compared.

Table 21.1 shows the data for the dyslexics (which will also be found in the Summary Chart in Chapter 6) along with the control data collected by Miss Watts. The cross-lateral subjects (right-handed, left-eyed and left-handed, right-eyed) have been grouped together and, as in the Summary Chart, the abbreviations R (= 'right'), L (= 'left') and M (= 'mixed') have been used, with the first letter of each pair signifying handedness and the second letter eyedness. Percentages are given in brackets.

Table 21.1 Figures for handedness and eyedness of dyslexic and control subjects					
	RR	*RL* *LR*	*LL*	*MR* *ML*	*RM* *LM*	*MM*
Dyslexic subjects	122(55)	44(20)	9(4)	35(16)	11(5)	2(1)
Control subjects	36(58)	18(29)	2(3)	6(10)	0(0)	0(0)

If we now pool all those who were right-handed and right-eyed and designate as 'UHE' (= unusual handedness or eyedness) all the others the figures are as shown in Table 21.2.

Table 21.2 Comparison of those dyslexics and controls who were right-handed and right-eyed with the rest

	RR	UHE
Dyslexic subjects	122	101
Control subjects	36	26

From this table it is plain that there is not a significantly larger proportion of left-handers or UHE subjects in the dyslexic group (Note 21.1), and indeed, though the result is not statistically significant (Note 21.2), there is actually a slightly larger proportion of cross-lateral subjects in the control group! The lack of association between dyslexia and unusual handedness has been reported in a number of other studies (Note 21.3); the belief that there is some simple association between them must now be regarded as highly questionable. That more sophisticated tests of 'cerebral dominance' (itself no easy concept) could yield different results is not in dispute, particularly in view of what is known about the role of the left hemisphere in speech (Note 21.4), but if 'handedness' is understood in its standard sense it is dangerous to assume that a disproportionate number of dyslexics show unusual handedness.

There remains the possibility that there is an enlarged proportion of mixed handers in the dyslexic population. If once again we pool the figures into a four-cell table the results are as shown in Table 21.3.

Table 21.3. Comparison of dyslexics and controls in respect of mixed handedness

	'Mixed'	Others
Dyslexics	48	175
Controls	6	56

These differences just fail to reach the 5% level of significance (Note 21.5). Even if they are genuine, however, the interpretation is not obvious. Certainly they do not permit any comprehensive theory of dyslexia in terms of 'poorly developed dominance', since at most such a theory would be applicable only to a relatively small proportion of dyslexics (22% in this particular sample).

Even more important, however, is the consideration that inconsistency of hand or eye preferences in the tasks given is very slender evidence on which to base statements about 'dominance'. Dyslexics show uncertainties in all sorts of ways; it is not clear that the inconsistencies shown in these two tests by a small proportion of dyslexic subjects are evidence for anything more than typical 'dyslexic muddle'. One of the subjects, incidentally, who was 'mixed' at both the handedness and the eyedness tests was the problematic S208 (see Chapter 5) who indeed was liable to show confusion in a variety of ways.

There is a further belief about dyslexia which seems to me to merit examination and which can be checked by the available data. This belief is that to understand dyslexia it is appropriate to use the analogy of the mirror. It is sometimes suggested or implied that when dyslexics confuse left and right or 'b' and 'd' the central nervous system some-how signals the mirror image of the correct answer. Orton's concept of 'strephosymbolia' has perhaps given credibility to this view; the impli-cation is that it is an important fact about certain errors that the response is the mirror image of the correct one.

If this were true one might expect there to be more confusions over left and right and more b–d errors in those with UHE or in those of mixed handedness or eyedness than in other dyslexic subjects. The data in the Summary Chart make possible a test of this hypothesis. There were in fact 149 of the 223 subjects who scored 'plus' on the Left–Right test and 34 who scored 'minus' (40 scoring 'zero'). If these are classified according to handedness and eyedness the results are as shown in Table 21.4.

Table 21.4 Relation of handedness and eyedness to 'plus' and 'minus' on the Left–Right test

	RR	RL LR	LL	MR ML	RM LM	MM
'Plus' on L–R test	81	25	8	26	7	2
'Minus' on L–R test	20	8	1	4	1	0

If we again pool the figures in respect of those with UHE the results are as shown in Table 21.5.

Table 21.5 Comparison of the right-handed, right-eyed group with the UHE group in respect of 'plus' and 'minus' on the Left–Right test

	RR	UHE
'Plus' on L–R test	81	68
'Minus' on L–R test	20	14

As is plain from inspection this result is not statistically significant (Note 21.6). Similarly if we compare the 'mixed' handedness group with the rest the results are as shown in Table 21.6.

Table 21.6 Comparison of the 'mixed' handedness group with the other groups in respect of 'plus' and 'minus' on the Left–Right test

	'Mixed'	*Others*
'Plus' on L-R test	35	114
'Minus' on L-R test	5	29

Again this result is non-significant (Note 21.7).

Figures for b–d confusion tell the same story. In this case the Summary Chart shows that there were 74 subjects for whom there was first-hand evidence of b–d confusion and 78 where no such confusion was reported (with 71 scored as 'zero'). If these subjects are similarly classified according to handedness and eyedness the results are as shown in Table 21.7.

Table 21.7 Relation of handedness and eyedness to b–d confusion

	RR	*RL* *LR*	*LL*	*MR* *ML*	*RM* *LM*	*MM*
b–d positive	36	16	4	16	2	–
b–d negative	46	16	2	10	4	–

If we again pool the figures in respect of the UHE group the results are as shown in Table 21.8.

Table 21.8 Comparison of the right-handed, right-eyed group with the UHE group in respect of b–d confusion

	RR	*UHE*
b–d positive	36	38
b–d negative	46	32

The result is again non-significant (Note 21.8). Similarly, if we compare the mixed handedness group with the rest, the results are as shown in Table 21.9.

Table 21.9 Comparison of the 'mixed' handedness group with the other groups in respect of b-d confusion

	'Mixed'	*Others*
b–d positive	18	56
b–d negative	14	64

This result is again non-significant (Note 21.9). We may therefore conclude that there is no tendency for either the UHE subjects or the 'mixed' group subjects to be more prone to b–d confusion than other dyslexic subjects.

The evidence in this chapter has been almost entirely negative. Dyslexic subjects are no more prone to UHE than are controls; at most the evidence shows slightly more inconsistency of response in a few of them when given particular tests of handedness and eyedness. In addition, the subjects in the UHE and 'mixed' groups are no more prone than other dyslexic subjects to have difficulty with the Left–Right test or to show b–d confusion.

Indirectly, therefore, the results give limited support for the view that difficulties over left and right and over 'b' and 'd' are labelling difficulties, since in that case there would be no particular reason to associate them with UHE in any form. That dyslexics sometimes confuse letters that are, in fact, the mirror images of each other is not in dispute. Whether this behaviour, however, has anything to do with unusual handedness or eyedness is doubtful, and there is reason to think that analogies with mirror phenomena are not as important as was once supposed.

Chapter 22
Struggles and
Misunderstandings

The next two chapters will be concerned with some of the social aspects of dyslexia. I shall try to show (1) that the family's problems can be exacerbated if the child's dyslexia is misunderstood, and (2) that, conversely, a carefully explained diagnosis can give a fresh orientation and new hope.

Much of the evidence in the present chapter is derived from what the parents told me. Not surprisingly, therefore, I have sometimes wondered whether they were guilty of exaggeration and whether, had I consulted the teacher or other official whom they mentioned, I would have received a very different story. On the other hand, there was a remarkable consistency in the information given: the same kinds of cavalier treatment were reported by many different families, and their accounts regularly gave the impression of 'ringing true'. Even, therefore, if there has been some degree of distortion (and I am by no means convinced that this is so), any wholesale discounting of what was said seems out of the question. On some occasions, too, I was able to see written reports where professional workers had put their views in writing, and in these cases there can clearly be no question of any misrepresentation.

As a first illustration, here is a letter from the mother of S59:

His headmaster thinks he is below average in intelligence, which I do not accept. After seeing a programme about 'dyslexia' on the television a couple of Sundays ago, I 'phoned an educational psychologist who does not like the term dyslexia, nor for that matter does T's headmaster. When I asked how T was going to get on at senior school in a year's time and what facilities would be available to help T the educational psychologist was very vague and woolly. I have been led to believe T's difficulties would gradually disappear, but especially since seeing the TV programme, I am convinced that this is not so. These children have to contend with a great deal of frustration and I feel it would help them to understand themselves better if their true handicap was explained to them.

Reference to the Summary Chart in Chapter 6 show that T's intelligence rating was given as Y, with scaled scores of 17 and 17 on two WISC sub-tests – figures which scarcely square with the statement that he was 'below average intelligence'.

I received the following further information after the assessment:

One of T's teachers ripped out his work in front of the entire unit (100 children) and made such an exhibition of the affair that T was reduced to tears... When we called to see the Headmaster they defended themselves by saying that T was too easily distracted, he could do better if he tried harder and his work was inconsistent. When they read your report they shook their heads as if to say 'this can't be right'. They were willing to accept that T's spelling age was 7.6 and his reading age was 9.8 but as for the rest they were not prepared to accept your findings at all. Well, as far was we were concerned the only course was to try and help T at home and just hope that one day the message would get through to them.

Here are parts of a letter from the mother of S109:

I have been particularly concerned by his present teacher's assessment which described him as lazy, stupid, a child who gave up very easily... He has just finished 'Watership Down' and declared it brilliant. I feel if he can appreciate and grasp a reasonable level of literature there exists the possibility that it is wrong for a teacher to label him as stupid.

Reference to the Summary Chart shows an intelligence rating of Z, with two passes at Superior Adult II despite his being aged only 11.

Similarly the mother of S56 said at the start of the assessment: At (name of town) he saw a Dr — who said he's just slow. 'He's slow' – we've been getting the story for so long.

In the case of S118 his mother told me that he had been called 'lazy', 'lethargic' and 'confused' at school, and was gaining a reputation for being 'charming but prone to idleness and scruffy work'. She also told me that although her daughter was said to be 'scholarship material' she herself believed that the boy was the brighter of the two; this view was partially supported by the results of the intelligence test which I gave him, where he obtained a rating of Y. She herself was a qualified teacher, and at one point – speaking of her own experience – she said: 'At no point in his mother's training course was dyslexia mentioned, and among our many acquaintances who are teachers most know next to nothing about it'.

When S132 was brought for assessment at age 11 his mother told me that they had been trying to get help since he was aged 8, while the mother of case S127 said 'It's been running for six years. They said he'd grow out of it'. Similarly the mother of S53 said 'We are always told not to worry, that it is bound to come in time'. A letter from the father of S47 said:

His primary school teachers have for the past two years been advising 'Don't worry'. But as the problem persists, we feel the time has come to seek further advice. Local channels – family doctor and health visitor – have been explored with negative result.

In similar vein the mother of S111 told me that her daughter 'has been going to the Local Educational Psycologist (sic) for 4 years with no improvement in her reading'.

Lack of proper help was also mentioned in a letter from the mother of S163.

He has been described in all school reports as 'lazy', however he is very willing and helpful. He feels inadequate and resorts to irresponsible and antisocial behaviour in order to impress. Last year, because of this behaviour, we consulted the Child Guidance Clinic at —. Although we asked if he could be Dyslectic, he (the doctor) would not comment on dyslexia. Despite his difficulties he is not receiving any remedial attention at school.

A letter from the father of S241 underlines the same point:

At his primary school I mentioned dyslexia to the headmistress who assured me that his reading problems were entirely due to lack of effort and concentration. His form master... has told me that there is a definite inherent disability evident from his written work... I wrote to the BMA Nuffield Library who sent me 3 books on dyslexia, which further confirm my original diagnosis of my son's problem. Unfortunately I have no idea of a remedy.

Ironically enough, it was sometimes the parents who – despite not being trained teachers – recognised that the help which was offered to the children was inappropriate. Thus the mother of S82 wrote to me after the assessment saying 'She (the teacher) suggests that E must write her spellings out several times and learn them. This I know will not help'.

It was sometimes possible for me to see the teachers' comments in school exercise books. One of the disturbing features was the lack of *constructive* comment. For example, in a book belonging to S72 I found the following account of a chemistry lesson:

What we first did was get a fetter funl and some cotter woo and blod the megl and put sand in. Then we got some buy want and put it on the top. Then we wotch it come froo. It come froo clener. But it was not clenunuf.

The comment from the teacher was 'A lot of spellings to correct'. On another occasion the boy wrote:

Now we got some washud up lquwer and put some water with it. The we bloo budl with it. We bloo the (illegible) of the busn berner...

His teacher's comment was, 'Make more effort with your spellings'. Some writing by S71 was characterised as 'Lazy, untidy work', while S213 was told 'Very careless. Take more care with spelling', and a comment in the exercise book of S158 was 'Your work is full of spelling mistakes'.

Sometimes there was evidence not just of adverse comment but actually of cruelty. Thus I was told by his mother that S43 had been made to sit outside the headmaster's door as a punishment, and that one teacher had threatened him with the cane and made him stand in the corner, saying that he should wear the dunce's cap.

A similar lack of sensitivity had apparently been shown by the teacher of S117: we had reached the stage in the assessment where she had been asked 'nineteen, take away seven' and had given the answer as 'eleven'; when I asked her how she did her calculations she said, 'I usually use my fingers. Mr — pulls your hair if you can't do it straight away'.

Another disturbing feature was the adverse criticism of parents which I sometimes read in teachers' reports. Thus a teacher wrote of S162, 'He is an only child and the mother tends to be over-protective... Just as lazy about his written work'. I also read that he was 'a spoiled only child around whom home life revolves...very difficult to motivate'.

The following is also a distressing example of what appears to be a total misunderstanding of a dyslexic child's needs. The mother of S232 told me as follows:

N's class teacher took the view that N 'needed a good thump' to knock some sense into him so he would get on with some work. His difficulties in other aspects of school work, particularly arithmetic became increasingly apparent, but his teachers failed to make any allowance and as a result he became increasingly despondent. He finds memorising of tables quite impossible and has great difficulty in copying or remembering numbers... We discovered that his teacher gave up trying to teach him maths and during maths periods gave him a book to read. As you may imagine this was not a success as he found it quite impossible to concentrate sufficiently to read a book whilst a lesson was being taken on an entirely different subject, and he was then punished for being unco-operative.

One of the obstacles which many parents experienced was the entrenched attitudes of those who insisted that the child's difficulties were due either to tensions within the home or to inadequacies on the child's part such as lack of self-confidence or lack of motivation. The following, for instance, is an extract from a letter written by the mother of S20.

The educational psychologist said that C is not dyslexic but that all his difficulties stem from being jealous of his sister... Apparently a remedial teacher
has seen C and reported to the headmaster that he is a very average child
with an IQ of 100 whose only problem is that he is completely lacking in
self confidence.

The mother of S159 reported that her son had been said by his
teacher to have an 'emotional blockage'. Of S38 the educational psychologist had written:

I think this is the sort of child who would learn to read much faster in
response to psychotherapy than any form of remedial teaching. She certainly has a major antipathy now to anything connected with the printed word
and she also clearly has a very confused sense of identity.

The following are extracts from an educational psychologist's report
on S14.

A has a very low opinion of himself. He is probably naturally reserved and
even withdrawn but his lack of animation and poor confidence need not
necessarily follow from his introverted personality... I have seen his parents
who have also consulted me over A's brother P (S108). I have hinted (sic) to
them strongly (sic) that I feel that home attitudes may have contributed to
A's problems and have encouraged them to do what they can to reassure
him and restore his confidence... A will do well in school subjects when his
own attitudes and motivation are improved... A needs to know that he has
nothing to fear in the challenge that reading presents. He knows of his
brother's difficulties in this area and his parents have observed that there is
a little animosity between them. A is choosing not to try rather than try and
fail which in this family is probably more anxiety provoking than in many
others.

I find it hard to comment on this report. If one regards the two
brothers as dyslexic, then clearly the picture is quite a different one. It
has certainly been my experience that some dyslexic children 'choose
not to try rather than try and fail' and that as a result the impression is
given that their 'attitudes and motivation' are at fault. But the way to
bring about the appropriate change is to explain to them the nature of
their dyslexic handicap, so that 'failure' is not the terrible thing that it
seemed to be and the defensive strategy of 'not trying' is recognised as
unnecessary. It is not the search for underlying motives, as such, which
makes the above report misguided, but rather the failure to recognise
that the boy's behaviour was the response to a dyslexic-type handicap.
This leads to unconfirmed speculations about the family being less able
than some other families to tolerate anxiety and perhaps to the attaching of too much significance to the alleged 'animosity' between the two
brothers. Moreover, if one uses the dyslexia concept, this immediately
makes sense of the fact that *both* brothers were dyslexic, since the

condition is known to run in families, whereas as far as the writer of
the report is concerned this important aspect of the situation is
ignored. Finally, in the absence of any suggestion of dyslexia, A's 'low
opinion of himself' becomes just an isolated and inexplicable fact
(unless indeed one searches for further speculative explanations in
terms of sibling rivalry or parental expectations), whereas if both he
and his parents recognise that the 'low opinion' is the natural consequence of the dyslexic handicap the way is open for constructive help.
This report is therefore an interesting – albeit sad – example of how
lack of the dyslexia concept can lead to a wrong view of the situation.

Sometimes the use of the word 'dyslexia' appears itself to have exacerbated controversy. Thus the mother of S36 told me that when she
mentioned dyslexia to her doctor he said 'This is a modern thing like a
slipped disc'. Similarly I was told that an educational psychologist had
explicitly declared that S174 was 'not dyslexic', while the parents of
S242 were told that she 'can't be dyslexic' on the grounds that her
reading age was the same as her chronological age. They reported,
however, that she was regularly in trouble for poor spelling, and that
once, when she had taken four hours over some homework, the
teacher had supposed that she had 'scribbled it off in five minutes'.

An educational psychologist who spoke to me on the telephone
about S226 said that he was very cross with a psychiatrist who had diagnosed the boy as dyslexic and that he 'had no business to do so'. He
also spoke of 'emotional pressures' on the boy and asked me not to
use the word 'dyslexia' in my report as it might affect his chances of
getting help. Sometimes there was no firm denial that the child was
dyslexic, but nothing was done about it. For example, the mother of
S252 wrote to me saying:

> Very little notice was taken when we informed the school she was dyslexic. I
> doubt whether they believed in such a thing, and she continued to work
> uncomplainingly, though never reading for pleasure.

The parents of S147 said that they had been told by T's headmaster
that he was 'sure there was nothing wrong', but mother added, 'The
school did not want to know'.

Sometimes the reactions on the part of the school appear to have
been positively hostile. Thus the mother of S180 told me (and her
report was confirmed in a letter to me from a mutual acquaintance)
that at school her son was 'pulled out of the class' and made to read
aloud, with the comment, 'Your mother says you're dyslexic. You
aren't'. The following is a teacher's report on S111:

> When D first arrived at school she quickly informed the group that she was
> 'dyslexic' (writer's inverted commas). She was quite happy to use this as an

excuse not to work... D usually takes a long time to start writing with excuses such as her pen having just broken or just run out. On such occasions D needs firm persuasion, anything less produces further delays. Because of these frequent time-wasting procedures D rarely leaves herself enough time to complete her work.

A report from the educational psychologist said:

It is difficult to avoid the conclusion that D's problem is any more profound than sheer laziness and lack of motivation.

Once again it is not so much the facts that are in dispute as the way in which one interprets them. It is of course a common strategy among dyslexic children to resort to 'time-wasting devices' when they are in an unsympathetic environment, and many dyslexic adults will confirm this; but the obvious way to make sense of such behaviour is to recognise that the child is trying to avoid a stressful situation in which his lack of skill will be shown up with resultant humiliation. Similarly it is no doubt the case that some undiagnosed dyslexic children show 'lack of motivation'; but this is understandable if the child is placed in circumstances where he knows that he will fail. To describe a child simply as 'poorly motivated' gives no indication of what can be done to bring about a change, whereas to describe him as 'dyslexic' gives a different view of the situation: there are in that case all kinds of things which can be done to help – specialist tuition, discussion of compensatory strategies, and, above all, explanations which make clear to the child that he is not just 'stupid' and that his difficulties over reading and spelling and in other areas are not his fault.

Sometimes the failure to acknowledge that the child is dyslexic is accompanied by not only an unsympathetic attitude but by teaching methods which are now known to be unsuitable. The following are extracts from a letter addressed to S12 from a senior remedial teacher (though it may have been intended primarily for his mother):

H, you must get quite clearly in your mind that there is no good reason or excuse why your spelling should not be far better than it is. You are capable of becoming at least average in spelling ability, in my opinion, almost certainly above average.

Whether you achieve this depends on three things.
1. The first thing is to get clear in your mind that success depends entirely on your own efforts...
2. Having fallen behind on reading, spelling and speed of completing your written work, the only way you can hope to catch up is by doing some work regularly every day... The hardest part is to make yourself do at least ten minutes work every day out of school time for the next year or two.
3. The first thing you must set yourself are (sic) a series of clear targets which you will aim to achieve each week, or each day... In addition to setting targets, you must work out the most effective method for teaching your-

self. I believe that you have been using inefficient methods, otherwise you
would be having no difficulty...

Your target should be to collect a minimum of ten words every week from
your school written work, which you have had difficulty with in spelling correctly... By writing words repeatedly, you can, in time, transfer all the words
you need to your automatic muscle memory. All that is needed is time,
determination, and revision... Finally, H, do not expect to read through
these notes once and understand everything in them. We spent an hour
together a little while ago and I made all these suggestions then. I bet a
pound to a penny you have forgotten most of what I said then. Read these
notes every week for the next month or two... I will call into your school
occasionally to ask how you are getting on. I hope you will be able to report
that this method is working well.

It is perhaps worth spending a few moments indicating how the use
of the concept of dyslexia would have led to a different view of the situation. (1) One would not use the expression 'no reason or excuse' but
would make clear that there is a very obvious reason why the boy was
having difficulty, namely because he is dyslexic: he has a constitutionally caused handicap which is not his fault. (2) One would agree that he
could be as good or better at spelling than other boys of his age, but
one would not expect him to achieve this by his 'own efforts'; such an
expression merely adds to the pressure in an unconstructive way.
(3) One would not say that he had 'fallen behind', but rather that such
progress as he had in fact made was something to be commended.
(4) It is not 'the hardest part' for a dyslexic person to make an effort. In
many cases what has gone wrong is that their efforts have resulted in
such a small amount of success. (5) To expect a dyslexic boy of this age
to 'work out the most effective method' for teaching himself seems
ludicrous if we reflect that dyslexia-centred methods have evolved into
their present form only after many decades of work by experienced
adults (Note 22.1). (6) If what is advocated is 'writing words repeatedly' without any explanation of the links between sounds, muscular
movements and the letters on the page, it is hard to see why 'muscular
memory' should be more effective than memory for auditory or visual
representation of letters. (7) Time, determination and revision are certainly needed, but the thought of an 8-year-old dyslexic boy reading
through the proffered notes is an appalling one. Given his memory limitation, he would indeed forget any parts which he had managed to
understand. (8) An 'occasional' visit to the school by a remedial teacher
is totally inadequate. (9) The whole tone of the letter is critical rather
than reassuring; had the measures in fact been adopted their failure
would have intensified the boy's feelings of guilt and humiliation.

One can usefully describe acceptance of the concept of dyslexia as
'getting the message'. Without the concept certain things about a
child's behaviour may be puzzling (for example his anomalous failure
in learning to spell or his lack of self-confidence) and some indeed may

be exasperating (for example his mistaking the time of his music lesson or misremembering the telephone number that he was given), but there would be no suggestion that these things are related. Once the concept of a constitutionally caused limitation (dyslexia) is brought in, however, the different parts of the picture fall into place. It is not that for some inexplicable reason the child lacks confidence and therefore has not learned to spell; on the contrary he is lacking in confidence because a constitutionally caused limitation has made learning to spell difficult. Similarly it is not some unexplained cussedness which caused him to mistake the time of the music lesson or misremember the telephone number; these mishaps are the result of the same constitutional limitation which also caused the weak spelling. The evidence reported in this chapter indicates the additional pressures which are put on a dyslexic child and his family if these links are unrecognised.

Chapter 23
Effects of Diagnosis

As was indicated in Chapter 2, the final stage of the assessment usually consisted of a discussion between myself, the child and his parents.

In most cases I started by giving the results of the reading and spelling tests, the intelligence test and the dyslexia test. Although this information was intended primarily for the parents, it also gave the child a chance to understand why I had asked particular questions. The majority of my subjects listened attentively during the discussion, and even those younger ones who appeared to have 'switched off' would sometimes become alert again when some aspect of their case was being discussed which appeared to interest them.

In the case of older children I would refer to their 'strengths and weaknesses' with an indication of what exactly their handicap involved. To the 7- and 8-year-olds I would say much the same thing in rather simpler words, for example, 'We'll be talking about the things that you are good at and the things that you are less good at'. I did not hesitate to use the word 'dyslexia' even with younger children if it seemed likely to help them, though it was important to explain what it meant; for example I might say, 'It doesn't mean you are stupid or lazy but there are some few things, like reading and spelling, which you will find more difficult than some of the other boys (or girls) in the class'. At no point was it my intention to impose a diagnosis which the child or his parents could not accept or understand. Frequently I might say, 'Does this make sense to you?' or 'Does this seem to you to be a correct view of the situation?' (Note 23.1).

It was also an important point of principle never to give misleading information or false reassurance. Even during testing I would never tell a subject that he had 'done well' if this was not the case. It was possible to be constructive and encouraging without having to pretend that there were no difficulties ahead. Where there had been some striking success – for example on a difficult item from the intelligence test – I would call the parents' attention to this; and indeed during the testing I would sometimes say to the subject, 'Would you like to try this very difficult one? It is really for older people'. This kind of procedure makes it possible to *show* him that he is not stupid, as opposed to just *telling* him (Note 23.2).

Secret fears that they were stupid, or even mad, were regularly found among my subjects, and it was sometimes possible to bring these fears into the open. For example, it transpired that S127 had earlier been worried that he was, in his words, a 'nut-case'; and when his mother described how he and some slower children had been 'loaded' together (i.e. put in the same 'band' at school) he commented 'Some *were* nut-cases' (Note 23.3).

Sometimes I was able to make clear that I understood the subject's feelings of frustration. For example, in the case of S167 his mother had reported that he used to fly into a rage and 'resented being told to pull his socks up'. I therefore started the discussion by saying, 'I am sure he must have had a miserable time earlier on', and later indicated that he might have underestimated his own ability. Another procedure which I sometimes found useful was what I call the 'prophylactic warning'. This involves making clear to the subject that there are still, unfortunately, people who are unsympathetic to the notion of dyslexia and that he must not mind too much if they start saying to him that he is stupid, lazy, or 'playing up'. Since this was always said in the presence of the parents my hope was that the whole family would cooperate in trying to offset any damage which might otherwise be caused by unimaginative and unsympathetic handling. I was also implicitly conveying to the child that at least his parents understood the problem or, if there had previously been misunderstandings within the family, that these misunderstandings could now be regarded as a thing of the past. Finally, this kind of warning was an indication that I myself understood the position; it was perhaps an additional reassurance that such a warning should come from someone who was outside the family and was in a position to speak authoritatively. It was once reported to me, after I had appeared in a television programme on dyslexia, that a young dyslexic boy had said to his parents, 'Thank goodness there are some grown-ups who know how you feel'. If the child realises that there are people who understand his problems, this may well help him not to take too seriously the strictures of the unsympathetic.

Sometimes, too, it was possible for me to show how the dyslexia had contributed to family tensions. For example, S183 came to see me with his stepfather and they made clear when I spoke to them after the assessment that they had quarrelled in the past. I was able to interpret the dyslexic difficulties as a source of the misunderstanding between them and it was plain that, with these difficulties explained, there was the chance of a fresh start and new understanding between the two of them.

In all cases I followed up the discussion by sending a written report in which I summarised the main points of the assessment. Many of the letters which I received after the assessment were something more than conventional expressions of gratitude; there seems little doubt that suitable discussions with dyslexic children and their families can result in significant changes in behaviour. The extracts which follow illustrate the kind of thing which I have in mind (Note 23.4).

The mother of S47 wrote:

Since his visit to Bangor S is much happier; his difficulty has at last been recognised, and he is cooperating readily in our efforts to help him overcome it.

A month after the assessment the mother of S61 telephoned me and I noted down the following remarks:

I used to cry myself to sleep, as I could see there was something wrong, but they would only say he was lazy. When I asked him he said, 'I needn't worry any more about being called lazy'. I really am very grateful.

Soon afterwards she said in a letter, 'As I mentioned on the 'phone there is a remarkable change in G's attitude and he's happier than we have seen him for a long time'.
The mother of S62 wrote:

He is, and has been since (date of assessment), a much more relaxed and happy boy, with lots of self confidence which has taken away his need to be aggressive with his little brother and sisters. This has made the whole family more relaxed.

The mother of S67 wrote:

We all came away feeling as though a load had been lifted from us; most especially M. I know he has worried for so long about what was wrong with him and to be told he is an able intelligent boy who has a problem called dyslexia which with a lot of effort and the right sort of help he can overcome is to him a tremendous relief. You must have received many similar letters!... My big regret is that I didn't take things into my own hands earlier and thus saved M such a struggle and so much worry.

S75 was reported by his mother to have been singing in the car on the way home, and to have said:

I'm so glad I've been to see Professor Miles. Now I know I'm not stupid.

S95 wrote to me at the age of 21, ten years after his assessment, saying that he had just successfully completed a 2-year BTech HND course.

I am now in my thired week at BBC...as an engineer. In your report I belive that you said simething to the effect that – 'I see no reason why (Brian) should not fulfil his ambition to join the BBC'. If I am correct, then you are a very good judge! Finally I would like to thank you & all that took part in 'checking me over', as it was THE turning point in my life.

The mother of S107 wrote:

As you can imagine, we all feel happier in our minds knowing what the problem is.

The mother of S125 wrote:

I can't tell you how much more relaxed he is now, and how much your advice has helped both my husband and I, and also J's teachers.

The father of S137 wrote:

Your discussion with my wife and the formal report are a great comfort to us and to G.

The parents of S139 sent a joint letter many years after the assessment.

She is now well established as a Staff Nurse at — Hospital...She has been married for over two years. There is no doubt in our minds that her visit to you was of absolutely crucial importance, in terms of your specific recommendations and even more in terms of its effect on her self-confidence.

The mother of S146 wrote:

M seems to be tackling his problems in a much more relaxed manner since his visit to you... I can never thank you enough for your help with M and explaining to us his problems thus enabling us to have a very happy relationship with him.

After S147 had been accepted at a sympathetic school his father wrote:

T is now well upon his way and such success he will undoubtedly now make of life will certainly in large part be due to you.

The mother of S155 wrote:

Your report on W has been tremendously helpful... All in all we have been most fortunate in that your report has sparked off interest and help from the other departments whose teachers have W in their classes... We have a lot to thank you for.

The mother of S192 wrote that her son 'appears to be a very much happier boy, more settled and relaxed'.

The mother of S193 wrote:

I cannot say how relieved we were to hear your diagnosis – for though we had felt T to be bright, the last few years at school, and our early attempts to find him work, had been very discouraging. Now we feel we have a new lease of life. T has gone off to — College of Education in good heart and with a very different attitude to work from what we have been seeing up to now.

The tutor of S200, who was at a College of Education, wrote:

It was very clear from the way he spoke in the car on our journey home last Friday that C's morale had been considerably boosted by his visit to Bangor.

The mother of S189 and S204 wrote:

Both boys came away feeling less despair than for a long time and more assured that they were not idiots doomed to failure.

The father of S212 wrote:

We are very grateful to you for the time and trouble you gave to J's case. The psychological encouragement has been a real reward for his own personal efforts to overcome his difficulty and has vindicated our feeling that he was not as backward as we had been led to believe.

The mother of S218 wrote:

D is in such elated form – it is quite obvious that his session with you lifted a long endured burden: he now feels exonerated and his personal dignity has been restored. I cannot thank you enough.

The mother of S221 wrote (many years later):

I remember my visit to your unit very clearly as a turning point for my 19 yr old son... As a result of your report, he came to terms with a disability that had increasingly frustrated us, and which had caused him and me to feel guilty and to blame ourselves and each other!...As you see, I am very proud of him and very grateful for the findings and advice you gave us on that fateful day in Bangor.

The mother of S241 wrote:

The school is still making S do French – his report comes 'could do better with more consistent effort'. However S has now accepted that he must at least show willing to please his French teacher and, thanks to you, we understand and pay no attention to his poor results. We have noticed a remarkable change in S during his 4 years at school. During the first year he was miserable because the boys made fun of his dreadful spelling – he

became white and introverted. Then you came along, assessed his problem
and he know what was wrong. He still had an uphill fight and since children
are cruel and attack the weakest member was still made miserable at times,
but at least the family understood, supported and encouraged while making
it clear he himself had to fight his battles.

Chapter 24
New Developments*

Since this book was first published in 1983 many new developments have taken place. It is not possible to do justice to all of them and in this chapter I shall refer only to those which are directly relevant to the theme of the book.

First, it is now possible to study brain activity by a wide variety of techniques (Note 24.1). In this connection I should like to single out for special mention the work of Dr Albert Galaburda and his colleagues at Harvard University. It has been possible for these researchers to carry out post mortem examination of the brains of individuals known to have been dyslexic in their lifetime (Note 24.2). A panel of experts has been used to examine the data on individual cases, and a subject is counted as 'dyslexic' only if the experts are in full agreement over the diagnosis (Note 24.3).

The part of the brain which has received special attention is the planum temporale, which is part of the temporal lobe. Eight brains have so far been examined, all of which showed structural abnormalities, in particular ectopias (intrusions of cells from one layer to another) and dysplasias (disorganisations of cells within a cell layer).

Now earlier research had shown that in the great majority of brains the plana in the two hemispheres are asymmetrical and different in size. What was particularly striking about all the eight brains was that there was symmetry of the two plana and approximate equality of size. Dr Galaburda and his colleagues are cautious in their interpretation of this finding, but their tentative suggestion is as follows:

> Indirect evidence suggests that asymmetry of the planum results from the greater pruning down of one of the sides during late fetal life and infancy, a process that implicates asymmetry of developmental neuronal loss. Symmetry, on the other hand, reflects failure of asymmetrical cell loss to occur. The exuberant growth of the otherwise smaller side in the symmetri-

---

*Chapters 24–32 were written for the second edition.

cal cases might produce complex qualitative alterations in the functional
properties of the system (Note 24.4).

This is to suggest that in dyslexics there may be an unusual balance
of skills – a point to which I shall return later in the chapter.

One further research paper by members of the Harvard team
requires mention. The authors are Margaret Livingstone and colleagues
(Note 24.5). The central theme of the paper is the difference between
the magnocellular and parvocellular pathways in the visual system. 'In
primates', the authors write, 'fast low-contrast visual information is carried by the magnocellular subdivision...and slow, high contrast information...by the parvocellular division'. It was found that when five
dyslexic adults were compared with suitably matched controls they differed on certain physiological measures when low-contrast stimuli
were presented but did not do so when high-contrast stimuli were presented. (These measures involved the presentation of visual stimuli by
means of a pattern generator and the recording of responses by means
of electrodes placed on the skull.) This suggested that there might be
an abnormality in the magnocellular system of dyslexics. It was then
found that in the brains of five of the dyslexics who had been studied
post mortem by Dr Galaburda and his colleagues the parvocellular layers were not unusual, but that there was considerable disorganisation
in the magnocellular layers, with the cell bodies appearing smaller. The
authors consider the possibility that other cortical systems besides the
visual have a fast and a slow sub-division and that dyslexia specifically
affects the fast sub-divisions.

Research by William Lovegrove (Note 24.6) has led to similar conclusions. Instead of using the terms 'magnocellular' and 'parvocellular'
Lovegrove speaks of the 'transient' and the 'sustained' channels of the
visual system; on the basis of a number of experiments he concludes
that in the case of dyslexics it is the transient system which is deficient
and that this makes it difficult for them to handle information which is
presented at speed. At the end of his paper he suggests that there may
be 'auditory analogues' of the deficits in the visual transient system.
This suggestion is very similar to that made by Livingstone and her colleagues.

Some years earlier Paula Tallal (Note 24.7) had been able to demon-
strate that dysphasic children (children with major speech problems)
often have difficulty in coping with auditory and other information
when it is presented at speed. When the same tests were repeated with
reading disabled children she found that some of them (presumably
those who by the criteria offered in this book would count as 'dyslexic') had similar problems – and significantly were also weak at reading
nonsense words. She wonders if in these cases it is a weakness at rapid
processing of speech sounds which is at the root of their difficulties.

Whereas serious deficits in the rate of processing the acoustic stream may
lead to serious developmental language disorders, the more subtle deficits
found in some of the reading impaired children we studied may be related
to inabilities to learn the letter-to-sound correspondences involved in phonics skills (Note 24.8).

This conclusion is in line with the widely held view that the central
problem for dyslexics is a weakness at the *phonological* level. It is to
this area that we must now turn.

'Phonology' is usually defined as the science of speech sounds in so
far as they convey meaning. What has been suggested is that dyslexics
do not easily acquire the names (or 'spoken representations') of stimuli
in the environment. The point has been succinctly put by Frank
Vellutino who speaks of 'a subtle language deficiency' and characterises
the phonological weakness as 'the inability to represent and access the
sound of a word in order to help remember the word' (Note 24.9).
At the risk of over-simplification one could perhaps say that, on this
view, the central difficulty for dyslexics is one of 'verbal labelling'
(Note 24.10).

Further evidence suggesting a weakness at the phonological level
has been summarised by Hugh Catts (Note 24.11). Many dyslexics are
weak at segmentation – that is, at dividing words up into their con-
stituent phonemes (Note 24.12). They may also be weak at synthesising
separate phonemes into a single word, for instance the sounds 'c', 'a',
and 't' into 'cat'. Another interesting way of breaking up words is into
onset and rime: in the case of 'cat' the 'c'-sound is the onset and the
'at'-sound the rime. There is reason to think that most children find
rimes easier to distinguish than separate phonemes (Note 24.13).
Difficulty in recognising that words rhyme, as documented in Chapter
18 of this book, is now agreed to be part of the picture (Note 24.14);
there is also reason to think that many dyslexics are weak at the recall
of auditorily presented nonsense words (Note 24.15).

Uta Frith has put forward a model according to which the learning
of reading and spelling can usefully be divided into three stages, which
she has termed the logographic, the alphabetic and the orthographic.

Logographic skills refer to the instant recognition of familiar words. Salient
graphic features may act as important cues in this process...Alphabetic skills
refer to knowledge and use of individual phonemes and graphemes and
their correspondences...Orthographic skills refer to the instant, analysis of
words into orthographic units without phonological conversion (Note
24.16).

Using the Frith model, one might say that dyslexics are held up
at the alphabetic stage and that it is for this reason that they need
systematic training in making links between letters and sounds (Note
24.17).

The acquisition of such links is commonly known as 'paired associate learning'. For example, if nonsense sounds are 'paired' with nonsense shapes there is good reason to think that dyslexics will normally require more exposures to the 'pairs' than non-dyslexics before they are able to name the shapes correctly (Note 24.18). A sound, of course, ceases to be nonsense when it has become paired with a shape, since it is then the 'name' of that shape; a 'verbal labelling' deficiency will therefore show itself when sounds that are initially nonsense have to be treated as words. It is also interesting to note that when a child learns to talk this, too, is a case of paired-associate learning: what are originally meaningless sounds gradually become associated with things and events in the environment; in due course the child recognises that a particular occasion is appropriate for the uttering of particular words. If dyslexics need more 'pairings', however, before the appropriate associations are made, one would expect them to be late talkers; there is good reason to think that this is in fact the case (Note 24.19).

There is also reason to believe that, whether or not the person is dyslexic, words acquired earlier in life take less time to retrieve than words acquired later (Note 24.20). Following up this idea my colleague, John Done, and I gave a picture naming task to dyslexics and suitably matched controls between the ages of 12 and 14. Pictures of familiar and less familiar objects were presented on cardboard, and by means of a voice-key it was possible to determine how long the subjects took to find the correct name. Some experiments with younger children enabled us to assign an 'age of acquisition' to a wide range of words; and the results with the 12- to 14-year-olds supported the claim that words such as 'octopus' and 'bagpipes', which we knew to have a late age of acquisition, did, indeed, take both groups longer to name than words with an earlier age of acquisition such as 'tree' and 'bicycle'. What we also found was that, regardless of age of acquisition, the dyslexics took consistently longer than the controls to produce the name. The differences in response time led us to suggest that the age of word acquisition for dyslexics was on average about 10 months later than that for controls (Note 24.21).

The relatively long time needed by dyslexics for word retrieval can be used to explain why they are relatively weak at the recall of auditorily presented digits. It is widely agreed that immediate memory – or what is now called 'working memory' – is 'time-based': in other words, on the assumption that the items are disconnected, how many items we can remember is a function of how long it takes to say them (Note 24.22). Now, given that dyslexics tend to need more time than non-dyslexics to retrieve verbal labels, it follows that they will make fewer retrievals per unit time; in that case what is commonly called their 'memory span' will necessarily be smaller. Moreover, given that the problem is one of verbal labelling, there will be the same difficulty whether the stimuli are presented auditorily or in any other way; this makes sense of the fact that dyslexics were found to be weaker even than spelling-age-matched controls when digits were presented visually (Note 24.23).

Mention should also be made of some research which is being carried out by Rod Nicolson and Angela Fawcett, of Sheffield University (Note 24.24). In an initial set of experiments 23 dyslexics and eight suitably matched controls, all aged between 12 and 13 years, were required to carry out a variety of tasks involving balancing on a beam. There was, not surprisingly, no difference between the two groups. When further tasks were superimposed, however, for instance counting backwards (with the level of difficulty adjusted to the needs of each child) or pressing the left of two buttons if a high tone sounded and the right, if a low tone sounded, the dyslexics' balancing performance was impaired.

The authors initially used these findings to argue in favour of what they call the 'dyslexia automatisation deficit' (DAD) hypothesis – that skills in dyslexics do not easily become automatic. However, the exact interpretation of their data is open to question, as they themselves would agree. One possibility is that a verbal labelling deficit theory, though it accounts for many of the phenomena of dyslexia, is incomplete. It would be particularly interesting if tasks could be discovered which do not involve verbal labelling yet at which dyslexics perform less well than non-dyslexics.

It is not in dispute, of course, that there are some automatic skills – driving a car is an obvious example – at which dyslexics can be fully competent. What is particularly exciting about the DAD hypothesis is the number of possible experiments which it generates. For instance, it would be interesting to find out whether the driving of dyslexics is affected more than that of controls if a highly complicated secondary task is superimposed. It is a matter of familiar experience that in difficult traffic situations even a non-dyslexic driver may sometimes say, 'Don't talk to me'; it would be interesting to find out more about what particular tasks complicate the situation for dyslexics. However that may be, Nicolson and Fawcett have not only encouraged researchers to take the concept of 'automaticity' seriously; they have invited us to consider carefully what happens when different tasks are superimposed.

Research also continues into the genetics of dyslexia (Note 24.25). There can, of course, be no doubt that in some families a genetic factor is at work (compare Chapter 20); my personal view is that in those studies where concordance in monozygotic twins has *not* been found this is due to faulty selection of subjects. However that may be, there is still the puzzling fact that the same pattern of difficulties sometimes arises when others in the family are affected and sometimes when they are not.

Finally, I should like to return briefly to the neurological findings mentioned earlier in the chapter. They have two consequences which are particularly relevant to the theme of this book. In the first place they make sense of the widely held view that dyslexics are likely to show an unusual balance of skills. Despite their weaknesses in the mechanics of reading and writing, they may show remarkable creative powers in other areas, including art, literary composition, architecture, engineering and a variety of constructional skills. This kind of creative ability is thought normally to be a function of the right cerebral hemisphere and the ability to deal with language and symbols analytically to be a function of the left. The word 'normally' is important here, as there are known to be exceptions and the area is one in which it is all too easy to be simplistic (Note 24.26). It is possible, therefore, that the different 'functional properties' of the dyslexic's cerebral organisation, to which Galaburda and his colleagues refer, show themselves in this unusual balance of skills. If so, then in standard cases dyslexics will show unusually powerful 'right hemisphere' skills while their 'left hemisphere' skills will tend to remain relatively weak.

In a recent book (Note 24.27) Thomas West has taken up the idea of an imbalance of skills in a remarkably interesting way. He provides a series of biographical sketches of various individuals who have shown unusual powers of creativity but have, as it were, paid the penalty by being slow readers and poor spellers, or in general by showing weakness at the analytic aspects of language. His examples include Albert Einstein, Thomas Alva Edison and W.B.Yeats. Not all of those about whom he writes were dyslexic in the 'classic' sense, but West is able to show that they all had the unusual *balance* of skills that is typically found in dyslexics. Part of his argument is that many of the tasks which in the past have called for analytic language skills will from now on be performed by computers. It is therefore, on his view, a serious fault in our educational system that it is weighted heavily in favour of those who possess such skills. They are the people who pass conventional examinations – and then become teachers and expect all their pupils to be like them! In contrast, those who are weak on the literacy side but have exceptional creative talents may sometimes be insufficiently appreciated. If West is right, some radical re-thinking of educational objectives is called for.

In Chapter 18 of the first edition of this book, under the heading 'Art and Craft', I wrote: 'One must...suppose...that those talents which are least affected by the handicap will be the ones which tend to flourish' (see pp. 145–146 of this edition). I now believe this to be an over-simplification. In the time since the above was written, I have met many dyslexics who showed outstanding ability in the areas in question; in the light of the Harvard research and West's biographical sketches, I do not believe that this is merely a product of their environment – that it was simply absence of success on the literacy side which led them into areas where the literacy requirements were less demanding. On the contrary, I think it can be said that their distinctive talents, when these exist, are no accident: their cerebral organisation is such that success in certain areas is just what would be expected.

There is a second consequence of the Harvard research. If Galaburda and his colleagues are right, then the physiological changes which lead to dyslexia are found in late fetal life and early infancy; in that case, if one is to pick out a child as dyslexic, one need not wait for reading or spelling failure to occur.

What is interesting is that recognition of dyslexia at a very young age has been found to be possible, at least for someone with the appropriate experience. The following is an extract from an article written by Jean Augur, who not only has had many years' experience as a teacher of dyslexics but has encountered the condition in her own family (Note 24.28).

> My grandson spoke very clearly at an early age. He was even able to remember and recite rhymes and jingles with incredible accuracy. When only three he pointed to 'M' on a car number plate and said, 'That's Macdonalds'. He had made the connection between the 'M' of the Macdonald's logo, even though the latter is different in shape from the letter on the car number plate. At four this child knew that 'cat', 'fat', 'sat' and 'hat' rhyme, and said 'They all end with the same letters'. No dyslexic profile there in my view. Now five-and-a-half and at school, this child is reading without difficulty, and can spell many three letter words correctly...My little granddaughter has an early family lisp. She chatters incessantly, but it is not always clear what she is saying. She mixes up lots of words and phrases e.g. 'tebby-dare' for 'teddy bear', 'Mishyell' for 'Michelle', 'cobblers' club' for 'toddlers' club'. She confuses 'in' with 'out', 'up' with 'down'. She has difficulty labelling, so that when asked to name a certain colour when the latter is indicated to her she cannot, but when that colour is named for her, she can pick it out in a range of colours when asked to do so. She prefers activities with a technical or 3-dimensional content. In view of our family history I am watching her with great care.

The issue of early recognition of dyslexia is one which requires further research. It nevertheless seems safe to say, in our present state of knowledge, that a distinctive pattern of oral language can be found in the dyslexic well ahead of the time when he attempts to cope with written language.

The following, then, is a tentative account of how the manifestations of dyslexia arise. For neurological reasons – connected with deficiencies in the magnocellular system – there may be an anomaly of development which sometimes gives rise to an unusual balance of skills. This anomaly is sometimes, but not always, the result of hereditary factors. Reasoning is unaffected, and in some areas such as art and engineering there may be exceptional talent. There are weaknesses, however, which may show themselves as early as age 3 in spoken language and there-after when the child is required to deal with written language. Many of these weaknesses are overcome by practice and suitable training, but the processing of symbolic material at speed remains difficult.

From the point of view of the present book, one of the key concepts is that of a deficiency in verbal labelling. In the next chapter an attempt will be made to show how the typical responses of dyslexics to items in the Bangor Dyslexia Test make sense if one assumes that a deficiency in verbal labelling is at the root of their problem.

Chapter 25
Theoretical Basis for the Bangor Dyslexia Test

When the items in the Bangor Dyslexia Test were first tried out they had no firm theoretical basis. I was in no doubt that they were in some way connected, since there was a consistent pattern of responding in subjects who differed widely in both age and background. It was far from clear, however, what lay behind the connection or what was causing what.

If, however, as was suggested in the last chapter, dyslexics are weak in the area of verbal labelling, this could make sense of why they find the items in the Bangor Dyslexia Test difficult and why the various compensatory strategies described earlier in the book were necessary. I shall therefore consider the items of the test in turn from this point of view.

(1) The Left–Right item

There is good reason to think that commands such as 'Touch my right hand with your left hand' are difficult for dyslexics not because of 'directional confusion' as such but because the *labels* 'left' and 'right', which are used to describe direction, are confusable.

It is perhaps worth asking in this connection why there is not the same difficulty in sorting out, say, 'red' from 'green' or 'horse' from 'cart'. The answer appears to lie in the lack of consistency with which the words 'left' and 'right' are used. A red object does not turn into a green one if one looks at it from a different angle, nor does a horse turn into a cart. Yet the wall of a room, for instance, is on the left if one faces one way and on the right if one faces the other. Such inconsistency creates some degree of difficulty even in the case of non-dyslexics; I suspect that what is happening in the case of dyslexics is that their weakness at verbal labelling is superimposed on this initial difficulty. Experience suggests that the great majority of them, provided, of course, that they are of suitable age and experience, are able to cope with the single commands, 'Show me your right hand' and 'Show me your left ear' (Note 25.1). What exposes their weakness is the request to carry out the dual task – distinguishing their own left and right and, superimposed on this, distinguishing the tester's left and right. The task is further complicated by the fact that three different parts of the body have to be distinguished – hand, eye and ear. In itself this addition makes only minimal memory demands, but, although it is not a matter which I have systematically investigated, I think it likely that if the demand related only to, say, the hand the task would be considerably easier and hence less likely to pinpoint the distinctive weakness of the dyslexic.

If one's memory becomes overloaded various different strategies are possible. One of these is to ask the person to repeat what they said, while another is verbal rehearsal – that is, muttering the words under one's breath as an aid to memory. Both are strategies which everyone uses from time to time. It seems likely – though, once again, further research would be needed to establish the point more securely – that in this particular context dyslexics use them more frequently than controls. The weakness at verbal labelling could in that case be seen as the 'deciding straw' which makes 'RR' responses (request for the question to be repeated) and 'EQ' responses (echoing the question) a useful way of compensating for an initial limitation.

It was pointed out in Chapter 10 that in order to identify left and right on the tester's body some subjects turned round in their seats or, in less extreme cases, imagined themselves to be turning round. In this connection I have elsewhere used the formula 'Doing is a substitute for naming' (Note 25.2). If we now assume that searching for the appropriate verbal label is more difficult for dyslexics than for non-dyslexics, it follows that this strategy is of help to dyslexics precisely because it lessens the amount of such searching. It is not, of course, a strategy that is likely to occur to any large number of dyslexics, but the fact that it happens at all makes sense if one assumes that verbal labelling is the basic problem.

(2) The Polysyllables item

To explain the difficulties experienced by dyslexics in the repetition of some polysyllabic words, for instance 'preliminary' and 'statistical , it may be helpful in the first place to turn to the evidence from phonology (Note 25.3). To produce the 'm' sound the two lips need to touch each other, while to produce the 'n' sound the tongue has to be placed on the alveolar ridge. It follows that to articulate the words 'preliminary' and 'anemone' what is required is to move at speed between places of articulation which are close together. The same goes for the 'ph', 'l', and 's' sounds in 'philosophical'. In the case of 'statistical' the most common error is to say 'satistical'; it is possible that in failing to repeat this word accurately the dyslexic is at the same stage as some younger children. It is known that a consonant cluster followed by vowel and consonant is harder to articulate than consonant–vowel–consonant, and it therefore makes sense that the first 't'-sound should be omitted. The second 'st' is different ('stati*st*ical') because the 't' begins a new syllable ('sta-tis-tic-al') and in this position in the word the 'st' is not perceived as a cluster. The initial 'st' is also in an unstressed syllable, and phonemes in unstressed syllables are always more vulnerable than phonemes in stressed ones.

What is involved seems to be that a distinctive dyslexic weakness (difficulty in finding the right word) is particularly shown up if at the same time a task has to be carried out which is also difficult for non-dyslexics.

Now if one takes a dyslexic person *slowly* through, say, the word 'preliminary' ('Say "*pre*"; say "*pre-lim*"; say "*in*"; say "*in-ary*": say "*pre-lim-in-ary*"' – with pauses where the hyphens are shown) they will very probably be successful; on the other hand I have regularly found that they revert to failure if they then try to say the components too quickly (Note 25.4). This finding makes sense if one postulates some kind of fault in the magnocellular system, as a result of which coping with the components of words such as 'preliminary' at speed presents dyslexics with a distinctive problem. Unless they slow down their speech rate, they are at risk of saying the syllables of the word in the wrong order; this in its turn may lead to the 'false match for order' (see Chapter 9) which is often found in dyslexics' spelling.

(3,4) The Subtraction and Tables items

Weakness at verbal labelling also affects some aspects of mathematics. In particular, there is reason to think that dyslexics have a smaller repertoire of number facts at their disposal than do non-dyslexics. This is something which has already been mentioned in Chapter 15, but the discussion there can now be supplemented.

By 'having a number fact at one's disposal' I mean being able to give the answer to a particular calculation sum 'in one' – to be able to do so 'automatically'. (This is another area where the difficulty of dyslexics in acquiring 'automatic' responses shows itself; compare the references to the work of Nicolson and Fawcett described in the last chapter.) Thus most readers of this book will be able to say 'in one' that $8 \times 7 = 56$ or that $44 - 7 = 37$; these number facts are available for immediate use. If, however, they were asked, 'What is 27×23?' or 'What is $491 - 327$?', they would be unable to give the answer 'in one' but might say something like, 'Give me a moment or two and I will work it out'. Now there is reason to think that the 'threshold' – the point at which one has to say, 'Give me a moment and I will work it out' – is reached by dyslexics with lower numbers than it is for non-dyslexics. This was certainly found to be the case in a study in which dyslexics between the ages of 12 and 14 were tested on their immediate knowledge of multiplication number facts (Note 25.5). It was not, of course, that they had no number facts at all: many were able, in particular, to give immediate answers in the case of the 5 x, 10 x, and 11 x tables, and on these three tables the differences between them and the controls were less. Similarly in the case of '6 – 3' I have always found that the very great majority of dyslexics are able to say 'three' with no hesitation or working out. In contrast, 19 – 7 is interesting because it falls around what may be called the 'critical area' where most non-dyslexics of suitable age can give the answer 'in one' whereas a significantly larger number of dyslexics are unable to do so. It now seems that in choosing this item for inclusion in the Bangor Dyslexia Test I had stumbled somewhat fortuitously on a good example of a sum which is at the right level of difficulty for differentiating the two groups.

It remains to ask, 'Why use fingers?' and 'Why use marks on paper?' A likely answer seems to be this. One must assume that the dyslexics' greater success with the 5 x, 10 x, and 11 x tables was because these tables are, in a special sense, 'regular'; it follows that, provided the algorithm is known, much less is needed by way of memorisation. Now there is one wholly dependable regularity in the number system, namely that *the numbers go up in ones*. If therefore a person does not know 'in one' that 19 – 7 = 12 an obvious compensatory strategy is to deal with the numbers one by one. This is precisely what using fingers or marks on paper achieves. There is in fact reason to believe that a similar strategy is used by non-dyslexic children at a younger age (Note 25.6).

Now it can also be said that the acquisition of number facts is a task which requires paired associate learning. We need to learn, for example, that 2 x 3 has to be associated with 6, that 9 – 7 has to be associated with 2, and so on. It therefore makes sense of the data to say that dyslexics can, indeed, eventually acquire number facts but that they need more 'paired associations' before they are able to do so. Since the training which they receive varies considerably from one individual to another one would expect there to be considerable variety among them both in their knowledge of number facts and in their use of compensatory strategies when such knowledge is lacking. This is precisely what we find, as is shown by the evidence reported in Chapters 15 and 16.

Now, as was noted in Chapter 24, Nicolson and Fawcett showed that if a relatively difficult task, such as counting backwards, is superimposed on an easier one, such as balancing, the easier task may be affected (Note 25.7). Now reciting tables in the traditional way requires the person to cope with several tasks simultaneously. Not only are there difficulties in keeping track of the 'preamble' ('one six is...two sixes are...' etc.), as was pointed out in Chapter 16; as a result of pressure the subject may make a variety of other slips, such as breaking into the 'wrong' table or saying 'eight sixties' in place of 'eight sixes'. With suitable practice the responses become automatic, and a non-dyslexic child who has had this practice simply 'sails through' tables without even stopping to think. For dyslexics, on the other hand, one may surmise that any skill which involves considerable linguistic complexity, such as reciting tables, does not easily become automatic and breaks down under pressure.

(5,6) Months Forwards and Months Reversed
(7,8) Digits Forwards and Digits Reversed

Learning the months of the year is in some ways comparable with learning the alphabet and learning the days of the week. Mention was made at the end of Chapter 14 of occasional difficulties, even on the part of older dyslexics, in giving the days of the week, and Note 14.5 refers to the problems experienced by some dyslexics in learning the alphabet. The facts which require theoretical explanation are that among older dyslexics it is only a very small number who have difficulty with the days of the week, while many more have difficulty with the months of the year, and it is probable that quite a number have difficulty in saying the alphabet (Note 25.8). The key factors seem to be the length of the series and the number of opportunities for learning it. In the case of the days of the week, there are only seven separate units and children are regularly exposed to them. In the case of the alphabet there are 26 separate units, and it is likely that some dyslexics and not others will have been required to learn them and that some will have succeeded in learning them as a result of the 'chanting' method (Note 14.5). In general, one can say that if an individual has a weakness at verbal labelling the links between separate members of a series will not be easily formed: to associate two items may not be all that difficult, or even three or four. Beyond that, however, the extra time required for retrieving the names will significantly reduce the efficiency of immediate memory, for reasons given in the last chapter. Basically, therefore, difficulty with months of the year and difficulty with recall of digits – along with difficulty in learning the days of the week and learning the alphabet – can be brought under the same explanatory principle: slow retrieval makes the learning of items in a disconnected series difficult, and success will be a function both of the length of the series and of the opportunities for learning it. Since these last two factors may be very different in the case of different dyslexics it is not surprising that we find considerable variety.

When the items have to be said in reverse order (Months Reversed and Digits Reversed) we once again have the situation where an extra task is superimposed. The initial weakness therefore becomes compounded.

(9) b–d confusion

Confusion over 'b' and 'd' is also something which can be explained in terms of a verbal labelling deficit. Much has been made in the past of the fact that 'b' and 'd' are mirror images of each other. It is not clear, however, *pace* Orton, that mirror images as such present dyslexics with any distinctive problem. We need also to remember that there are two additional complications in the case of 'b' and 'd', namely that they have to be paired with two auditorily confusable sounds and that both these sounds are articulated in the forward part of the mouth. It is possible, therefore, that this combination of difficulties is liable to affect anyone, whether dyslexic or not. Why many dyslexics continue to confuse 'b' and 'd' may be that, superimposed on these other difficulties, is a weakness at verbal labelling, and it is this weakness which is distinctive to dyslexia.

Although few dyslexic adults confuse 'b' and 'd' in either reading or writing, there is evidence that they need more time than non-dyslexics in order to distinguish the two. Some years ago (Note 25.9) I set up an experiment in which a 'b', a 'd', a star (*) and a plus sign (+) were juxtaposed; underneath was a printed sentence. For example the subject might be presented with

*

\+

The star is above the plus

or

b   d

The b is to the right of the d

The subject then has to press one of two keys: 'Y' for 'yes' if the sentence is true or 'N' for 'no' if the sentence is false. (For the first of the above examples the correct answer is 'yes'; for the second it is 'no'.) The subjects were students aged 19 and over; it was found that the dyslexics took very much longer than the controls, especially when 'b' and 'd' were part of the stimulus. If 'b' and 'd' had been presented singly, I am sure the differences between dyslexics and non-dyslexics would have been much less. What the results show, in my opinion, is that one can pick up distinctive difficulties – even in older dyslexics – if one gives the subject a verbal labelling task in timed conditions in a context where other difficulties have also to be surmounted.

On one occasion I was giving this test to a very sophisticated dyslexic adult who told me part way through the experiment that he had just devised a new strategy which would enable him to respond more quickly. He had started, as had other subjects, by assuming that it was necessary to distinguish *both* 'b' and 'd' *and* 'left' and 'right'. Using the new strategy he had only to distinguish 'left' and 'right'. He examined the stimulus in the bottom left corner without naming it; if the word 'left' appeared he compared this stimulus with the stimulus immediately above; if the word 'right' appeared he compared it with the stimulus above and on the right. Then, if there was a match he pressed the 'yes' key and if there was a mismatch he pressed the 'no' key. Readers who adopt his strategy with the two examples given above will find that it works! What at the start had been a naming task ('Is it a "b" or a "d"?') was now something much easier, namely a matching task; the only naming was the identification of 'left' and 'right'. Needless to say his response times from then on were very much faster. This is a striking example of a compensatory strategy on the part of a dyslexic by which he reduced the amount of verbal labelling in order to speed up his performance.

(10) Familial incidence

There is now no doubt that in some cases of dyslexia a genetic factor is involved (Note 25.10); if there are known to be affected relatives this is, of course, a highly significant part of the diagnosis. This item therefore needs no further theoretical justification.

Chapter 26
Data from a Large-scale Survey in Britain

Co-authors Dr M.N.Haslum and Professor T.J.Wheeler

This chapter contains data derived from the Child Health and Education Study (CHES) which started in 1970 (Note 26.1). The subjects were all those children in England, Scotland and Wales who were born during the week 5–11 April 1970. Data were collected at the time of their birth and again in 1975. Thereafter there was a further follow up during 1980 when they were aged between 10 and 11. As a part of the investigation an attempt was made to obtain valid information on the subject of dyslexia.

The educational tests used were: (1) a test of single word reading, (2) an adapted version of the Edinburgh Reading test (Note 26.2), (3) a spelling test in the form of a dictation, (4) a mathematics test, and (5) a Pictorial Language Comprehension test. In addition the children were given the Similarities and Matrices tests from the British Ability Scales (Note 26.3).

The single words were of graded difficulty, starting with 'play' and ending with 'desultory'. The Edinburgh Reading test called for both word recognition and comprehension; for example, in one section the children were given a combination of words and asked to cross out the one that did not belong (for instance in the case of the words 'Why are you been late?' the word to be crossed out was 'been'). The spelling test contained both regular and irregular words and a small number of nonsense words (e.g. 'prunty', 'blomp'). The mathematics test covered a wide range of items, 72 in all, the child in each case being required to mark the appropriate 'box' from a choice of five; among the questions were '5 – 3 = ...', 'Round off 3109 to the nearest hundred, please', and 'What units do we use to measure the capacity of the bottle?' (where a bottle of cola was presented). The Pictorial Language Comprehension test initially involved pictures of four different objects; when the tester said a name (e.g. 'aeroplane') the child had to point to the correct picture out of four; in later items the tester read out a full sentence (e.g. 'No house has a chimney'), and again the child had to point to the correct picture.

In the Similarities test the child had to say how three things were alike and then produce a fourth of the same kind (as it might be 'horse', 'cow', 'sheep'...; 'they are animals, and another one is "pig"'). The Matrices test was of the usual kind: the child needed to recognise relationships between figures and then choose from a number of alternatives the correct figure to fill a vacant space.

As possible indicators of dyslexia, we used the Recall of Digits test from the British Ability Scales and the Left–Right, Months Forwards and Months Reversed items from the Bangor Dyslexia Test (see Appendix I). All these will be referred to in what follows as the 'dyslexia' items (Note 26.4).

Following common practice among researchers, we treated it as a necessary condition for dyslexia that the child should be an 'underachiever' – that is, that he should be weaker at reading or spelling than might have been expected from his intelligence. We decided that the most satisfactory measure of intelligence was to combine the Similarities score with the Matrices score, and in what follows this figure will be referred to as the 'intelligence score'. This procedure did not commit us to belief in 'IQ' in the traditional sense but only to a recognition that differences in reasoning power may be associated with different outcomes on educational tests. For this purpose it was important to choose test items which did not place dyslexics at a disadvantage (compare Chapter 2); there is reason to think that by using these two items we would be satisfying this requirement (Note 26.5).

Basically what is needed in picking out dyslexics is evidence of incongruity. From the arguments presented in Chapter 24, it seems that the dyslexic has an unusual *balance* of skills; a discrepancy between intelligence score on the one hand and reading or spelling score on the other seemed a good way of measuring this imbalance. We specified that this discrepancy had to be at least a certain size (Note 26.6).

Now children can underachieve for a variety of reasons. It follows that if dyslexics are a separate group one needs to specify criteria for distinguishing them from other underachievers. This we did in terms of the number of 'pluses' and 'zeros' on the four dyslexia items. At the time of writing the exact specification has not been decided, but we have in mind that to qualify as a dyslexic a child would need to have at least the equivalent of two 'pluses' out of a possible four.

The tests were administered by class teachers and scored by the survey team. The number of children tested was 12905, along with a further 200 who, on grounds of severe educational retardation, were given a 'special pack' which contained a set of easier tests as well as the standard survey tests. In research on this scale there will be a certain amount of 'noise' in the data; for example one cannot be sure that all teachers administering the tests followed the instructions with 100% accuracy. There are, however, no good reasons for supposing that anything went seriously amiss.

There are many ways in which it will be possible to treat the data in the future. In this chapter we shall limit ourselves to two. First we shall present some population norms for the Bangor Dyslexia Test; secondly we shall present some evidence which bears on the issue of its validation.

Norms for Recall of Digits already exist (Note 26.7). Up to now, however, there have been no adequate norms for the Left–Right, Months Forwards and Months Reversed tests. Table 26.1 shows what these norms are for 10-year-olds.

Table 26.1 Performance of 12 905 10-year-olds on three items from the Bangor Dyslexia Test

		No.	%
Left–Right	−	9760	76.2
	0	1639	12.8
	+	1408	11.0
	(Missing	98 (0.8%))	
	Total	12 905	
Months Forwards	−	9160	73.2
	0	2390	19.1
	+	971	7.8
	(Missing	384 (3.0%))	
	Total	12 905	
Months Reversed	−	7078	57.7
	0	3575	29.1
	+	1615	13.2
	(Missing	637 (4.9%))	
	Total	12 905	

From these, figures it may be inferred that in any similar group of 10-year-olds one can expect about 11% to come out as 'plus' on the Left–Right test, about 8% to come out as 'plus' on Months Forwards and about 13% to come out as 'plus' on Months Reversed.

As they stand, however, the figures do not indicate what part is played by intelligence. For interest, therefore, we have prepared a further table from which all children whose combined score on the Similarities and Matrices tests was less than 90 have been excluded. Norms for this restricted range of children are given in Table 26.2

Table 26.2 Performance of 9341 10-year-olds on three items from the Bangor Dyslexia Test (children of low intelligence excluded)

		No.	%
Left–Right	–	7698	82.7
	0	875	9.4
	+	740	7.9
	(Missing	28 (0.3%))	
	Total	9341	
Months Forwards	–	7193	78.2
	0	1507	16.4
	+	499	5.4
	(Missing	142 (1.5%))	
	Total	9341	
Months Reversed	–	5837	64.0
	0	2422	26.6
	+	857	9.4
	(Missing	225 (2.4%))	
	Total	9341	

As the percentages of 'pluses' in all three items are smaller than those in Table 26.1, it is arguable that lack of intelligence may contribute to a 'plus' response.

Secondly, we were also interested in the possibility of using the data from the Child Health and Education Study in order to check if the four 'dyslexia' items could be validated. What is involved is not, of course, any kind of independent yardstick, since the validity of such a yardstick would itself be open to question (Note 26.8). The argument which follows is based on the fact that there is, at the very least, one part of the definition of dyslexia about which there can be no disagreement.

Whatever the word is taken to mean, everyone would agree that it implies educational disadvantage. If, therefore, the four 'dyslexia' items are what they purport to be, then those who come out as 'plus' on them will tend to be more educationally disadvantaged than those who do not. This means that one would expect them, overall, to obtain lower scores on educational tests than those who score 'zero' or 'minus'.

Now, as was indicated above, five educational tests were used in the study– a Word Recognition test, the Edinburgh Reading test, a Spelling test, a Mathematics test and a Pictorial Language Comprehension test. We therefore checked whether there was an association between positive indicators on the dyslexia items and low scores on the educational tests. We also checked if there was an association with the child's gender or age. Age had to be taken into account because testing took place throughout the year 1980 and there was therefore a gap of about nine months between the oldest and youngest children tested.

The statistical technique used (that of stepwise regression) is somewhat complex and for more details the reader is referred to the relevant literature (Note 26.9). A key concept is that of *variance*. Individual scores vary and the variance is a measure of the extent to which they are scattered around the average. If there is an association between any two tests (call them 'test A' and 'test B'), then a significant proportion of the variance of test A will be accounted for by the influence of test B.

To over-simplify, a check was made as to what part, if any, was being played by the different variables (Recall of Digits, Gender etc.) in contributing to the variance in each of the five educational tests. All the variables were entered into an equation in such a way that the influence of each could be calculated separately.

The results of the analyses are set out in Tables 26.3 and 26.4.

Table 26.3 Association between dyslexia indicators and educational performance.

	Regression coefficient	Explained variance (%)	Change (%) in explained variance
1. Word Recognition test			
Recall of Digits	−0.29	8.53	8.53*
Months Reversed	−0.27	13.87	5.34*
Left–Right test	−0.15	14.99	1.11*
Months Forwards	−0.21	15.93	0.96*
Gender	0.02	15.99	0.06†
2. Spelling test			
Months Reversed	−0.30	8.67	8.67*
Recall of Digits	−0.23	14.93	6.26*
Months Forwards	−0.25	16.57	1.64*
Left–Right test	−0.15	17.58	1.01*
Gender	0.13	18.23	0.65*
3. Edinburgh Reading test			
Months Reversed	−0.30	8.70	8.70*
Recall of Digits	−0.27	14.09	5.39*
Left–Right test	−0.19	16.06	1.97*
Months Forwards	−0.20	16.83	0.77*
4. Mathematics test			
Recall of Digits	−0.28	8.00	8.00*
Months Reversed	−0.26	12.80	4.80*
Left–Right test	−0.19	14.98	2.18*

Table 26.3 (contd)

	Regression coefficient	Explained variance (%)	Change (%) in explained variance
Gender	–0.07	16.03	1.05*
Months Forwards	–0.19	16.87	0.84*
Child's age	–0.04	16.97	0.10*
5. Pictorial Language Comprehension test			
Recall of Digits	–0.17	2.76	2.76*
Gender	–0.11	4.01	1.25*
Months Reversed	–0.11	5.12	1.11*
Left–Right test	–0.11	5.94	0.82*
Months Forwards	–0.08	6.09	0.15*
Child's age	–0.02	6.12	0.03*

Notes: * $p<0.001$; † $p<0.005$. A negative figure under 'gender' implies higher scores by boys, a positive figure higher scores by girls.

The first column in Table 26.3 shows the regression coefficients. These indicate how much the word recognition test score, for example, changes for unit increase in the variables in the equation. In the case of this test, it can be seen from the analysis that there is a much greater change associated with Recall of Digits and Months Reversed than there is for the other variables. It can also be seen that whilst the gender of the child has an influence on word recognition performance (a positive value indicating that girls had higher scores than boys), it is tiny compared with the influence of the dyslexia indicators. This is also true for performance on the Spelling, Edinburgh Reading and Mathematics tests.

Technical details of the second and third columns ('explained variance %' and 'change in explained variance %') need not be given here. If, however, we look at the results for the word recognition test we see that five of the items, including gender but not age, were contributing significantly to the variance, that Recall of Digits accounted for the highest percentage of variance (8.53%) and that Months Reversed accounted for a further 5.34%. The middle column shows that Recall of Digits and Months Reversed were accounting in conjunction for 13.87% of the variance. As a check it can be seen that the entry in the middle column always represents the sum of the entries in the right-hand column that have occurred up to that point.

It is worth noting that the greatest total variance explained was for the spelling test (18.23%) and that the explained variances for the Word Recognition, Edinburgh Reading and Mathematics tests were similar (15.99%, 16.83% and 16.97%, respectively), whereas the explained variance for the Pictorial Language Comprehension test was very much less (6.12%).

If we ask why this should be so, the answer seems to lie in the distinctive nature of the Pictorial Language Comprehension test. As we have seen, in the items of this test a word or a sentence is presented orally to the subject who then has to respond by pointing to one of four pictures, namely the one described by the word or sentence. Since dyslexics appear to show no particular weakness at comprehension as such (compare the data on 'memory for sentences' in Chapter 18) and since the response does not involve word finding or writing, there is little in the task that would be expected to present dyslexics with difficulty. A small decrement might perhaps be expected if on occasions a dyslexic 'loses the thread' of what is said to him, but one would not expect a large decrement, nor, indeed, did we find one. In contrast, we would expect all four 'dyslexia' items to be associated more strongly with weakness at spelling.

As it stands, however, the above analysis is incomplete. If it is to be fully compelling we also need to take into account differences in the children's intelligence level. A further analysis was therefore carried out in which we considered, not the actual scores at word recognition and spelling, but the 'residuals' – that is to say, the scores in so far as they were different from what would have been predicted in the light of the child's intelligence. The results are set out in Table 26.4.

It will be seen from this table that, even when the influence of intelligence is removed, a significant amount of variability in both the word

Table 26.4 Association between dyslexia indicators and underachievement on the Word Recognition and Spelling tests

	Regression coefficient	Explained variance (%)	Changes (%) in explained variance
1. Word Recognition residual			
Months Reversed	−0.18	3.08	3.08*
Recall of Digits	−0.17	5.32	2.24*
Months Forwards	−0.16	6.12	0.80*
Left–Right test	−0.05	6.16	0.04*
2. Spelling residual			
Months Reversed	−0.19	3.69	3.69*
Gender	0.16	5.72	2.03*
Recall of Digits	−0.13	7.36	1.64*
Months Forwards	−0.11	8.36	1.00*
Left–Right test	−0.02	8.39	0.03†

Notes: * $p<0.001$; † $p<0.005$.

recognition and spelling tests is still accounted for by the dyslexia items.

It should also be noted that the most powerful predictors of educational attainment consistently turn out to be Recall of Digits and Months Reversed. It is difficult to be sure what exactly this signifies, but both items involve 'memory' in some form – the one requiring the ability to give an immediate verbal response, the other the ability to retain items in sequence over a period of time. Exactly what kinds of memory task are and are not easy for dyslexics remains a matter for further research.

What the present analysis shows is that all four dyslexia items are negatively associated, independently of each other, with four different measures of educational achievement (and to some extent with a fifth). If they were not measures of *something* these associations would be hard to explain. Although the choice of items for inclusion in the Bangor Dyslexia Test originated largely on the basis of 'hunch' (see Chapter 3), the above analysis suggests that this 'hunch' was not entirely without justification. Further attempts at justification will be offered in the chapters which follow.

Chapter 27
Further Data from Britain

Co-author Sula Ellis

The data which are presented in this chapter were collected as part of an investigation into speed of calculation in dyslexics (Note 27.1). They are included here because of their relevance to the validation of the Bangor Dyslexia Test.

If the test is a valid indicator of dyslexia, it follows that children who on independent grounds are believed to be dyslexic will score more 'pluses' on it than non-dyslexic children of the same chronological age. In addition, if dyslexia genuinely represents a deficit or anomaly and is not just the effect of late development, then these children will also score more 'pluses' than younger children matched for spelling age.

In this chapter we shall describe how both of these predictions were put to the test.

So as not to beg any questions we shall refer to those whom we believed to be dyslexic as the 'test group'. They will be distinguished from controls matched for chronological age (CA controls) and from controls matched for spelling age (SA controls). The major decision that we had to take was how best to pick them out – given, of course, that the Bangor Dyslexia Test could not be used for this purpose if we were to avoid circularity.

We regarded a reading test as unsatisfactory for two reasons, first because there is now convincing evidence that children can have dyslexic-type problems and still be adequate readers (Note 27.2), and secondly because some children are poor readers not for the constitutional reasons implied by the word 'dyslexia' but simply through lack of intelligence or lack of opportunities to learn. In the case of a spelling test the first of these two difficulties is avoided, since if a child is spelling up to his age level it is arguable that at least the existence of dyslexia in his case is somewhat problematic, and unless subjects are in very short supply there is no need to risk contaminating one's statistics with results from doubtful cases. The second difficulty is avoided if one gives the spelling test to subjects who are of adequate intelligence and are known to have been in an environment where opportunities to learn were present. In so far as this was achieved in the present study, it is safe to claim that members of the test group were dyslexic in the required sense.

To avoid possible complications due to gender differences and because of the greater availability of male dyslexics, it was decided to restrict the investigation to the study of boys.

The initial procedure was that one of us (SE) visited four schools, all of which made provision for dyslexics and one of which accepted dyslexics only. The children in these schools were given the S_1 spelling test (Note 27.3) and either the Raven Standard Progressive Matrices (SPM) (Note 27.4) or the Raven Coloured Matrices (Note 27.5) according to their age. We stipulated that no boy should be eligible for inclusion in any of the three groups unless he came out as at least average (50th percentile) for his age on the appropriate Raven Matrices test. This ensured that all subjects were of adequate intelligence. In addition, because all four schools were in the private sector, we felt justified in assuming that all the children would have been given the chance to learn to spell. It followed that those selected for the test group were poor spellers despite adequate intelligence and opportunity. This created the strong presumption that all or most of them were dyslexic. It should also be remembered that it was the policy of all four schools to accept children who had been diagnosed as dyslexic; although we are in no position to know the precise criteria for dyslexia adopted in particular cases, there is at least a presumption that as a result of the schools' selection policies the boys whom we assigned to the test group were dyslexic in the required sense. Another advantage of drawing our subjects from private schools was that we felt justified in assuming that any differences that existed in socio-economic status would be constant across our three groups.

Now if one uses a restricted age group there is a danger that one may be tempted to over-generalise from the results. The initial tests were therefore given to any available boy between the ages of 7 and 14 years. We then specified that the criterion for membership of the test group should be a spelling age on the Schonell S_1 test at least 24 months behind chronological age, while in the case of the CA and SA controls the criterion was that spelling age should be within six months of chronological age or better. This procedure gave us a 'pool' of 133 subjects.

Drawing on this 'pool', we divided the test group and the CA controls into two separate bands, namely those aged 13 and 14 years and those aged 10 and 11 years. There were 15 boys in the older test group, along with 15 CA controls and 15 SA controls, and there were 10 boys in the younger test group along with 10 CA controls and 10 SA

controls. The SA controls had, of course, to be considerably younger
than members of the other two groups, and in the case of the 10- and
11-year-old dyslexics we in fact needed to go as low as age 7 to find
suitable 'matches'.

Table 27.1 gives the particulars of the three groups of 13- and 14-
year-olds and table 27.2 the particulars of the three groups of 10- and
11-year-olds.

Table 27.1 Older age level: number of children (*n*) and mean chronological and
spelling ages in months for each of the three groups. Standard deviations are
given in brackets

Group	n	Chronological age	Spelling age
Test group	15	166.73 (± 7.27)	129.67 (± 10.95)
CA controls	15	168.73 (± 4.85)	167.00 (± 5.74)
SA controls	15	114.20 (± 10.95)	129.00 (± 11.72)

Table 27.2 Younger age level: number of children (*n*) and mean chronological
and spelling ages in months for each of the three groups. Standard deviations
are given in brackets

Group	n	Chronological age	Spelling age
Test group	10	128.80 (± 2.71)	90.10 (± 4.87)
CA controls	10	126.60 (± 7.96)	143.60 (± 13.39)
SA controls	10	89.60 (± 3.07)	90.40 (± 4.41)

The Bangor Dyslexia Test was administered by SE in a quiet room
within the school and scored in accordance with the instructions in the
manual. If any b–d confusions occurred on the S_1 test, or if the boy or
one of his teachers reported such confusion, the result was scored as
plus. Checks for familial incidence were carried out via the boy himself,
via his teachers and via the school records; if all these sources proved
negative, this item was scored as minus.

Frequency distributions of 'pluses' are given in Tables 27.3 (older
age group) and 27.4 (younger age group). Each 'zero' response has
been scored as half a 'plus'.

In the case of the older children, it can be seen that the lowest score
in the test group was 4.5. This meant that there was no overlap with
the CA controls and a single case of overlap with the SA controls, one
boy in the latter group having a score of 5.5 (Note 27.6). Statistically
these differences are highly significant (Note 27.7). In the case of the
younger children, it can be seen that there was no overlap between the
test group and either of the other two groups – again a result which
statistically is highly significant (Note 27.8). None of the CA controls in

Table 27.3 Frequency distribution of 'pluses' on the Bangor Dyslexia Test, older age group

No. of 'pluses'	Test group	CA controls	SA controls
0–0.5	–	–	2
1–1.5	–	7	3
2–2.5	–	4	3
3–3.5	–	4	4
4–4.5	3	–	2
5–5.5	5	–	1
6–6.5	3	–	–
7–7.5	3	–	–
8–8.5	1	–	–

Table 27.4 Frequency distribution of 'pluses' on the Bangor Dyslexia Test, younger age group

No. of 'pluses''	Test group	CA controls	SA controls
0–0.5	–	–	–
1–1.5	–	4	2
2–2.5	–	4	–
3–3.5	–	2	6
4–4.5	–	–	–
5–5.5	–	–	1
6–6.5	–	–	1
7–7.5	2	–	–
8–8.5	5	–	–
9–9.5	3	–	–

either group had more than three 'pluses', though besides the score of 5.5 in the older group of SA controls there were two scores of 4.0, while in the younger group of SA controls there was one score of 5.0 and one of 6.5.

Since there were independent criteria for supposing that the boys in the two test groups were genuinely dyslexic, and since they consistently obtained more 'pluses' than did the CA controls, it can be claimed that the Bangor Dyslexia Test did, indeed, distinguish dyslexics from non-dyslexics. Moreover, since these boys also scored more 'pluses' than the SA controls, and since this result held up in both groups, there is also support for the view that the difficulties experienced by dyslexics cannot simply be attributed to late development.

Chapter 28
Data from Greece

Co-author Andriana Kasviki

The data reported in this chapter were part of a wider enquiry, the purpose of which was to determine whether there was evidence for dyslexia in Greece (Note 28.1). This enquiry involved, among other things, the testing of children on a Greek version of the Bangor Dyslexia Test. As a result it was possible to provide data which could be submitted to an analysis similar to that reported in the last chapter. This would comprise comparisons between a test group (those whom we believed to be dyslexic), controls matched for chronological age (CA controls), and controls matched for spelling age (SA controls).

The Bangor Dyslexia Test was therefore translated into Greek (see Appendix IV for the Greek version). The translation gave rise to two main problems. The first was that of finding suitable Greek equivalents for the words 'preliminary', 'philosophical' etc. which occur in item 2. It was clear that a simple translation of these words would not necessarily achieve what we were aiming at. The English words contain special combinations of the letters 'm', 'n', 's', 't' etc. and there was no guarantee that the Greek equivalents would be words of comparable difficulty. This, of course, is a problem whatever the language into which the test is translated; as will be seen in Chapters 28 and 29, it also arose when the test had to be translated into German and Japanese. In the case of translation into Greek we were able to use the existing Greek words 'philosophikos', 'anemone' (which is the same as the English word), and 'statistikos'; although the Greek words for 'preliminary' and 'contemporaneous' were not ideal, the final list of words turned out to be usable.

The second problem was that the Greek alphabet has no letters which correspond in all respects (visual appearance, sound, place of articulation etc.) with the English letters 'b' and 'd'. However, the symbols ϐ and ϑ (approximately 'v' and 'th') are auditorily confusable and the places in the mouth where they are articulated are very close together. It was therefore decided to check on whether there were any cases of confusion between these two letters. Six words which gave the opportunity for such confusion were selected from school reading books and all subjects were asked to read them. Similar confusions in the spelling test were also noted. Any child who showed confusion at either reading or spelling was scored as 'plus'.

In order to rule out possible cases of mental handicap, all children in the study were given the Raven Standard Progressive Matrices (SPM) (Note 28.2). By means of a suitable table, their scores were converted into IQs, and it was decided to exclude from the study any child whose IQ was less than 90. The scores in fact ranged from 92 to 135. No one was included who was not a native Greek speaker and a check was made with the teachers that none of the children in the study suffered from significant physical or emotional problems.

As there are no standardised tests of spelling in Greece it was necessary to make our own selection of suitable words. Thirty-seven single words were selected, including both regular and irregular ones, along with five non-words and three three-word sentences (Note 28.3). 'Spelling score' was defined as the number of words or sentences correctly spelled; this was out of a possible maximum of 45.

Three hundred and fifty children were given the spelling test, their ages ranging between 7 years 0 months and 11 years 0 months. Ten schools were chosen at random from various middle-class areas in Athens; all were in the state system and the children were of similar socio-economic background.

The three groups were selected on what were basically the same principles as those described in the last chapter. Since, however, there are no schools in Greece catering specifically for dyslexics and since there were no independent criteria in terms of which a diagnosis of dyslexia could be checked, we selected for inclusion in the test group those 47 children in the age range 9 to 11 years who obtained the lowest scores on the spelling test. If there were dyslexics in Greece at all, it was clearly among the underachievers at spelling where they would be found, though this procedure does not allow for there being non-dyslexic underachievers. The CA controls were matched on the SPM with the test group but were different in that they were adequate spellers. The SA controls were younger children, age range 7 to 9 years, matched for spelling score with the children in the test group. Thirty-two of the children in the test group were boys, 15 were girls. This gives approximately a 2:1 ratio, which is smaller than that reported in many studies of literacy difficulties.

With regard to the 'familial incidence' item in the Bangor Dyslexia Test, it was possible in the case of the test group to interview members of their families, and in eight cases out of the 47 there were reports of someone else in the family being affected. In the case of the other two groups it was necessary to consult the teachers' records, and in no case was there any positive evidence. In view of the overall uncertainty with regard to this item, it was decided to score the Bangor Dyslexia Test out of 9 (with 'familial incidence' omitted) instead of out of 10.

Particulars of the three groups are given in Table 28.1.

Table 28.1 Particulars of the three groups				
	n	*Mean age*		*Mean spelling score*
Test group	47	119.23	(± 4.03)	9.19 (± 5.66)
CA controls	47	119.47	(± 4.14)	28.02 (± 5.95)
SA controls	47	98.68	(± 4.81)	9.08 (± 2.32)

n = number of children in the group; age is given in months, and 'spelling score' indicates the number of words correctly spelled out of a maximum of 45. Standard deviations are given in brackets.

The logic of the argument is the same as that set out in Chapter 27. If dyslexia is genuinely an anomaly and if the Bangor Dyslexia Test picks out dyslexics in the required sense, the prediction is that the test group will show more 'pluses' not only than the CA controls but also than the SA controls. A frequency table in respect of number of 'pluses' for each group is set out in Table 28.2.

Table 28.2 Distribution of 'pluses' out of a possible nine for test group, CA controls and SA controls			
No. of 'pluses'	Test group	CA controls	SA controls
0–0.5	–	8	–
1–1.5	–	13	1
2–2.5	–	12	13
3–3.5	–	6	18
4–4.5	–	8	15
5–5.5	6	–	–
6–6.5	11	–	–
7–7.5	16	–	–
8–8.5	8	–	–
9	6	–	–

It can be seen from this table that no-one in the test group had fewer than 5 'pluses', while no-one in either of the other two groups had more than 4.5. This is in contrast to the comparisons reported in Chapters 27 and 29, where the groups showed a small amount of overlap. Overall it is necessary to suppose that extraneous factors (in particular lack of the appropriate experience) can occasionally lead to a significant number of 'pluses' on the Bangor Dyslexia Test in the absence of dyslexia; but the present data show that this is not inevitable.

Table 28.3 gives the mean number of 'pluses' for each of the three groups.

Table 28.3 Mean number of 'pluses' for test group, CA controls, and SA controls on the Bangor Dyslexia Test (out of a possible 9). Standard deviations are given in brackets		
Test group	6.70	(± 1.85)
CA controls	2.15	(± 1.36)
SA controls	3.39	(± 1.08)

The mean of the test group is significantly different from the means of the other two groups (Note 28.4).

Forty children in the test group confused ℓ and ϑ, compared with two CA controls and eight SA controls. Detailed examination of the results of the spelling test showed that even when the SA controls made errors they were more likely than the test group to represent the sounds correctly (Note 28.5). This gives support to the idea that all or most of the poor spellers in the test group were dyslexic in the required sense, since difficulty in learning sound–symbol associations is agreed to be a common characteristic of dyslexia.

If this is correct, it can be claimed not only that dyslexia exists in Greece but that a Greek version of the Bangor Dyslexia Test differentiates dyslexics both from age-matched controls and from younger children matched for spelling age.

Chapter 29
Data from Germany

Co-author Claudia de Wall

A German translation of the Bangor Dyslexia Test will be found in Appendix V. We have entitled it *Der Bangor Legasthenie Test* (abbreviated in what follows to BLT). 'Legasthenie' is the standard German word for 'dyslexia' (Note 29.1). In what follows we shall report on some pilot studies in which the BLT was tried out in Bochum, Germany.

Before presenting our findings, however, we think it may be of interest to indicate what changes were needed to the English version of the test and why.

For the most part the translation was straightforward. As with the Greek translation, however, the Polysyllables item created problems. We began by looking for German words that were like the English words in being awkward to pronounce; various words were tried out, for instance 'abandonieren', 'Agamemnon' and 'eliminieren'. It transpired, however, that all of them were too easy for good and bad spellers alike, and there seemed little future in attempts of this kind.

It then occurred to us that the objectives of the test could be satisfactorily met if in place of real words we substituted nonsense words. This has two advantages. In the first place, if real words are used those children who are familiar with the word in question are at a different starting point from those who are not, and their results are not therefore strictly comparable. Secondly, if one uses nonsense words it is possible to control the way in which the different phonemes (units of sound) are combined; indeed it would be possible in the long term to devise nonsense words which could be used internationally. If, as was suggested in Chapter 25, what the test is tapping is the ability to deal at speed with phonemes whose places of articulation are close together, then the best substitute for the present words would be nonsense words chosen precisely so as to meet this requirement. This, however, would have been a major research undertaking; for immediate purposes we decided that it would be best if the item were simply omitted.

We also found it necessary to introduce two changes in the method of scoring, one in the Tables item, one in the Digits Forwards and Digits Reversed items.

In the case of the Tables item, one of the instructions in the English version is that if the subject asks whether he may leave out the 'preamble' ('one six is...', 'two sixes are...' etc.) this is scored as 'plus'. In Germany, however, when children recite tables the normal procedure is not to include the preamble. In the pilot study over 60% of the children, including controls as well as those believed to be dyslexic, started to recite without it. It was therefore decided that this response on its own should not count as a 'plus'. In the main experiment the tester (C de W) added to the instructions the phrase 'and please do not forget to say "one times", "two times"'. If in spite of this a request to leave out the preamble was still made the response was scored as 'zero', and if two or more reminders had to be given it was scored as 'plus' .

In the case of the Digits Forwards and Digits Reversed items, we found that the scoring system in the English version of the test was too strict for German children: in the pilot study over 70% of the controls came out as 'plus'. An attempt was therefore made to discover German norms for tests involving the recall of digits. Data are in fact available for a Digits Forwards item, 2,567 children having been tested from Germany and 531 children from Austria, Switzerland and South Tirol (Note 29.2). As an approximate guide one can say that the typical German-speaking child aged between 7 and 12 years is likely to be able to recall five digits correctly and to fail at six. In the English version, however, a plus score can be avoided by children aged 9 to 12 years only if at least one series of six digits is passed.

It is possible that the differences between German-speaking and English-speaking children are a consequence of the 'word length effect'. It has been found that if a list contains longer words fewer are remembered than if it contains shorter words (Note 29.3). In addition it would appear that the crucial factor is the time needed to say the word (Note 29.4). In the present case it is possible (though detailed research would be needed to establish the point) that German digits take longer to say than English ones. Whether or not this is the case, we were left in no doubt that a change in the scoring system was needed.

It was also thought that there might be advantages in reverting to the system which is used in many 'digit span' tests (Note 29.5). This involves awarding one point for each correctly repeated series of digits. The main difference is that, if this method is adopted, one does not automatically award a plus if there is failure at a shorter string of digits and success at a longer one. The assumption in the existing method is that this kind of inconsistency is a distinctive characteristic of dyslexics – sufficiently distinctive to be useful in picking them out. This, however, may not be the case and with the new method an early failure is not necessarily a dyslexia indicator if it is compensated for by later successes. The point is one which could usefully be taken into account in future versions of the English test.

If a child passed the first trial for a given number of digits, two points were awarded and it was not thought necessary to give a second trial. Since there are seven Digits Forwards items and four Digits Reversed items the maximum possible score for the former is 14 points and the maximum possible score for the latter is 8 points.

The following system of scoring was then adopted:

(a) Digits Forwards
Ages 7–8: score as plus if the subject obtains fewer than 5 points
Ages 9–12: score as plus if the subject obtains fewer than 6 points
Ages 13 and over: score as plus if the subject obtains fewer than 7 points
(b) Digits Reversed
Ages 7–8: score as plus if the subject obtains no points
Ages 9–12: score as plus if the subject obtains fewer than 3 points
Ages 13 and over: score as plus if the subject obtains fewer than 5 points

Two studies have been carried out to date (Note 29.6). The first involved 13 children from the Institut für Legastheniker Therapie in Bochum and 29 controls from schools in the Bochum area (Note 29.7). The age range was between 9 years 6 months and 14 years 6 months. As this was only a pilot study no detailed check was attempted on the diagnosis of dyslexia by the therapists at the Institute, and in the case of the controls it was considered sufficient to select them if the therapist was satisfied that dyslexia was excluded (Note 29.8).

In the course of the study the problem of scoring the Tables item came to light, as did the problem of scoring the Recall of Digits. It also became plain that more work was needed on the Polysyllables item. The overall result was encouraging, however, since those whom we believed to be dyslexic scored more pluses and fewer minuses overall than did the controls, and when the scores on the items were examined separately it was found that there were statistically significant differences in the case of Left–Right, Subtraction, Tables and Months Reversed.

The second study was an attempt to replicate the findings of the first in a more systematic way. The logic of our enquiry was the same as that reported in the last two chapters. We compared the test group (those whom we believed to be dyslexic) not only with controls matched for chronological age (CA controls) but with controls matched for spelling age (SA controls). As has already been pointed out, this procedure is a check on whether the difficulties of the dyslexic can be understood simply in terms of late development or whether the evidence forces us to regard them as manifestations of some kind of deficit or anomaly. If members of the test group perform no differently from SA controls either view is tenable; if on some tests they perform less well then it is not enough to think simply in terms of late development.

So as to remove any possibility of the results being affected by low intelligence, all children were given the Raven Standard Progressive Matrices (SPM) (Note 29.9), and no one was included in the study unless their score on the SPM was at the 50th percentile (average for their age) or above it. To pick out dyslexics we relied primarily on a spelling test (Note 29.10). We knew that all the children had had a reasonable opportunity to learn to read and write; it followed that if we picked out those who were poor spellers despite this opportunity and despite their having adequate intelligence then at least the great majority of them would be dyslexic in the required sense.

In the spelling test the maximum possible score was 100 (Note 29.11). No-one was included in the test group with a score of over 54; no-one was included among the CA controls with a score of under 59, and no-one was included among the SA controls who was spelling at less than grade level. No attempt was made to match the subjects for gender. The test group were taken from the Special Needs Department of a Realschule ('O'-level high school); the CA controls were from the same school, and the SA controls were from a primary school in Bochum.

It was not possible to obtain data on familial incidence or on b–d confusion, and since the Polysyllables test was not scored (see above) the maximum number of pluses on the BLT for any one individual was 7.

Particulars of the three groups are given in Table 29.1.

Table 29.1 Particulars of the three groups

Group	n	Age (months)		Spelling	
Test group	8	141.75	(± 4.24)	42.88	(± 8.07)
CA controls	8	136.25	(± 2.68)	77.00	(± 11.41)
RA controls	8	113.25	(± 3.63)	44.63	(± 9.55)

n = number in the group; age is given in months, and 'spelling' indicates the score on the spelling test. Standard deviations given in brackets.

Table 29.2 gives the distribution of pluses on the BLT for each of the three groups out of a maximum of 7. As before, a 'zero' response has been scored as half a 'plus'.

Table 29.2 Distribution of pluses on the BLT out of a maximum of 7 for test group, CA controls and SA controls

No. of 'pluses'	Test group	CA controls	SA controls
0–0.5	–	3	1
1–1.5	–	2	1
2–2.5	2	3	2
3–3.5	3	–	3
4–4.5	2	–	1
5–5.5	1	–	–

The test group therefore had many more pluses than the CA controls and marginally more pluses than the SA controls (Note 29.12) though not at a fully convincing level of statistical significance (Note 29.13).

If, therefore, we are justified in assuming that all or most of the test group were dyslexic (see above), then it can be claimed that the German equivalent of the Bangor Dyslexia Test did indeed pick out dyslexics. That dyslexia represents a deficit rether than delayed development is not fully established by the present data, but if they are supplemented by the data reported in Chapters 27 and 28 the conclusion must be seen as highly probable.

Chapter 30
Data from Japan*

Co-authors Professor Jun Yamada and Adam Banks

The Japanese writing system is unique in that three types of script – syllabic hiragana and katakana and logographic kanji (of Chinese origin) – are used complementarily. The first two systems, hiragana and katakana, are easy for most children to learn, and by the end of their first year of primary school, when they are between 6 and 7 years old, they are expected to have mastered both of them. Hiragana and katakana are both speech–sound-based systems in which each character represents a syllable (or more precisely *mora*) such as や or ヤ for /ya/. Hiragana are used to represent grammatical function words and katakana to represent words borrowed from other languages. They are easy to learn because each kana represents a more fixed and stable linguistic unit than a phoneme and because a one-to-one correspondence system is well maintained. On the other hand, each kanji represents a morpheme (Note 30.1), for example 矢 for /ya/ meaning 'arrow'. Kanji tend to be easier to learn than individual kana because each kanji form is associated with a speech word that is meaningful for learners. Pupils are taught 996 kanji by the time they leave primary school. On the face of it, therefore, one would expect potentially dyslexic children to have relatively little difficulty in reading a text written in Japanese (Note 30.2).

This chapter is concerned with two questions: first, whether there are in fact any dyslexic children in Japan, and secondly, if so, whether the Bangor Dyslexia Test is a useful instrument for identifying them.

To answer the first question, two timed tests of oral reading were given. The decision to test under timed conditions seemed to us important. From the evidence cited in Chapter 24, there is reason to think that few tasks which others can do are necessarily impossible for dyslexics provided they put in sufficient time and practice; the problem is that of carrying out these tasks at speed. From an examination of our results (see below) there are grounds for confidence that we have been able to pick out genuine dyslexics – grounds which we would not have had if the tests had been carried out in untimed conditions.

In the first test the child was asked to read out loud a passage taken from a story book for primary school children which uses both kana and simple kanji; in the second test the passage to be read was written only in katakana. The reason for giving both tests was that we suspected that there might be some dyslexics who were successful in reading the ordinary text but whose dyslexia would be shown up if they had to read a passage written solely in katakana. As was noted above, katakana are basically used to represent words borrowed from other languages; a passage written solely in katakana is therefore more difficult to read.

The length of the first passage was 280 characters and the length of the second 188 characters. The subjects were 125 4th graders (69 boys and 56 girls) aged between 9 years 3 months and 10 years 2 months. All were typical pupils at a typical Hiroshima school, with the exception of two who were said by the teachers to be mentally handicapped. The results for these two children have not been included in our data.

Testing was carried out on an individual basis in a school classroom. Both in this test and in the Bangor Dyslexia Test (see below) the tester manually recorded each of the child's responses, while at the same time the responses were tape-recorded for later analysis.

The results of the two reading tests are set out in Table 30.1 in terms of time needed for reading 100 characters of the ordinary text and 100 characters of the katakana text.

Table 30.1 Mean time in seconds per 100 characters in the two passages. Standard deviations are given in brackets

Ordinary text:	27.6	(± 10.0)
Katakana text:	49.9	(± 18.7)

To pick out possible dyslexics it was therefore necessary to look for scores that 'stood out' as being massively different from the mean. For this purpose two standard deviations seemed a reasonable cut-off point. We in fact found eight children who satisfied this criterion on at least one of the two texts. Five of them satisfied it on both and even the three that did not do so fell very little short, as can be seen from Table 30.2.

Table 30.2 Time needed in seconds for the eight slowest readers to read 100 characters from the ordinary passage and 100 characters from the katakana passage

Subject no.	Sex	Ordinary text	Katakana text
1	B	48	93
2	B	68	95
3	G	57	79
4	G	48	103
5	B	57	96
6	B	40	95
7	G	43	96
8	G	60	123

In column 2 'B' = boy, 'G' = girl.

The overall distribution of scores was a normal curve with a 'hump' at the lower end (see Figure 30.1 for the distribution in the case of the katakana test).

Those whom we picked out had shown themselves over two separate tests to be slow at decoding; this slowness is agreed to be an important characteristic of dyslexia (compare Chapter 24). In addition,

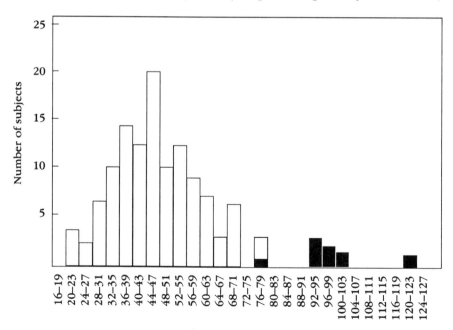

Figure 30.1 Seconds per 100 characters. Scores of probable dyslexics are shown in dark type

observations during testing suggested that these children were more prone than the others to mid-word pauses, to incorrect intonations and to transpositional errors.

An untimed test of reading, in whatever language it is given, may of course pick out a number of 'false negatives' – that is, children who are in fact dyslexic (in the sense of showing other signs of dyslexia) but have learned to become adequate readers. In the present conditions, however, we were testing whether the child could read *at speed*; it is arguable that a person who can not only read adequately but can do so at speed cannot be disadvantaged to any significant extent by dyslexic problems. Our procedure did not wholly rule out the risk of false negatives – those whose slow reading was primarily the consequence of environmental factors, such as social deprivation or absence from school, rather than of constitutional ones. In the schools where we carried out the investigation, however, it appears unlikely that such factors were operating on any significant scale (Note 30.3). It therefore seems justifiable to regard these eight children as dyslexic and to use the remaining 117 as controls.

The fact that there was not a higher proportion of boys is perhaps surprising in view of what has been reported elsewhere (Note 30.4). However, the figure of eight children in a sample of 125 is in line with many of the estimates in western countries (Note 30.5).

The answer to our first question must therefore be in the affirmative. There are dyslexic children in Japan who on tests which require rapid decoding do not simply constitute the extreme tail of a normal distribution.

Our second question was whether the modified version of the Bangor Dyslexia Test can be used to identify them. This would be the case only if the eight dyslexics scored more 'pluses' overall than the other children in the study.

Various modifications were made to the Bangor Dyslexia Test, the intention being to catch the spirit of the original rather than include exactly the same items. A complete version will be found in Appendix VI (Note 30.6). For purposes of the present research, however, it could not be given in full because the school could allow us only limited time. We therefore restricted ourselves to five items (Note 30.7).

Item 1 was a shortened version of the Left–Right test, with no follow-up questions. One point was awarded for each correct answer, with 10 points therefore as the maximum. If 7 or more answers were given correctly the result was scored as 'minus'; if there were 4, 5, or 6 correct answers it was scored as zero, and if there were 3 or fewer correct answers it was scored as 'plus'.

Item 2 involved reciting the 7x and 8x tables. The main innovation here was that the performance was timed. If the mean score for the two recitations was under 40 s the result was scored as 'minus'; if it lay between 40 and 59 s the result was scored as 'zero', while if it was 60 s or more the result was scored as 'plus'.

In item 3 the child was asked to count backwards in threes from 96 and, in a second task, in threes from 88. If the mean score for the two trials was less than 40 s the result was scored as 'minus'; if it lay between 40 and 59 s the result was scored as 'zero', while if it was 60 s or more the result was scored as 'plus'.

In item 4 the child was asked to say five sounds from the syllabary backwards, namely 'ta', 'chi', 'tsu', 'te' and 'to'. The syllabary comprises eight other sounds as well. All schoolchildren are used to this string of syllables because they have overlearned them while learning the corresponding hiragana and katakana. If the task was completed in under 15 s the result was scored as 'minus'; times of 15 to 19 s were scored as 'zero', and times of 20 s or more were scored as 'plus'.

Item 5 was Digits Reversed. The digits were spoken by the tester at the rate of approximately 1 per second. The digits used were 284, 6529, 1827 and 3419. For each set two points were awarded if it was correctly repeated without hesitation; one point was awarded if it was correctly repeated but with hesitation, and no points were awarded if there was any error. The maximum possible score was therefore 8 points. A score of 4 or more was counted as 'minus', a score of 3 as 'zero', and a score of 2 or less as 'plus'.

In accordance with the usual policy in this book 'zeros' have been scored as equivalent to half a 'plus'. Table 30.3 shows the performance of the dyslexics on the five items.

Table 30.3 Performance on five items						
Case no.	L–R	Tab.	Counting backwards	Syllabary backwards	Digits Reversed	Total
1	0	–	+	–	0	2.0
2	–	+	+	–	+	3.0
3	+	+	+	–	0	3.5
4	–	–	–	+	+	2.0
5	–	+	+	+	+	4.0
6	+	–	+	+	+	4.0
7	–	–	+	+	0	2.5
8	+	–	+	+	+	4.0

Table 30.4 compares the number of 'pluses' obtained by these eight dyslexics in comparison with the 117 controls.

Table 30.4 Distribution of 'pluses' out of a possible five among dyslexics ($n = 8$) and controls ($n = 117$)

No. of 'pluses'	Dyslexics	Controls
0.0	–	10
0.5	–	12
1.0	–	23
1.5	–	18
2.0	2	17
2.5	1	20
3.0	1	8
3.5	1	1
4.0	3	5
4.5	–	2
5.0	–	1

The difference between the two groups was found to be highly significant (Note 30.8). The trend is therefore established, even though there are exceptions in individual cases. The most marked of these are the two dyslexics with only 2 'pluses' and the nine controls with over 3.5 'pluses'. These nine controls are, of course, only 8% of the total.

When we came to examine individual items, we found that they varied considerably in their predictive power. Table 30.5 shows the percentages in each group who scored 'plus' on a given item. (As usual, 'zeros' have been assigned half to 'plus' and half to 'minus'.)

Table 30.5 Percentages of dyslexics ($n = 8$) and of controls ($n = 117$) who scored 'plus' on the five items

	L–R	Tab	Counting backwards	Syllabary backwards	Digits Reversed
Dyslexics	44	38	88	63	81
Controls	32	33	47	36	33

It is plain from inspection that the Left–Right and Tables items are less efficient predictors than the other three. In the case of the Left–Right item it should be noted that the procedure was different from that used in the English version of the test: the results were scored on 'number of correct responses', no account being taken of hesitations, echoing the question, or requests for it to be repeated. In the case of the Tables item it is possible that the thoroughness with which Japanese children are taught their tables may account for the relatively small percentage of 'pluses' among the dyslexics compared with that found for dyslexics in Britain; but even if this is the case it would not account for the very minimal percentage difference between dyslexics and controls. The other three items appear to be good discriminators.

It can therefore be claimed both that dyslexia exists in Japan and that the Japanese adaptation of the Bangor Dyslexia Test discriminated the dyslexics from the non-dyslexics in three items out of five.

Chapter 31
Forty-eight Dyslexic Adults

The first edition of this book (1983) gives details of only five subjects aged 20 and over. Since 1978, however, I have carried out assessments on about 70 dyslexic adults. In a few cases the data were too incomplete to use, and there were also about a dozen cases who could more properly be placed in Group III (see Chapter 4) – those of limited intellectual ability and a few others who, despite having problems of some kind, did not present the typical dyslexic picture. The remaining 48 provide the subject matter of the present chapter.

I did not treat absence of a figure for intelligence, reading or spelling as a necessary condition for exclusion provided the person was doing a skilled job and had a history of late reading or other literacy difficulties (Note 31.1). If figures for intelligence were available inclusion was conditional on satisfying one or more of the following criteria: (1) at least one pass at the first grade of Superior Adult on the Terman–Merrill test (Note 2.7), (2) a score of at least 15 on the Advanced Progressive Matrices (Note 2.13), or (3) the holding down of a skilled job.

The notation in Table 31.1 is the same as that used in the Summary Chart in Chapter 6, where the symbols 'L–R', 'Pol.' etc. are explained. Data on handedness and eyedness are not included, since the evidence reported in Chapter 21 suggests that they are not relevant. The other main difference is in the 'int' (intelligence) column. Here an Arabic numeral represents a score on the Advanced Progressive Matrices, while a capital Roman numeral indicates the highest grade of Superior Adult on the Terman–Merrill test at which the subject obtained a pass (Note 31.2). The symbol 'u' has been added if the subject was attending university or had obtained a degree (Note 31.3).

It was difficult to obtain good evidence on whether the subject confused 'b' and 'd' or whether others in his family were affected. With the younger subjects I had relied largely on information supplied by the parents, whereas few in this age group were accompanied by their parents and on both matters many of them seemed very unsure. In the

227

absence of positive evidence, I recorded the b–d item as 'minus' and the 'famil' item as 'nk' (not known); it is possible that the figures under 'b–d' and 'Fam' in Table 31.1 are an underestimate (Note 31.4).

Now it is plain from Table 31.1 that many dyslexics, including university students, continue in adulthood to show 'pluses' on some items of the Bangor Dyslexia Test.

The difficulties and compensatory strategies for dealing with 'left' and 'right' were entirely similar to those reported in Chapter 10, except that, as one might expect among adults, there were many more references to car driving. For example S272 said, 'I still have to stop and think if someone says "Turn left" when I am driving'; S280 said, 'For my driving test I had "left" and "right" on my thumbs', while S290 said that she put a piece of Elastoplast on her finger. S305 described how her driving instructor 'went crazy' because she could not carry out the instructions 'right hand down' and 'left hand down'.

It should be noted that 'months of the year' is not all that effective a test for picking out dyslexic adults. By far the majority of the dyslexics came out as negative on both the Months Forwards and Months Reversed items. In the case of the subjects, aged 18 and under, whom I have assessed since 1978 the figures for Months Forwards were 78% 'pluses' at age 10, 58% 'pluses' at age 11, and 33% 'pluses' at age 12; in the case of Months Reversed the figures were 91%, 76%, and 60% (Note 31.5). This particular series of names is therefore something which many dyslexics do eventually learn, though it seems that they require many more 'exposures' to it than do non-dyslexics.

The male: female ratio is 44:14, which is 2.4:1. It is therefore less than that given for cases 1 to 257 (see Chapter 20) where it was 4.25, but I can think of no convincing reason why this should be so.

It is also worth commenting on some of the scores for intelligence, word recognition and spelling.

One of the striking things about the 'intelligence' column is the number of very high scores on the Advanced Raven Matrices. Three were of 30 or over and seven were between 25 and 29. Raven's norms for university students give a mean of 21 and a standard deviation of 4. A score of 25, therefore, puts the person in the top 16%, while a score of 29 represents the top 2.5% – not of the general population but of a *university* population. The Advanced Matrices test is unlike traditional examinations (other than those involving multiple choice) in that almost nothing is needed by way of decoding: to communicate one's response one has to retrieve the appropriate numeral from a choice of eight and write it in the correct place. No other kind of 'word finding' is called for, as it is in essay writing, and there need be no search for the most appropriate form of words. Also the patterns presented on the page are there, so to speak, in their own right; they do not 'stand for' something else, the phonological representation of which has to be

Table 31.1 Details of 48 dyslexic adults

Case no.	Sex	Age	Int.	R_1	S_1	DF	DR	LR	Pol	Sub	Tab	MF	MR	b–d	Fam	Total
265 u	M	19	18	87	61	+	+	+	−	+	+	0	−	−	+	6.5
266 u	M	19	27	98	88	−	+	+	0	0	0	0	−	−	0	4.5
267	M	19	29	100	90	+	+	−	−	+	+	−	−	−	nk	4.0
268	M	19	III	93	70	−	+	+	−	+	+	+	+	0	nk	6.5
269	M	19	I	25	17	+	+	−	0	+	+	−	−	−	nk	4.5
270	M	19	II	90	65	+	+	+	+	+	+	−	+	+	0	8.5
271	M	19	17	*	*	+	+	+	−	−	−	−	−	−	nk	3.0
272 u	M	19	III	95	77	+	+	+	−	−	+	−	0	−	nk	4.5
273	M	19	III	79	51	+	+	+	+	+	+	0	−	+	nk	7.5
274	F	20	III	31	21	+	+	+	+	+	+	−	+	0	0	8.0
275	M	20	III	34	17	+	+	0	0	+	+	+	+	0	nk	7.5
276	M	20	23	98	92	+	+	+	−	0	+	−	−	−	nk	4.5
277	M	20	19	96	56	+	+	+	−	+	+	−	+	−	nk	6.0
278 u	M	21	15	93	90	+	+	+	−	+	+	−	−	−	nk	5.0
279 u	M	21	31	92	91	+	+	+	−	0	0	−	+	−	nk	5.0
280	F	21	25	98	94	+	+	+	−	−	0	−	−	+	nk	4.5
281	F	21	22	*	*	−	−	+	0	0	+	−	−	+	+	5.0
282 u	F	22	25	86	86	+	+	+	0	−	+	0	−	−	nk	5.0
283 u	M	22	III	100	88	+	+	0	−	+	+	−	−	+	0	6.0
284	F	22	II	33	22	+	+	+	+	+	+	−	+	−	nk	7.0
285 u	F	22	20	91	74	+	+	+	−	−	0	−	−	+	+	5.5
286 u	M	23	26	94	74	+	+	+	0	−	+	+	−	−	nk	5.5
287 u	F	23	23	*	*	+	+	+	+	+	+	−	+	−	+	8.0
288	M	24	III	69	43	+	+	+	+	−	−	−	−	+	nk	5.0
289 u	M	24	*	*	*	+	+	+	+	−	−	0	−	−	0	5.0
290 u	F	24	31	*	*	+	−	0	+	−	+	−	−	+	+	5.5
291	M	24	WAIS	95	63	+	+	+	0	0	+	−	−	0	nk	5.5
292	F	25	III	90	77	+	+	+	0	−	−	−	−	−	nk	3.5
293 u	M	25	23	95	79	+	+	+	0	−	−	−	−	+	+	4.5
294	F	26	15	86	69	+	+	+	0	+	+	−	+	−	+	7.5
295	M	27	22	83	66	+	+	+	0	−	+	−	0	−	nk	5.0
296	M	28	*	33	13	+	+	+	+	0	+	+	+	−	nk	7.5
297	F	28	15	89	86	+	+	+	−	+	0	−	−	−	nk	4.5
298	M	29	III	61	40	+	+	+	0	−	0	−	−	−	0	4.5
299	M	30	II	71	39	+	+	+	+	−	+	−	−	−	nk	5.0
300	M	30	I	50	14	+	+	+	+	+	+	−	+	−	nk	7.0
301	F	33	II	29	16	+	+	+	+	+	+	−	−	+	nk	7.0
302	M	36	III	91	52	+	+	+	−	0	+	0	+	−	0	6.5
303 u	M	36	30	*	*	+	+	+	−	0	0	−	−	−	+	5.0
304	M	36	24	81	37	+	+	+	+	0	+	−	−	+	+	7.5
305 u	F	38	26	83	60	+	−	+	+	−	+	−	−	+	+	6.0
306	M	38	*	44	11	+	+	+	om	−	+	−	+	−	+	7.0
307 u	F	39	27	92	77	+	+	+	+	+	+	−	−	+	+	8.0
308	M	39	21	97	70	−	−	+	0	−	−	+	0	−	+	3.5
309 u	M	41	*	*	*	−	+	0	−	+	+	−	−	−	nk	3.5
310	M	42	I	81	63	+	+	+	+	−	+	−	+	−	nk	6.0
311	M	47	SPM	80	48	+	+	+	+	+	−	−	+	−	nk	6.0
312	M	59	II	96	*	+	+	−	−	+	−	−	+	−	+	5.0

retrieved. What is being tapped is skill at reasoning – the ability to recognise relationships – and not skill at finding the right words for communicating one's ideas to others. It has sometimes been suggested that dyslexics function more effectively when dealing with three dimensions than when dealing with two. I suspect, however, that it is not the number of dimensions as such that is relevant, but rather the fact that many of the things that we have to deal with in two dimensions are symbolic. Where a two-dimensional situation does not require the translation of symbols into their phonological representations, it would seem that dyslexics are at no disadvantage. Matrices tests are a good illustration of this point.

Many of the subjects obtained high scores on the Schonell R_1 word recognition test. This result underlines, yet again, how misleading it is to equate 'dyslexia' with 'reading difficulty'. If a person is able to recognise single words correctly in untimed conditions this does not exclude the possibility that other indicators of dyslexia are present (Note 31.6).

With regard to spelling I again thought it would be interesting to collect some control data. Politicians and others fulminate these days about how the standard of spelling is very low, and it occurred to me that it would be worthwhile to check if dyslexic students are any worse at spelling than other students. I therefore gave the last 30 words of the Schonell S_1 test to 42 second-year undergraduates who were reading for an honours degree in psychology. Table 31.2 gives a frequency distribution of scores. (The symbol 'f' indicates frequency.)

Table 31.2 Frequency distribution of spelling scores of 42 undergraduates, out of a maximum of 30

Score	f	Score	f
30	3	23	3
29	3	22	1
28	6	21	3
27	5	20	1
26	4	19	–
25	5	18	–
24	7	17	1

If it is assumed that these subjects could all have spelled the first 70 words in the test correctly the scores range from 87 to 100. In contrast 39 out of the 48 dyslexic subjects had scores of less than 85. It seems, therefore, that although some dyslexics learn to spell not too badly, the general trend is for them to be weaker than those who are poor spellers through lack of training. Typical mistakes on the part of the non-dyslexics were 'irresistable' for 'irresistible' and the wrong number of 'b's or 'g's in 'toboggan'. There was no faulty ordering of syllables and no evidence of lack of awareness of letter–sound relationships.

At this point I think it may be interesting to include a letter written to me by S302. Despite the immaturity of the handwriting this subject solved the really difficult 'tree' item at the top grade of Superior Adult on the Terman–Merrill test.

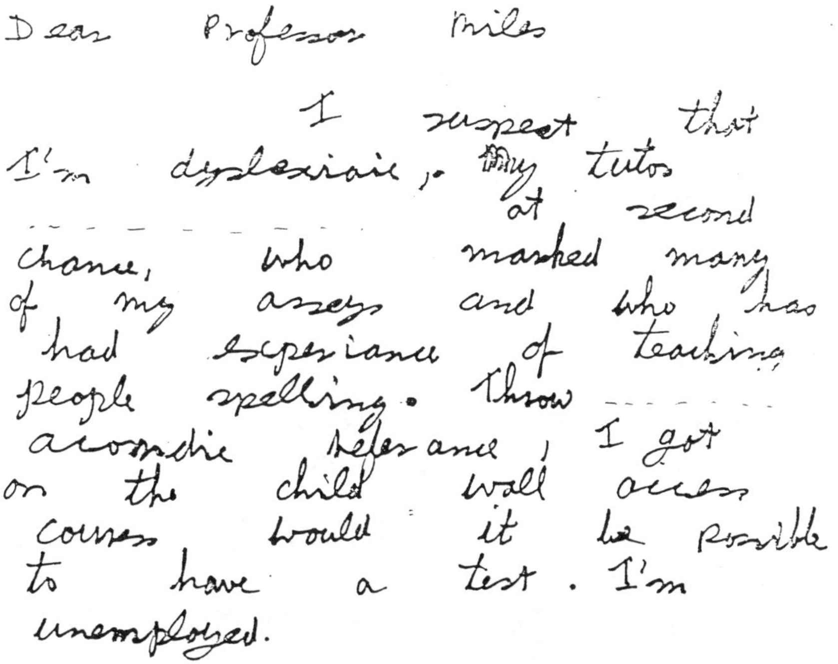
Dear Professor Miles
I suspect that I'm dyslexiaic, my tutor at second chance, who marked many of my asseys and who has had escperiance of teaching people spelling. Throw acomdic referance, I got on the child wall acess courses would it be possible to have a test. I'm unemployed.

Figure 31.1 Sample of writing by a highly intelligent dyslexic adult

Finally, the dyslexic adult is often extremely articulate. One can therefore learn a great deal from what they *say* about their dyslexia and their reactions to it. I regularly made a point of recording points of interest during assessments; I would like to end this chapter by quoting some of the things which my subjects mentioned during the course of the assessment. I do so under three heads: (1) accounts of the difficulties, (2) adverse social consequences of dyslexia, and (3) effects of diagnosis.

Accounts of the Difficulties

S265: 'I can get the ideas in my head but on a bad day they come out as gibberish.'
'I might write g-o-i-n-d- for "doing".'
'If a word has two syllables I put the first in before the second' (meaning 'I put the second in before the first').
'If I think hard the writing goes.'
'I learn chemical bonds by picturing.'

S266: 'Small words get me.' (He had spelled 'which' as 'wich', 'wicth' and 'wihitch'.)

S267: 'If I have to convert it into written speech or writing there is a break in the link...In trying to keep up the speed I can't keep up with the words.'

His father, in a letter to me, quoted his son as explaining his problem in communication as follows:

> When I think about something, words and thoughts come easily but concentrating on the actual mechanics of putting it down on paper means that I forget the subject involved. I find speech a two-way process whereby I think of a word and then try to speak that word or phrase. I find it difficult to think, speak and write that thought down.

S274: 'When I see, say, Mrs Smith's face in the shop I can write "Smith". If she rings on the 'phone and says "Smith" I can't write it unless I recognise the voice and put it to the face.'

S278: 'You can picture things in biological science whereas numbers are too abstract.'

S279: 'They [his tutors] didn't understand what I was getting at. It seemed obvious to me.'

S285: 'With a word processor you haven't got to concentrate on holding the pen correctly.'

S286: 'I couldn't do morse unless there was more time'.
'Someone would send me for a spanner on the starboard side and I would walk to port.'

S289, a history graduate, was taking a Master's degree in palaeography. The part of the course which he found particularly difficult was deciphering ancient text.

S290: 'I would say "stimulated" for "simulated".'
'Sometimes a newspaper looks like gobbledegook. I got the prospectus for Bangor and opened the Welsh side. I thought, 'God! this is difficult today – I can't make head or tail of it.'

S291: 'I find myself mentally two paragraphs in front of what I'm writing.'

S292 had been confused between 'density' and 'destiny'. She could not make out what was meant by the destiny of wines (Note 31.7).

S297: 'When you tell me "Tuesday" I have to think "Monday, Tuesday, Wednesday...I have to repeat the alphabet when I look up words in a dictionary.'

S303 (a musician) wrote to me after the assessment: 'I have found that storing images of the printed page won't work for me...Symbols are not simply lifted off the paper and acted upon; they must be read, sorted out, re-worked in the mind. In themselves they are useless' (Note 31.8).

S305: 'Every word that I write that is more than four letters – and even four letters if I haven't read them frequently – I have to say them letter by letter in my mind. It is fatal to interrupt me at home as I have to think of two things at once. If I write XYZ (the first three letters of her surname) and I am interrupted I have to start again.'

S309: 'I don't like symbols' (he cited '=', '<', and '>'), and I don't like chemical formulae.'

S310 (during the first item of the Bangor Dyslexia Test): 'Your rear and my left hand' (substitution of 'rear' for 'right').

Adverse Social Consequences of Dyslexia

These are well known (Note 31.9), but it may be helpful to include a few examples.

S270: 'I can't play poker; you've got to work it out' [that is, the numbers]. 'I can't play darts as I couldn't add up'...(In a letter) 'At the moument I find slight difficulty with my numbers, which is more critical as numbers of cows, for work which is most irratating. Do you have any suggestions. It is mostly seing a number then writing somthing diffirent'.

S280: 'When I give directions it's hopeless.'

S309 (who had been in the navy): 'The captain said to me, "What's the opposite to *north*?" and I couldn't do it.' (He in fact identified the points of the compass correctly in the Terman–Merrill 'direction' items but thought it likely that he would go wrong under stress.)

S310: 'Someone got me to sign papers...I filled in three forms with long chassis numbers (20 figures) – these had come in the wrong position...In a bank it is difficult to sign my name when the shop assistant is there...I have difficulty in reading long and lengthy legal documents...You pretend you have read it so as not to hold up a meeting.'

S311: 'I have no idea of time and have difficulty in reporting "days worked".'

Effects of Diagnosis

The information in this section supplements that given in Chapter 23. A common picture is of individuals who are seriously demoralised but whose life is transformed – to a greater or lesser extent – when the nature of their dyslexia is explained to them.

S273: 'That afternoon managed to boost and encorige a great deel more than anything eles has ever done...Thank you for exspressing an intrest in me and for all the help and sourport I have found as a rescult of my day in Bangor.'

A friend of S275 who had attended a course on dyslexia at Bangor wrote: 'The day he saw you gave him a real boost and psychologically, emotionally – whatever you want to call it – he has never really looked back since then. He started a small motorbike business...all he needed was that little boost to his confidence'.

The mother of S280 wrote: 'She has gained in confidence amd has more commitment since her visit to you.'

S281: 'I don't know how to tell you how grateful I am. You see I have always believed I was very slow and rather stupid.'

S283: 'I would like to say thank you for your very wise words...You really have helped me to understand the situation that I have been through.'

S287: 'It was amazing to know that something is wrong and I'm not a complete duffer. I'm sure that is a familure story.'

S292: 'I was very glad and relived after I met you to know at last what the problem was...so that I can help others especily children to get help and be reconised.'

S299: 'I came to see you about 2 years ago...I am fit and well and getting on with my life a lot better from when I saw you, after the results of the tests and finding out that I was not thick or stupied it give me a new lease of life, I can only dicrabe it as chains being cut from my body.'

S301: 'I went to adult literacy class. A gentleman spotted I was dyslexic. Before that I thought I was a fool.'

S303: 'I know that I will look back on the day as a reference point in my experiences. You have started my mind on several new paths at once and this is most exciting for me...I feel a new freedom.'

S305: 'Most of my journey down I was preoccupied with the fact that you may well have assessed me as well below average – I stood outside your door for several minutes trying to pluck up the courage to knock. I still have not fully come to terms with the findings of the assessment...For the best part of my life I have lived with what all I can explain as being a divided self image – one part of me believing myself to be quite stupid, and on the other hand I had what can only be explained as an unquenchable thirst for knowledge and the dream and hope of one day being able to help children and adults in less priviledged positions.' ... 'It is a fact that not one single poem would have come about if it had not been for the dyslexia assessment; for years words of poems were trapped in my head.'

Chapter 32
Conclusions

My main aim in writing this book has been to place on record some of the many interesting things which dyslexics have said and done, particularly during assessments. This has always seemed to me to be an essential first step, without which one could not proceed to adequate quantification or theorising.

Quantification did not turn out to be too much of a problem. The specification of hesitations, pauses, echoing the question, requesting that it should be repeated etc. as possible indicators of a 'plus' (or 'dyslexia-positive') response on the Bangor Dyslexia Test allowed clinical impressions to be recorded in a systematic way; thereafter it was not difficult to check whether such responses were as frequent in non-dyslexics as in dyslexics.

The fascination of the research, however, did not lie in efficiently answering questions whose importance was undisputed, but rather in trying to find out what questions were most worth asking. It would have been 'efficient' if I had spent time on obtaining further norms for the Bangor Dyslexia Test or if I had been able to ensure that the same test of intelligence was given to all subjects of a given age. As with any research project, however, there was a limit on the time that could be made available; I was unwilling to give such routine work a high degree of priority. Research projects such as those described in Chapters 26–30 seemed more exciting. Moreover, in writing personally rather than in the style of a scientific journal I have tried to share with the reader the story of how things actually were, not as they might have been if I had taken more care to be 'efficient'.

When the first edition of this book went to press there was no comprehensive theory which made sense of the variety of manifestations which I had described. Things are now very different. The most likely causal chain, as I indicated in Chapter 24, seems to me to be this: for genetic or other reasons certain individuals have a weakness in the magnocellular pathways of the visual and auditory systems, with the result that it is difficult for them adequately to synthesise sequences of sounds – including speech sounds – if they are presented at too fast a rate. This in its turn leads to what has been called a weakness at the 'phonological' level: dyslexics have more difficulty than non-dyslexics in associating things and events in the environment with their spoken equivalents. The consequence is the whole range of weaknesses which have been described in this book.

I envisage that a number of changes will be needed in the Bangor Dyslexia Test in the future. Now that technology makes this possible it would be helpful if responses to the Left–Right item could be timed and, as was indicated in Chapter 29, there is a case for substituting nonsense words based on phonological considerations in place of the existing polysyllables. When more is known about speed of calculation in dyslexics – a topic currently being investigated by Sula Ellis (Note 27.1) – the present Subtraction and Tables items may need to be changed, with items substituted which best differentiate dyslexics from non-dyslexics in terms of time needed to respond. The Months Forwards and Months Reversed items are suitable up to about age 12 but after this age they are less effective as discriminators, and this needs to be made clear in future versions of the test. Digits Forwards and Digits Reversed should be retained but scored differently, and information on b–d confusion and on familial incidence should continue to be sought. Reading of nonsense words should be introduced and all reading tests should be timed.

Re-thinking is also needed on the *purposes* of a dyslexia assessment. In particular we need to bear in mind the anatomical evidence (see Chapter 24) which suggests that the balance of skills may often be unusual in dyslexics. Although much research has been carried out into their weaknesses, there has been virtually none into the question of whether they have distinctive strengths (Note 32.1). Traditionally it appears to have been assumed that all one needed to do was to satisfy oneself that the person had 'adequate intelligence' as judged by his IQ figure and then check if his scores on tests of reading and spelling were 'discrepant'. In the early part of this book I paid some degree of lip service to the concept of IQ by using the term and then qualifying it by drawing a distinction between a 'composite IQ' (based on a composite of all items in a given test battery) and a 'selected IQ' based on selected items only. In recent assessments, however, I have abandoned all reference to IQ. I believe, on reflection, that the term has all kinds of misleading associations, and while I have no regrets at having departed at times from the standardised instructions when I have conducted the WISC and Terman–Merrill tests, I now regard the concept of a 'selected IQ' as a not very satisfactory compromise. Looking back, it seems to me that in checking for a discrepancy between IQ and reading or spelling score I was doing mostly the right thing – but for the wrong reason! (Note 31.2).

The key concept is not IQ but discrepancy. What one needs to discover from an assessment is whether the person has the imbalance of skills which is typical of the dyslexic. It is perhaps more helpful in place of 'IQ' to substitute the expression 'reasoning power' (since this does not imply any kind of permanent and fixed possession) and to ask if the subject's reasoning power is at variance with some of his other abilities, in particular his abilities at tasks which call for rapid verbal labelling. Most items in intelligence tests require verbal labelling of some kind, if only minimally, since at the very least the subject has to understand the question or the instructions and produce a response. If the labels are sufficiently familiar, however, and the conditions are untimed the evidence suggests that dyslexics are at no disadvantage. Thus if their oral vocabulary is adequate (as it normally is) their reasoning power may enable them to respond adequately to a Similarities item ('How are — and — alike?'); they may be successful in grasping what is required in a social situation, such as those which figure in the Comprehension sub-test of the WISC and, as was noted in Chapter 31, they may often be highly successful at matrices items. If, however, verbal labelling plays an important part in the test itself, as it does in reading and spelling tests, in the items of the Bangor Dyslexia Test, and in the Coding sub-test of the WISC, one would expect their difficulties to become apparent.

It is not surprising, therefore, that those researchers who have selected for study children whose reading or spelling scores are discrepant with their IQs have in fact succeeded in picking up quite a large number of dyslexics. A traditional intelligence test does indeed in large measure tap reasoning power, while tests of reading and spelling, particularly the latter, call for ability at verbal labelling. One is introducing less 'noise' into the situation, however, if one selects those items from traditional intelligence tests where the dyslexic has sufficient verbal labelling skills for the purpose in hand; this makes sure that his reasoning skills are not underestimated.

A further advantage of this approach is that it gives us a way of dealing with the persistently asked question, Can a child with a low IQ be dyslexic? On traditional assumptions there is no way of giving a satisfactory answer. The typical dyslexic is commonly supposed to be within the average range of IQ or higher; on the other hand it seems arbitrary and dogmatic to suppose that those with low IQs are somehow 'different' and therefore cannot ever be called 'dyslexic'. Once, however, we think in terms of an unusual balance of skills, the problem is solved. If reasoning ability is severely limited there cannot from the nature of the case be any imbalance.

More research is needed on comparative studies of dyslexia, particularly in countries which do not use the standard western writing systems. From the evidence presented in Chapters 28, 29 and 30 there is reason to think that suitably adapted versions of the Bangor Dyslexia Test can be used to detect difficulties in verbal labelling and that it is a 'robust' test in that it has been found useful in different parts of the world.

Finally, I have not limited myself in this book to the so-called 'cognitive' aspects of dyslexia – that is, to the study of dyslexics' strengths and weaknesses at learning and remembering. Individuals respond to their dyslexia in a variety of ways. One of the most common responses is loss of self-esteem – usually as a result of pressures imposed by an educational system that is ill-adapted to their needs. The Bangor Dyslexia Test can be used as a 'way in' to people – as a way of helping them to verbalise their feelings. For instance item 1 (concerned with 'left' and 'right') includes the question, 'Did you have difficulty when you were younger?' There is no reason why at this point, if it seems appropriate, a tester should not ask, 'Did they tease you about it?' or 'Did it make you feel a complete fool?'. It was a necessary part of the research that I should aim at studying 'real people' (Note 32.3); this meant not simply checking up on their cognitive skills or lack of them but on the question of how they verbalised to themselves about the situation – what they thought and felt. As is shown by the evidence cited in Chapters 23 and 31, if dyslexics are given an accurate account of both their strengths and their weaknesses this can lead to striking improvements in their self-confidence and self-esteem. For full understanding of dyslexia it seems to me important that such matters should not be overlooked.

Appendix I
The Dyslexia Test

During the period of the research minor amendments were made to the layout of the test-sheet. The wording remained the same, however, except for minimal changes. Where the instructions to the tester are not obvious they are given in brackets. When the test came to be marketed separately a few further changes were made, and the memory for sentences, handedness, eyedness and rhyming tests were omitted. The version that follows is the one used during the 1972–1978 research period and which supplied the information for the Summary Chart in Chapter 6.

Copies of *The Bangor Dyslexia Test* – as it is now called – are available from LDA, Duke Street, Wisbech, Cambs PE13 2AE, England. Thirty test sheets are supplied, along with a users' manual.

TEST ITEMS

Important

It is very important that someone who later reads this form should have a record of exactly what happened. Use of a tick is in order if the subject gives the correct response instantaneously, but please record all delays and hesitations and always indicate if the subject asks for the question to be repeated, echoes the question, or tries to reorientate himself by repeating what went before. (Use the abbreviations RR = request for repetition, EQ = echoed the question, and EP = epanalepsis, taking up what he has already said.) Please do *not* put a cross if the answer is wrong, but record as accurately as possible *what the subject said*. Where appropriate, record any supplementary questions which you yourself ask.

Name   Date

1. Left–Right (body parts)

Instruction	Subject's response
(a) Show me your right hand	
(Did you have difficulty when you were younger?)	
(b) Show me your left ear	
(c) Touch your right ear with your left hand	
(d) (Putting hands on table) Which is my right hand?	
(e) Touch my left hand with your right hand	
(f) Point to my right ear with your left hand	
(g) Touch my right hand with your right hand	
(h) Point to my left eye with your right hand	
(i) Point to my left ear with your left hand	
(j) Touch my right hand with your left hand	

Special strategies:

_____

_____

_____

2. Repeating polysyllabic words

I am going to say some words and I want you to say them after me:

preliminary

philosophical

contemporaneous

anemone

statistical

3. Subtraction

What is: 9 take away 2   _____

                 6 take away 3   _____

                 19 take away 7   _____

                 24 take away 2   _____

                 52 take away 9   _____

                 44 take away 7   _____

4. Tables

Did they teach you tables at school?   _____

Did you have difficulty with them?   _____

Say your – times table   _____

(Give at least three tables. These should normally be the 6 ×, 7 × and 8 ×, but failures at the 2 ×, 3 × and 4 × can of course be informative. In the case of children aged 7 or 8, give the 4 × only.)

5. Months Forwards

Say the months of the year   _____

6. Months Reversed

Now say them backwards   _____

7. Hand

Show me the hand you write (draw) with   _____

Show me how you clean your teeth   _____

Show me how you throw a ball   _____

(Record which hand is used)   _____

8. Eye

(Cut a small hole in a sheet of paper and, holding up a pencil in three different positions, ask the subject if he can see the pencil through the hole. Record which eye is used.)

9. Repeating digits

(Give the Digit Span test as described in the Wechsler Intelligence Scale for Children.)

10. Memory for sentences

(Use three of the sentences from the Terman–Merrill test, one from age iv, one from age xi, and one from age xiii. In the event of a near-miss give six to eight trials. Responses should be recorded verbatim.)

11. Rhymes

(Give the Rhymes item from the Terman–Merrill test. If the subject has difficulty ask:)

(a) Give me any two words which rhyme   _____

                                               _____

(b) I shall give you two words and ask you if they rhyme. You must say 'Yes' or 'no'.

Cat	Dog	_____
Cat	Sat	_____
Mouse	Elephant	_____
Mouse	House	_____
Fish	Dish	_____
Butter	Gutter	_____
Butter	Jam	_____
Egg	Bacon	_____

12. Familial incidence

	(a) Definitely	(b) Possibly	(c) No difficulties	(d) No evidence
Father				
Mother				
Brothers				
Sisters				
Other relatives				

(In the case of (a) and (b) please give as much detail as possible.)

Summary

Name

Date

Age

Reading age

Spelling age

Intelligence rating   Z   Y   X   W   V   U

Indicators
(Score as +, 0 or −)

    Digits Forward

    Digits Reversed

    Left–Right (body-parts)

    Polysyllables

    Subtraction

    Tables

    Months Forwards

    Months Reversed

    b–d confusion

    Familial incidence

Samples of spelling

Appendix II
Scoring the Dyslexia Test

Notes

1. The following symbols should be used:

+ = subject fails the test or satisfies the other specified criteria. This indicates a 'dyslexia-positive' response.

– = subject succeeds in the test without showing any of the specified criteria for 'dyslexia-positive'; his performance is therefore 'dyslexia-negative'.

0 = subject satisfies some of the less stringent criteria but his response cannot be scored unambiguously as dyslexia-positive or dyslexia-negative.

(In the Digits test the 'zero' category is not used. In other tests two or more responses scored as 'zero' count as 'plus'.)

2. In some cases a score of 'zero' is obtained by any two of a particular kind of response, e.g. two corrections or two pauses. In these cases a single correction and a single pause can in conjunction be scored as 'zero'.

3. For purposes of summing the total performance a 'zero' may be scored as half a 'plus'. From the index-figure (the total number of 'pluses') no conclusions about dyslexia can be drawn if the subject is too young (under about 8) or of limited ability (in traditional terminology, with IQ under about 90). In the case of other subjects with a history of reading or spelling problems discrepant with their intelligence, the index-figure is a rough guide as to the strength of the presumption that other dyslexic signs will manifest themselves. The scores in this column should not be assumed to be on an equi-interval scale, nor is the number of 'pluses' necessarily an indication of the degree of severity of the dyslexia. Its precise significance must be determined according to context.

4. The following abbreviations may be used on the test form:

hes. = the subject hesitated

RR = the subject requested that the question be repeated

EQ = the subject echoed the question

EP = the subject 'cued' himself in by repeating what he had said before (epanalepsis)

Digit Span

The first number represents the series-length of the highest success, the second number the series-length of the lowest failure. Any 'double inversion', i.e. a score in which the first figure is two more than the second, is scored as 'plus' – for example 53 – unless a weaker performance involving only a single inversion, in this case 43, would count as 'minus'. (Note: the criteria given below are those used for the research reported in this book. When *The Bangor Dyslexia Test* was published separately some changes were made.)

(a) Digits Forwards

Age	Any failure to reach	Any failure at	Examples of plus	Examples of minus
7	5	4	43, 44	55
8	5	4	45, 54	56
9	5	4	64	
10	6	5	54, 55	66
11	6	5	56, 65	67
12	6	5	75	
13	6	5		
14	6	5		
15	7	6	65, 66	77
16	7	6	67, 76	78
17	7	6	86	
18 and over	7	6		

(b) Digits Reversed

Age	Any failure to reach	Any failure at	Examples of plus	Examples of minus
7	3	2	32	33
8	3	2	23	34
9	4	3	33	44
10	4	3	34	45
11	4	3	43	55
12	4	3	53	54
13	4	3		
14	5	4	44, 45	55
15	5	4	54, 64	56, 65
16	6	5		65
17	6	5	55	
18 and over	6	5		

In the case of those aged 14 and over a failure at 'five digits reversed' should be scored as 'plus' only in the case of those in intelligence categories Z, Y and X.

Left–Right

Score as +:
1. Two errors or more
2. Consistent mirror image of correct answer
3. Subject turns in his seat (real or imagined)

Score as 0:
1. Report of earlier difficulty over left and right and/or report of special strategy (watch, scar, 'the hand I write with' etc.).
2. Hesitations in working out the answer in at least two items ('hes.')
3. Any two examples of echoing the question or asking for it to be repeated (e.g. 'my left with your right, was it?') (RR or EQ)
4. One error
5. Two corrections

Polysyllables

All ages: 4 or 5 errors, score as +
In other cases score as follows:

No. of errors	Age											
	7	8	9	10	11	12	13	14	15	16	17	18 and over
3	0	0	0	+	+	+	+	+	+	+	+	+
2	–	–	–	0	0	0	0	0	+	+	+	+
1	–	–	–	–	–	–	–	–	0	0	0	0

Subtraction

Score as +:
1. 3 or more errors or failures
2. Any use of concrete aids such as fingers or marks on paper

Score as 0:
1. 2 errors or failures
2. Special strategy
3. Any two examples of echoing the question or asking for it to be repeated (EQ or RR)
4. 2 hesitations (hes.)
5. 2 corrections

(A single error, hesitation, or correction is scored as –.)

Tables

(Age 9 and over)

Score as +:
1. Any 4 or more errors over the three tables
2. Any loss of place (or uncertainty, as exemplified by questions such as 'Was it six sevens I was up to?')
3. Any request to leave out the preamble (i.e. to leave out 'one six is...' 'two sixes are...' etc.)
4. Any consistent error (e.g. $6 \times 3 = 20$, $7 \times 3 = 23$)
5. Any change into the 'wrong' table (e.g. in the case of the 6 x, 6×7 are 42, 6×8 are 48, 8×8 are 64)

Score as 0:
1. Any 2 or 3 errors over the three tables
2. Any attempt to reorientate by repeating the previous product (EP) (e.g. 'four sixes are twenty-four, five sixes are... mm... let me see, four sixes are twenty-four, five sixes are thirty')
3. Any 2 slips or corrections (e.g. 'Eight eighties, I mean eight eights')
4. Any one 'skip', e.g. from 6×8 to 8×8
5. Any report of earlier difficulty

(Age 7 or 8)

($4 \times$ table only)

Score as +:
1. Any 2 errors or more

Score as 0:
1. 1 error
2. 2 pauses
3. Any two attempts to reorientate by repeating an earlier product (e.g. 'Four fours are sixteen, five fours are... Let me see... four fours are sixteen, five fours are twenty')

Months Forwards

Score as +:
1. Any 2 or more omissions
2. Any 2 or more inversions (e.g. 'October, September' for 'September, October')
3. Any uncertainty where to start
4. Any query about the importance of order (e.g. 'Do I have to say them in order?')

Score as 0:
1. Any 2 corrections
2. Any 1 omission (e.g. Leaving out September)
3. Any 1 inversion
4. Any report of earlier difficulty or special tuition

Months Reversed

Score as +:
1. Any 2 or more omissions
2. Any 2 or more inversions
Score as 0:
1. Any 2 corrections
2. Any 1 omission
3. Any 1 inversion

Note that in both Months Forwards and Months Reversed a single cor-rected error is scored as minus.

b–d Confusion

First-hand evidence is scored as plus; second-hand evidence is scored as zero and absence of evidence is scored as minus. (Note that the plac-ing of letters in the wrong order, e.g. 'on' for 'no' or 'was' for 'saw' may be a different phenomenon and should not be uncritically assimilated to b–d confusion.)

If a 'plus' is to be given the tester must himself have evidence of b–d confusion, whether by examining the child's written work or in listen-ing to him read. If a parent or teacher *reports* that the child has or had difficulty, this is scored as zero.

Familial Incidence

First-hand evidence is scored as plus; second-hand evidence is scored as zero and absence of evidence is scored as minus. Note that absence of evidence does not *exclude* familial incidence: in case of adopted children, for instance, relevant evidence may not be available, and in place of 'minus' it is preferable to write 'nk' (= 'not known'). If a 'plus' is to be given the tester must have unambiguous evidence that at least one other member of the family is affected. For example, if he or a col-league has actually tested a brother, sister, cousin etc. and found him to be dyslexic, this would count as 'plus'. In contrast a report e.g. by a parent that he (the parent) has similar difficulties is scored as zero. (As a rough guide, 'I was very late at learning to spell and I still can't remember telephone numbers' scores zero, but a single 'oddity' in iso-lation, e.g. 'I am bad at remembering names' is scored as minus.)

Appendix III
Performance of Control Subjects

The notation is the same as that used in the Summary Chart in Chapter 6. Data are not available, however, in respect of Digits Forwards, b–d confusion or Familial incidence and the maximum possible number of 'pluses' is therefore 7. For details of the selection of dyslexic subjects for comparison purposes see Chapter 7.

Table III.1 Performance of control subjects

Case no.	Sex	Age	Int.	S_1	DR	L–R	Pol.	Sub.	Tab	MF	MR	Index
1	F	7;5	X	34	–	+	–	+	+	–	+	4
2	M	7;5	Z	47	–	+	–	+	+	–	–	3
3	M	7;10	X	33	–	–	–	+	+	+	+	4
4	F	7;11	Z	23	–	+	0	+	+	+	+	5.5
5	M	8;0	Z	59	–	–	–	–	–	–	–	0
6	M	8;1	U	25	–	+	–	+	+	+	+	5
7	M	8;2	W	54	–	+	–	–	–	–	–	1
8	M	8;2	W	38	–	0	–	0	–	+	+	3
9	F	8;4	X	39	–	0	–	–	+	–	0	2
10	M	8;4	X	22	–	+	–	+	+	+	+	5
11	F	8;4	X	40	–	0	–	+	+	–	–	2.5
12	M	8;5	Y	45	–	+	0	+	0	–	+	4
13	M	8;5	X	29	–	+	+	–	+	–	+	4
14	F	8;6	X	46	–	0	–	0	+	–	–	2
15	M	8;6	W	30	–	+	–	0	+	0	+	4
16	F	8;6	W	50	–	+	–	0	+	–	+	3.5
17	M	8;7	X	29	–	+	+	+	+	–	+	5
18	M	8;8	Y	22	–	0	0	0	+	+	+	4.5
19	M	8;10	X	45	–	+	0	–	–	–	+	2.5
20	M	8;11	U	50	–	+	–	–	–	0	0	2
21	M	8;11	X	42	–	+	0	+	0	+	+	5
22	M	9;1	V	51	+	–	–	+	+	+	+	5
23	F	9;1	V	41	+	+	–	0	+	–	–	3.5

Table III.1 (contd)

Case no.	Sex	Age	Int.	S_1	DR	L–R	Pol.	Sub.	Tab	MF	MR	Index
24	F	9;2	W	55	+	+	0	–	–	–	–	2.5
25	M	9;2	V	53	+	0	–	–	+	+	+	4.5
26	F	9;4	W	42	+	+	–	–	+	–	–	3
27	M	9;6	X	46	–	+	–	–	0	+	+	3.5
28	M	9;6	W	44	–	–	–	–	+	0	+	2.5
29	M	9;7	W	53	–	–	–	–	+	–	0	1.5
30	M	9;7	X	59	–	0	–	–	+	–	–	1.5
31	F	9;8	U	34	+	0	–	0	+	+	+	5
32	M	9;8	V	46	+	+	–	0	+	–	–	3.5
33	F	9;8	X	50	–	–	–	–	–	–	0	1.5
34	M	9;9	Y	73	–	0	–	–	+	0	+	2.5
35	F	9;10	W	48	+	+	0	+	+	0	–	5
36	M	9;11	W	56	–	–	–	–	+	0	–	1.5
37	M	9;11	X	47	–	+	–	–	–	–	0	1.5
38	F	9;11	Y	43	+	0	–	–	–	–	0	2
39	M	9;11	W	55	+	–	–	0	+	0	–	3
40	M	10;1	U	48	+	–	–	0	+	–	–	2.5
41	F	10;1	V	43	+	0	0	0	+	–	+	4.5
42	M	10;1	Y	46	–	0	+	–	–	0	0	2.5
43	F	10;2	U	59	+	+	–	+	+	–	+	5
44	M	10;2	W	63	+	–	0	–	–	–	–	1.5
45	M	10;4	Y	54	–	–	–	–	–	–	–	0
46	F	10;5	X	85	–	0	–	–	–	–	+	1.5
47	F	10;6	Z	81	–	0	–	–	–	–	–	0.5
48	F	10;6	W	49	+	–	–	–	–	–	–	1
49	F	10;7	X	66	–	–	–	–	–	–	–	0
50	M	10;7	W	42	+	–	0	0	–	–	–	2
51	M	10;8	X	55	–	0	–	–	+	–	+	2.5
52	F	10;8	X	67	+	+	0	0	+	–	+	5
53	M	10;8	W	40	–	0	+	–	–	+	+	3.5
54	F	10;8	X	65	+	+	–	–	+	–	–	3
55	F	10;8	W	53	–	–	+	–	+	–	0	2.5
56	M	10;9	X	85	–	+	–	–	+	–	–	2
57	M	10;9	X	67	–	–	+	–	+	0	–	2.5
58	M	10;9	X	41	+	0	–	+	–	–	0	3
59	F	10;9	V	62	+	+	–	–	–	–	–	2
60	F	10;9	W	53	–	–	–	–	0	–	–	0.5
61	M	10;9	Y	66	–	–	–	–	–	0	–	0.5
62	F	10;10	Y	81	–	0	–	–	–	–	–	0.5
63	F	10;11	X	69	+	0	–	+	–	–	–	2.5
64	F	10;11	W	70	–	–	–	–	–	–	–	0
65	F	10;11	X	57	+	+	–	0	–	–	–	2.5
66	F	11;0	V	80	–	–	–	–	–	–	–	0
67	M	11;0	W	63	+	–	0	–	–	0	+	3
68	M	11;1	X	72	+	+	–	+	+	–	–	4

Table III.1 (contd)

Case no.	Sex	Age	Int.	S_1	DR	L–R	Pol.	Sub.	Tab	MF	MR	Index
69	F	11;1	U	71	+	–	+	–	+	–	0	3.5
70	F	11;2	Y	69	–	–	–	–	0	–	–	0.5
71	F	11;2	W	65	–	+	–	0	+	–	–	2.5
72	M	11;3	W	64	+	–	0	–	+	–	0	3
73	M	11;3	X	87	–	–	–	–	–	–	–	0
74	F	11;3	V	69	+	–	–	–	–	–	–	1
75	F	11;3	U	49	+	–	0	–	+	–	–	2.5
76	F	11;4	V	82	–	0	–	–	–	–	–	0.5
77	M	11;4	W	51	–	+	+	–	+	–	–	3
78	M	11;4	U	50	–	+	+	+	0	–	0	4
79	M	11;5	Y	70	–	+	–	–	–	–	–	1
80	F	11;5	V	50	+	–	0	0	+	–	0	3.5
81	M	11;6	X	54	+	+	+	–	+	–	–	4
82	M	11;6	X	74	–	–	–	–	–	0	0	1
83	F	11;6	W	61	–	0	–	–	–	–	–	0.5
84	M	11;6	Y	77	–	+	–	–	–	–	–	1
85	F	11;6	X	70	–	–	+	0	–	–	–	1.5
86	M	11;7	X	74	+	0	–	–	–	–	–	1.5
87	M	11;8	X	76	+	0	–	–	+	–	–	2.5
88	F	11;8	W	50	+	+	0	–				2.5
89	M	11;8	V	51	+	0	–	0		–	–	2
90	F	11;11	V	65	–	–	+	–	–	–	–	1
91	F	12;0	W	62	–	0	+	–	+	–	–	2.5
92	F	12;0	X	62	–	–	+	–	+	–	0	2.5
93	M	12;0	W	66	+	–	+	0	+	–	0	4
94	F	12;1	X	87	–	0	–	–	+	–	–	0.5
95	F	12;5	V	75	–	+	–	0	+	–	+	3.5
96	F	12;5	X	65	–	+	0	0	+	–	0	3.5
97	M	12;5	X	78	+	–	–	–	–	–	–	1
98	M	12;7	X	82	–	–	0	–	–	–	–	0.5
99	F	12;8	Z	63	+	–	–	–	0	–	–	1.5
100	M	12;9	Z	93	+	–	–	–	–	–	–	1
101	F	12;9	U	64	–	0	–	0	+	–	0	2.5
102	F	13;5	V	80	–	+	–	–	0	–	–	1.5
103	F	13;6	W	89	–	+	–	–	–	0	0	1.5
104	F	13;7	W	86	–	–	0	–	0	–	–	1
105	M	13;8	V	83	–	+	–	–	–	–	–	1
106	F	13;11	U	82	–	0	–	–	+	–		1.5
107	M	13;11	V	77	–	–	0	–	+	–		0.5
108	F	14;0	U	76	+	+	–	–	+	–	0	3.5
109	F	14;0	U	94	–	–	–	–	–	–	–	0
110	F	14;3	Z	97	–	0	–	–	–	–	–	0.5
111	M	14;3	W	79	+	0	–	–	+	–	0	3
112	M	14;5	V	79	+	0	–	–	0	–	–	4
113	F	14;7	X	87	+	0	–	+	+	0	–	4
114	F	14;8	W	96	–	+	–	–	–	–	–	1

Table III.1 (contd)

Case no.	Sex	Age	Int.	S_1	DR	L–R	Pol.	Sub.	Tab	MF	MR	Index
115	F	14;9	X	83	+	+	–	–	+	–	0	3.5
116	M	15;0	V	81	+	0	+	–	+	–	–	3.5
117	F	15;1	X	83	+	–	0	0	+	–	–	3
118	F	15;1	W	86	+	+	–	–	–	–	–	2
119	M	15;4	Y	96	+	0	–	–	–	–	–	1.5
120	M	15;4	W	95	+	+	+	–	–	0	0	4
121	F	15;5	X	97	–	–	–	–	+	–	–	1
122	M	15;6	X	90	+	0	0	–	+	–	+	4
123	F	15;9	W	95	+	0	–	–	+	–	–	2.5
124	F	15;11	X	92	–	+	–	–	+	–	0	2.5
125	M	16;0	W	91	–	–	0	–	–	–	–	0.5
126	F	16;4	Y	94	+	0	0	0	+	–	–	3.5
127	F	17;3	X	89	+	0	0	–	+	–	–	3
128	F	17;4	Z	90	+	0	–	–	–	–	–	1.5
129	M	17;6	Y	80	+	0	0	–	+	–	–	3
130	F	17;8	Z	97	–	–	0	–	–	–	–	0.5
131	M	17;11	Z	97	–	–	–	+	–	–	–	1
132	F	18;0	X	92	–	+	–	–	–	–	–	1

Appendix IV
Greek Version of the
Bangor Dyslexia Test

The Bangor Dyslexia Test

Professor T. R. Miles

Καταγραφοντας τις απαντησεις:

Να ειστε ακριβεις και επεξηγηματικοι κατα τη σημειωση των απαντησεων των υποκειμενων σε καθε ερωτηση. Θα χρειαστει να κρατατε σημειωσεις σχετικα με το τι ακριβως εγινε ωστε να αξιολογησετε την αποδοση τους.

Χρησιμοποιειστε ενα σημαδι (✓) στη περιπτωση που το υποκειμενο δωσει την σωστη απαντηση αμεσως, αλλα παρακαλω σημειωστε ολες τις καθυστερησεις και διστγμους και παντοτε σημειωετε εαν το υποκειμενο ζητα να επαναληφθει η ερωτηση, επαναλαμβανει ο/η ιδιος/α την ερωτηση, η προσπαθει να επαναπροσανατολισει τον εαυτο του/της επαναλαμβανοντας ο,τι ακουστηκε πριν. Μην βαζετε σταυρο εαν η απαντηση ειναι λαθος, αλλα σημειωστε με οσο δυνατον περισσοτερη ακριβεια ο,τι ειπε το υποκειμενο. Οπου χρειαστει αναγκαιο, σημειωστε τις συμπληρωματικες ερωτησεις που του ρωτησατε.

Χρησιμοποιειστε τις ακολουθες συντομογραφιες:

δισ = το υποκειμενο διστζει.
ΕΕ = το υποκειμενο ζητα επαναληψη της ερωτησης απο τον εξεταστη.
ΕΙ = το υποκειμενο επαναλαμβανει το ιδιο την ερωτηση.
ΕΠ = επαναληψη (στην περιπτωση της προπαιδειας), δηλ. το υποκειμενο γυριζει πισω μερικα σταδια για να αρχισει παλι απο την αρχη.

Περιληψη

Ονομα _____ Ημερομηνια _____

Ηλικια _____ Εξεταστηκε απο _____

Οι ενδειξεις για την αξιολογηση ειναι +, 0 η −

1. Αριστερο–δεξι (μερη του σωματος).
2. Πολυσυλλαβες λεξεις.
3. Αφαιρεση.
4. Προπαιδεια.
5. Μηνες εμπρος.
6. Μηνες αναποδα.
7. Ψηφια εμπρος.
8. Ψηφια αναποδα.
9. β–θ μπερδεμα.
10. Οικογενειακη συσχετιση.
Αριθμος 'θετικων ενδειξεων' απο το συνολο των 10 ερωτησεων.

1. Αριστερο–δεξι (μερη του σωματος).

Οδηγια	Απαντηση του υποκειμενου	Οδηγια	Απαντηση του υποκειμενου
α. Δειξε μου το δεξι σου χερι (Ειχες δυσκολια οταν ησουν μικροτερος/ης ;)		στ. Δειξε το δεξι μου αυτι με το αριστερο σου χερι	
β. Δειξε μου το αριστερο σου αυτι		ζ. Αγγιξε το δεξι μου χερι με το δεξι σου χερι	
γ. Αγγιξε το δεξι σου αυτι με το αριστερο σου χερι		η. Δειξε το αριστερο μου ματι με το δεξι σου χερι	
δ. (Ο εξεταστης τοποθετει τα χερια του στο τραπεζι) Ποιο ειναι το δεξι μου χερι;		θ. Δειξε το αριστερο μου αυτι με το αριστερο σου χερι	
ε. Αγγιξε το αριστερο μου χερι με το δεξι σου χερι		ι. Αγγιξε το δεξι μου χερι με το αριστερο σου χερι	

Ειδικες σημειωσεις:

254

Appendices

2. Επαναληψη πολυσυλλαβων λεξεων. Προκειται να πω μερικες λεξεις και θα ηθελα να τις πεις μετα απο εμενα.

Απαντηση του υποκειμενου
προκαταρκτικοs
φιλοσοφικοs
ταυτοχρονοs
ανεμωνη
στατιστικοs

3. Αφαιρεση. Ποσο κανει:

Απαντηση του υποκειμενου
9 μειον 2
6 μειον 3
19 μειον 7
24 μειον 2
52 μειον 9
44 μειον 7

4. Προπαιδεια   α) Εχεις διδαχθει την προπαιδεια στο σχολειο; _____ β) Ειχες καποια δυσκολια με αυτην; _____ Δωστε τουλαχιστον τρεις προπαιδειες. Αυτες θα πρεπει κανονικα να ειναι, η προπαιδεια του 6x, 7x και 8x, αλλα αποτυχιες στις προπαιδειες του 2x, 3x και 4x μπορουν φυσικα να ειναι διδακτικες. Στην περιπτωση παιδιων ηλικιας 7 και 8 χρονων, δωστε την προπαιδεια του 4x μονο.
γ) Πες μου την προπαιδεια του _____ .

Απαντηση του υποκειμενου	Απαντηση του υποκειμενου	Απαντηση του υποκειμενου

5. Μηνες εμπροs. Πες τους μηνες του χρονου (απο την αρχη προς το τελος).

6. Μηνες αναποδα. Τωρα πες τους απο το τελος προς την αρχη.

7. Ψηφια εμπρος. Χρησιμοποιειστε τις ακολουθες λεξεις: 'Προκειται να πω μερικους αριθμους, και οταν θα εχω τελειωσει, θελω να μου τους πεις οπως ακριβως τους ειπα.' Τα ψηφια θα πρεπει να διαβαζονται δυνατα με ρυθμο ενα ανα δευτερολεπτο. Δωστε τη δευτερη σειρα ψηφιων μονο εαν το υποκειμενο εχει αποτυχει η ειχε δυσκολια με την πρωτη σειρα. Σταματειστε οταν το υποκειμενο εχει αποτυχει και στις δυο σειρες ψηφιων σε ενα συγκεκριμενο μηκος σειρας.

Σειρα 1	Απαντηση του υποκειμενου	Σειρα 2	Απαντηση του υποκειμενου
9 3 2		4 8 7	
3 6 1 5		8 2 4 3	
9 4 7 2 3		5 6 4 1 2	
5 3 9 1 8 4		7 4 6 8 3 2	
1 7 5 6 3 7 4		2 1 4 8 1 2 9	
4 5 1 3 6 7 9 2		5 3 8 7 1 9 6 2	
4 9 6 2 5 1 3 6 7		1 6 9 5 4 7 3 9 6	

8. Ψηφια αναποδα. Χρησιμοποιειστε τις ακολουθες λεξεις: 'Προκειται να πω ακομα μερικους αριθμους, αλλα αυτη τη φορα οταν θα σταματησω θελω να μου τους πεις αναποδα (δηλ. απο το τελος προς την αρχη). Για παραδειγμα, αν θα πω 3–2–6, τι θα ελεγες εσυ;' Στη συνεχεια προχωρειστε στα μερη που ακολουθουν, με την οδηγια 'Τωρα προσπαθησε αυτα.' Δωστε δυο σειρες ψηφιων σε καθε μηκος σειρας και σταματειστε εαν το υποκειμενο αποτυχει και στις δυο.

Σειρα 1	Απαντηση του υποκειμενου	Σειρα 1	Απαντηση του υποκειμενου
2 8 4		3 7 1	
6 5 2 9		3 8 4 6	
1 6 5 8 2		3 4 7 1 9	
8 5 3 9 2 4		9 7 1 6 3 8	

9. β–θ μπερδεμα. Υπαρχει καποια ενδειξη οτι το υποκειμενο μπερδευει το 'β' και το 'θ' η τα μπερδευε σε μικροτερη ηλικια (κατω των 8 ετων);

ΝΑΙ   ΑΜΦΙΒΟΛΟ   ΟΧΙ

☐   ☐   ☐   (Σημειωστε (✓) ως καταλληλο)

10. Οικογενειακη συσχετιση. Υπαρχει ενδειξη απο καποιον/α αλλον/η στην οικογενεια οτι εχει παρομοιες δυσκολιες;

ΝΑΙ   ΑΜΦΙΒΟΛΟ   ΟΧΙ

☐   ☐   ☐   (Σημειωστε (✓) ως καταλληλο και υποδηλωστε λεπτομερειες)

Μεταφραση: Α. Κασβικη / Translated by A. Kasviki.

Appendix V
German Version of the Bangor Dyslexia Test

DER BANGOR LEGASTHENIE TEST Professor T. R. Miles

Es ist sehr wichtig, daß Sie sich vor Durchführung
dieses Tests das begleitende Handbuch sorgfältig
durchlesen.

Notieren der Antworten:

Notieren Sie jede Antwort genau und ausführlich; denn um
die Leistung umfassend beurteilen zu können, benötigen Sie
eine ausführlichè Beschreibung des Testablaufes.

Haken Sie eine spontan richtig gegebene Antwort ab, aber
notieren Sie alle Anzeichen, die auf ein Verzögern der
Antwort hindeuten: vermerken Sie, ob der/die Getestete die
Frage noch einmal hören möchte, Ihnen die Frage
nachspricht oder versucht, sich an vorangegangenen
Aufgaben zu orientieren. Auch ein Zögern beim Antworten
sollten Sie festhalten. Haken Sie eine falsche Antwort nicht
einfach als falsch ab, sondern versuchen Sie, die Antwort
der/des Getesteten so genau wie möglich festzuhalten. Es
kann sinnvoll sein, auch Ihre zusätzlich gestellten Fragen zu
notieren.

Benutzen Sie die folgenden Abkürzungen:

zö für die Testperson zögert beim Antworten
wh für die Testperson möchte die Frage nochmals hören
eh für die Testperson "echot" die Frage
or für die Testperson orientiert sich an Vorangegangenem

ÜBERBLICK DER ERGEBNISSE:

Name_____ Datum_____
Alter_____ getestet von_____

Indikatoren bewertet mit +, 0, −

1. rechts- links (Körperhälften)
2. Mehrsilbige Pseudoworte
3. Subtraktion
4. Einmaleins
5. Monate vorwärts
6. Monate rückwärts
7. Zahlen nachsprechen vorwärts
8. Zahlen nachsprechen rückwärts
9. b-d Verwechslungen
10. Auftreten in der Familie

☐ 1. Rechts- Links (Körperhäften)

Instruktion	Antwort	Instruktion	Antwort
a. Zeige mir deine rechte Hand. (Hattest du damit Schwierig-keiten, als du jünger warst?)		f. Zeige mit deiner linken Hand auf mein rechtes Ohr.	
b. Zeige mir dein linkes Ohr.		g. Berühre meine rechte Hand mit deiner rechten Hand.	
c. Berühre dein rechtes Ohr mit deiner linken Hand.		h. Zeige mit deiner rechten Hand auf mein linkes Auge.	
d. (VersuchsleiterIn legt die Hände auf den Tisch) Welches ist meine rechte Hand?		i. Zeige mit deiner linken Hand auf mein linkes Ohr.	
e. Berühre meine linke Hand mit deiner rechten Hand.		j. Berühre meine rechte Hand mit deiner linken Hand.	

Spezielle Strategien:

☐ 2. Wiederholen mehrsilbiger Pseudoworte *Ich spreche dir ein paar ausgedachte Worte vor und möchte, daß du sie mir nachsprichst.*

Antwort

▢ 3. Subtraktion   *Was ist*

	Antwort
9 minus 2	
6 minus 3	
19 minus 7	
24 minus 2	
52 minus 9	
44 minus 7	

▢ 4. Einmaleins   a. "Hast *du das kleine Einmaleins in der Schule gelernt?"*_____ b. *"Hattest du damit Schwierigkeiten?"*_____Fragen Sie mindestens drei Blöcke ab. Normalerweise sollte es das 1x6, 1x7 und 1x8 sein, aber Versagen beim 1x2, 1x3 oder 1x4 können natürlich sehr aufschlußreich sein. Fragen Sie 7- und 8jährige Kinder nur nach dem 1x4. c. *"Sage das Ein-mal ...... auf und vergiß nicht, jedesmal das 'ein mal' zu sagen."*

Antwort	Antwort	Antwort

▢ 5. Monate vorwärts - *"Sag' die Monate eines Jahres auf!"*

▢ 6. Monate rückwärts   *"Nun sage sie einmal rückwärts auf."*

▢ 7. Zahlen nachsprechen vorwärts   Geben Sie folgende Instruktion: *"Ich werde dir jetzt ein paar Zahlen vorsprechen. Sobald ich fertig bin, möchte ich, daß du sie genauso nachsprichst."* Lesen Sie eine Zahl pro Sekunde laut vor. Geben Sie die Zahlen der Serie 2 nur dann vor, wenn bei Serie 1 ein Fehler gemacht wurde oder Schwierigkeiten auftraten. Der Test ist beendet, wenn bei einer Ziffernlänge beide Serien falsch wiedergegeben werden.

SERIE 1	Antwort	SERIE 2	Antwort
932		487	
3615		8243	
94723		56412	
539184		746832	
1756374		2148129	
45136792		53871962	
496251367		169547396	

▢ 8. Zahlen nachsprechen rückwärts   Geben Sie folgende Instruktion: *"Ich werde dir wieder einige Zahlen vorsprechen, aber diesmal möchte ich, daß du sie mir rückwärts nachsprichst. Wenn ich z.B. 3-2-6-sage, was würdest du dann antworten?"* Ist die Antwort richtig und die Aufgabe begriffen, fahren Sie mit beiden Serien zu einer Ziffernlänge fort. Der Test ist beendet, wenn beide Serien falsch wiedergegeben werden.

SERIE 1	Antwort	SERIE 2	Antwort
284		371	
6529		3846	
16582		34719	
853924		971638	

▢ 9. b-d Verwechslungen   Gibt es Anzeichen, daß der/die Getestete b und d verwechselt oder dies nach dem achten Lebensjahr noch getan hat? (Zutreffendes bitte ankreuzen!)

       ja   vielleicht   nein

▢ 10. Auftreten in der Familie   Gibt es weitere Familienmitglieder mit ähnlichen Schwierigkeiten? (Zutreffendes bitte ankreuzen und u.U. näher ausführen.)

       ja   vielleicht   nein

Appendix VI
The Bangor–Hiroshima
Dyslexia Test

バンガア・ヒロシマ難読症診断テスト　　　実施日
　　　　　　　　　　　　　　　　　　　　氏名

1　左右認知
　　1）　右手を出して。
　　2）　左耳を見せて。
　　3）　左手で右耳を触って。
　　4）　私の右手はどっち。
　　5）　右手で私の左手を触って。

　　6）　左手で私の右耳を指さして。
　　7）　右手で私の右手を触って。
　　8）　右手で私の左耳を指さして。
　　9）　左手で私の左手を触って。
　10）　左手で私の右手を触って。

2　多音節反復
　　1）　preliminary /priliminari/
　　2）　philosophical /filosofikal/
　　3）　statistical /statistikal/

3　九九
　　1）　6の段
　　2）　7の段
　　3）　8の段

4　数を2つ跳ばしで逆に数える
　　e.g., 100, 97, 94, 91, ...
　　1）　96から（75まで）　[96,93,90,87,84,81,78,75]
　　2）　88から（67まで）　[88,85,82,79,76,73,70,67]
　　3）　95から（74まで）　[95,92,89,86,83,80,77,74]

5 系列処理
   1） 月曜日から日曜日まで早く言って。
   2） では、それを逆に言って。
   3） たちつてと、と言って。
   4） では、それを逆に言って。
   5） なにぬねの、と言って。
   6） では、それを逆に言って。

6 数字反復
   0） 932
   1） 3615
   2） 94723
   3） 539184
   4） 1756374

7 数字逆反復
   0） 284
   1） 6529
   2） 1629
   3） 34719
   4） 971638

Notes

Chapter 1

Note 1.1. Throughout this book I shall refer to the persons whom I assessed as 'subjects'. Other possibilities were considered but rejected. Thus 'children' would have been misleading, since many of them were adolescents and some were adults; 'patients' would have implied a medical rather than an educational assessment, while 'assessee' or 'person-being-tested' would have been unbearable. (Nor would it have been practicable to follow the lead of that delicately nurtured Dickensian, Mr Podsnap, who invariably referred to his daughter as 'the young person'.) 'Subject', however, is the standard word used by psychologists when they report on their research and it has the merit of being both brief and accurate.

Note 1.2. The Bullock Report, *A Language for Life* (HMSO, 1975) states on p. 587 that the term dyslexia 'is not susceptible to precise operational definition'. No reasons are given for this curious and dogmatic statement.

Note 1.3. This book is, of course, concerned with *developmental* dyslexia rather than with any form of acquired dyslexia, and when the words 'dyslexia' and 'dyslexic' are used the qualifying adjective 'developmental' should be understood throughout. For an account of recent developments in acquired dyslexia see (1) M. Coltheart, K. E. Patterson and J. C. Marshall (eds), *Deep Dyslexia*, London: Routledge and Kegan Paul, 1979; (2) K.E. Patterson, J.C. Marshall and M.Coltheart (eds), *Surface Dyslexia: Neuropsychological and Cognitive Studies of Phonological Reading*, London: Lawrence Erlbaum,1985.

Note 1.4. See W. Pringle Morgan, 'A case of congenital word-blindness', *British Medical Journal*, 2, 1896, p.1378.

Note 1.5. See J. Hinshelwood, *Congenital Word-Blindness*, London: H. K. Lewis, 1917, especially Chapter 2, pp.43–51.

Note 1.6. See J. Hinshelwood, *Congenital Word-Blindness*, London: H. K. Lewis, 1917, Chapter 2, p.63 and Chapter 3, pp.64–74.

Note 1.7. See S. T. Orton, *Reading, Writing and Speech Problems in Children* and *Selected Papers*, Austin, Texas: PRO-ED, 1989. Orton is widely recognised as a great pioneer, particularly in view of the breadth and astuteness of his observations. His basic *theory* of dyslexia, however, is less than convincing – in particular his proffered explanation of b–d confusion in terms of the failure of the two halves of the brain to elide the two 'engrams' (or traces) of letters which are mirror-images of each other. This idea has generated some decidedly dubious speculations about the role of left-handedness and mirror-images in dyslexia. For further discussion see Chapters 9 and 21.

Note 1.8. See M. MacMeeken, *Ocular Dominance in Relation to Developmental Aphasia*, London: University of London Press, 1939.

Note 1.9. See M. MacMeeken, *Ocular Dominance in Relation to Developmental Aphasia*, London: University of London Press, 1939, p.27.

Note 1.10. See P. Blanchard, 'Psychoanalytic contributions to the problems of reading disabilities', *Psychoanalytic Study of The Child*, 2, 1946, 163–187.

Note 1.11. See T. R. Miles, 'Two cases of developmental aphasia', *Journal of Child Psychology and Psychiatry*, 1961, 48–70.

Note 1.12. See in particular M. Critchley, *The Dyslexic Child*, London: Heinemann Medical Books, 1970, and M. and E. A. Critchley, *Dyslexia Defined*, London: Heinemann Medical Books, 1978.

Note 1.13. See S. Naidoo, *Specific Dyslexia*, London: Pitman, 1972.

Note 1.14. See *Children with Specific Reading Difficulties* (Report of the Advisory Committee on Handicapped Children), London: HMSO, 1972.

Note 1.15. See Note 1.2, above.

Note 1.16. See *Special Educational Needs* (Report of the Committee of Enquiry into the Education of Children and Handicapped Young People), London: HMSO, 1978.

Note 1.17. See, in particular, E. Simpson, *Reversals*, London: Gollancz, 1980, and S. Hampshire, *Susan's Story*, London: Sidgwick and Jackson, 1981.

Note 1.18. On Helping the Dyslexic Child, by T.R.Miles, was published by Methuen Educational Books in 1970. *More Help for Dyslexic Children*, by T.R. and E.Miles, was published by the same publishers in 1975. The two books were revised in 1983 and published together as *Help for Dyslexic Children*, London: Routledge, 1983.

Chapter 2

Note 2.1. I myself received no money for carrying out the assessment as this formed part of my research work for the university, but those families who could afford it paid small sums to the Dyslexia Unit funds. This point requires mention, since arrangements for payment could in principle have influenced what happened during the assessments, though I have no reason for thinking that it did so in any relevant way.

Note 2.2. See F. J. Schonell and F. E. Schonell, *Diagnostic and Attainment Testing*, Edinburgh: Oliver and Boyd, 1952, p.42.

Note 2.3. For convenience I have used the old norms, since they were the only ones available when the research started. The differences between old and new norms are in fact not large enough to have any significant effect on my arguments.

Note 2.4. See F. J. Schonell and F. E. Schonell, *Diagnostic and Attainment Testing*, Edinburgh: Oliver and Boyd, 1952, p.71.

Note 2.5. In a sense, no doubt, a child who writes 'bancing' for *dancing* knows how to spell the word. One could argue, for instance, that if he had not been asked to write but had been told to spell 'dancing' by choosing from a pool of letters placed in front of him he might have answered correctly. In this case, as in some others, a dyslexic person may perform some components of a task but not others, and how to score his performance will then depend on which components one chooses to regard as important. In this particular case the difference in score would have been minimal whichever ruling had been given.

Note 2.6. Nor, of course, is it sensible to coach a child on the particular words which occur in a spelling test. Each word is, in a sense, representative of a population of words of similar difficulty, and if a word is specially taught one is therefore misleading oneself by sampling that population in a biased way.

Note 2.7. See L. M. Terman and M. A. Merrill, *Measuring Intelligence*, London: H.K. Lewis & Co., 1961.

Note 2.8. The instructions for this item are quite explicit: 'The subject is not allowed to use pencil and paper' (L. M. Terman and M. A. Merrill, *Measuring Intelligence*, London: H.K. Lewis & Co., 1961, p.134). Although departure from these instructions resulted in a wealth of interesting material, it was important not to present the scores as though they had been obtained under the conditions laid down in the manual.

Note 2.9. See *The Wechsler Intelligence Scale for Children*, by D. Wechsler. The original version was published by the Psychological Corporation, New York, in 1949. A revised version, the WISC(R), to which I changed over towards the end of the research, was published by the National Foundation for Educational Research, Slough, in 1976. Throughout the book I shall follow common practice in speaking of the 'WISC'. There will also be occasional references during the book to the 'WAIS' (Wechsler Adult Intelligence Scale), Psychological Corporation, New York, 1957.

Note 2.10. See T. R. Miles and N. C. Ellis, 'A lexical encoding deficiency II', in G.Th. Pavlidis and T. R. Miles (eds), *Dyslexia Research and Its Applications to Education*, Chichester: John Wiley & Sons, 1981 (especially pp.230 *et seq.*).

Note 2.11. I cannot resist referring to the situation where a very bright 9-year-old (S34), after testing, said to his mother 'What's my IQ?' and received the admirable answer, 'Thanks very much, but we're not entering the IQ stakes today'.

Note 2.12. It is sometimes said that because of their 'language' difficulty dyslexic children are likely to score lower on the Verbal than on the Performance half of the WISC. This has not been my experience. Dyslexic children of school age are not necessarily weak at tasks involving oral language, and in any case the division of the WISC into 'verbal' and 'performance' does not seem to me to be of any major theoretical significance.

Note 2.13. See J. C. Raven, *Advanced Progressive Matrices*, London: H. K. Lewis & Co., 1965.

Note 2.14. I originally used A, B, C, D, E and F. By convention, however, these letters represent grades and suggest by implication that a person with an A is more meritorious than a person with a B, and so on. In contrast Z does not at present imply anything more meritorious than U. Admittedly it is hard to escape the widely held view that high reasoning ability is to be admired, but at least one can avoid a notation in which such an assumption is 'written in' without examination.

Note 2.15. I have managed to collect data in respect of 11 dyslexic children, aged between 7 and 9, to whom a full-scale WISC was given, exclusive of the Digit Span and Mazes items. The mean difference between each subject's 'composite' IQ (based on the results of these 10 items) and the 'selected' IQ (based on extrapolation from the results on Similarities, Vocabulary, Comprehension, Picture Completion, Block Design and Object Assembly) was found to be 9 points. This figure may, of course, vary at different ages and at different IQ levels and may be greater in the case of the Terman–Merrill test. Where a full-scale WISC had already been given to one of my subjects, with a resultant 'composite' IQ, I assigned a grade-label one higher than that corresponding to the same level of 'selected' IQ.

Note 2.16. Raven gives a norm of 21 for university students, s.d. 4. Since it seemed reasonable to suppose that subjects obtaining grades X, Y and Z would have the necessary intellectual skills for taking a university degree, I decided to equate the range of scores 17–21 with grade X. If 26 or higher is then treated as very exceptional (grade Z), this leaves the range 22–25 for grade Y. These are of course approximations but not, I think, wholly meaningless ones.

Note 2.17. The norms for the Wechsler scale are so arranged that 'average for age' is set at 10, with a standard deviation of 3 units. Thus a score of 13 is one standard deviation above the average and therefore equivalent to an IQ of 115, while a score of 16 is two standard deviations above the average and therefore equivalent to an IQ of 130. Any child scoring above 7 or 8 is therefore within the average range or above it. The Terman–Merrill is scored somewhat differently. Each test item is assigned to an age-level, with a range between 2 and 14 years; above this level there are four groups of items, labelled respectively Average Adult, Superior Adult I, Superior Adult II, and Superior Adult III. In the Summary Chart I have used Roman figures to indicate the age-level of the subject's highest passes if these were at the 14-year level or below and at higher levels I have used the abbreviations AA, SA I, SA II, and SA III.

Chapter 3

Note 3.1. With hindsight I believe the position to be somewhat more complicated than this. There is reason to think that any inexperienced

language user is likely to be slow at a variety of 'information processing' tasks such as those included in the dyslexia test (compare N. C.
Ellis and T. R. Miles, 'Visual information processing as a determinant of
reading speed', *Journal of Research in Reading*, 1, 2, 1978, 108–120).
The dyslexic person is different not because of the slowness of his performance as such but because he remains slow despite constant practice. A person whose first language is not English would also be
expected to have difficulty with some of the items in the dyslexia test,
just as anyone except a native speaker would be expected to display
some degree of 'dyslexic'-type behaviour if the items were presented in
French. Data are in fact available which show how a student who had
just started to learn Russian needed considerably more time before she
could correctly name an array of six visually presented Russian letters
in comparison with the time which she needed to name English letters
and digits. This time decreased considerably, however, after a few
weeks. In contrast, a dyslexic student, presented with similar English
letters and digits, made some improvement after a few weeks but
reached a limit of 525 ms which he was unable to improve upon. See
T.R. Miles, 'On the persistence of dyslexic difficulties into adulthood',
in G.Th. Pavlidis and D.F. Fisher (eds), *Dyslexia: Its Neuropsychology
and Treatment*, Chichester: John Wiley & Sons, 1986.

Note 3.2. See T.R. Miles and T.J. Wheeler, 'Towards a new theory of
dyslexia', *Dyslexia Review*, 11, 1974, 9–11.

Note 3.3. I have been particularly influenced on this matter by the writings of E. Tulving who has systematically investigated the presence of
'cueing' in recall tasks. See, for instance, E. Tulving and S. Osler,
'Effectiveness of retrieval cues in memory for words', *Journal of
Experimental Psychology*, 77, 1968, 593–601.

Note 3.4. The data collected by Pollard were later used in a more systematic way. See Chapter 7 and Appendix III.

Note 3.5. When the Bangor Dyslexia Test came to be published this
rather complicated scoring system was abandoned. See T.R. Miles, *The
Bangor Dyslexia Test*, Cambridge: LDA, 1982.

Note 3.6. I am grateful to Gillian Morgan for this information.

Note 3.7. In the case of adults this somewhat stringent criterion had to
be modified (see Chapter 31).

Note 3.8. In view of the largely negative evidence on handedness and
eyedness (see Chapter 21) this item was not included in the published

version of the Bangor Dyslexia Test. The Memory for Sentences and Rhymes tests were also excluded, as it was not clear that either would produce a good 'return' for the time spent in administering them.

Note 3.9. In saying this, I am of course not disputing that, in the context of a particular piece of research, a research worker needs to specify with full precision how his dyslexic and control subjects were selected; indeed without such a specification the research could not be replicated. Such an operational definition should not be regarded as immutable, however, since methods of classification may change in the light of advancing knowledge.

Note 3.10. What are legitimate ways of treating the 'dyslexia index' figure statistically seems to me a difficult question. One can presumably say that a subject with an index figure of 6 'did more dyslexic things' than a subject with an index-figure of 3, and indeed that he did *twice* as many such things. As a consequence it therefore seems legitimate to calculate the mean number of 'pluses' for dyslexic (or allegedly dyslexic) subjects and controls in order to make comparisons between them, as is done in Chapter 7. Any implication, however, that a subject with an index-figure of 6 is 'twice as dyslexic' as a subject with an index-figure of 3 should of course be resisted, and even the validity of using the index-figures to give a rank-order of probability of dyslexia seems to me questionable, since the exact value of a particular index-figure may depend in part on extraneous factors such as the amount of compensatory teaching which the subject has received. Indeed from the clinical point of view it is perhaps safest to regard the index-figure simply as an aid to diagnosis. For a positive diagnosis stronger additional evidence is needed if the figure is low than if it is high, while for a negative diagnosis stronger additional evidence is needed if it is high than if it is low.

Chapter 4

Note 4.1. Somewhat over 300 files were taken from the Department and heaved into a caravan where, during a period of study leave, I was able to work without interruption. I decided not to make use of material obtained before 1972, and a few further files were discarded because there had been only brief consultation and not a full assessment. Two cases, one boy and one girl, were also omitted because they came from a predominantly Welsh-speaking background and spoke English only as a second language.

Note 4.2. See M. and E. A. Critchley, *Dyslexia Defined*, London: Heinemann Medical Books, 1978, Chapter 9.

Note 4.3. In one of these cases a young man aged 20 had recently discharged himself from a mental hospital and was either unwilling or unable to attempt the items in the dyslexia test.

Note 4.4. The fact that only 24 out of my 291 subjects (8%) were classified as belonging to Group III is in part, of course, a function of the referral system. It was known that I and my colleagues carried out educational rather than medical assessments, and those needing chiefly medical help would therefore mostly have gone elsewhere. The smallness of the percentage figure also suggests that the typical or pure cases of dyslexia are not difficult to identify, since there would be no point in seeking an assessment at Bangor unless there was some suspicion of a dyslexic problem. In addition, there is no support in my experience for the suggestion that there are parents who have taken refuge in the erroneous belief that their child is dyslexic as a way of avoiding having to face other problems. For what it is worth, not one of my 291 cases came in this category.

Note 4.5. For references and a further discussion of this point see Note 20.8.

Note 4.6. It is perhaps worth recording (see Chapter 12) that S126, who scored only two 'pluses' at the time of testing, produced some written work at the age of 18 in which 'd' had been written for 'b'. This seems to me a striking confirmation of the original diagnosis. In contrast, a recent re-examination of the file of S21, who scored 2.5 pluses at age 8, has made me think that she should have been placed in Group II.

Note 4.7. The 34 subjects for whom there were incomplete records are, of course, also part of the same 'pool'.

Chapter 5

Note 5.1. George Pavlidis, personal communication. For further details of the work of Pavlidis in investigating the eye movements of dyslexic subjects see G. Th. Pavlidis, 'Sequencing, eye movements and the early objective diagnosis of dyslexia', in G. Th. Pavlidis and T. R. Miles (eds), *Dyslexia Research and its Applications to Education*, Chichester: John Wiley & Sons, 1981. For a brief review of more recent research in this area see Chapter 5 of T.R. and E. Miles, *Dyslexia: 100 Years On*, Milton Keynes: Open University Press, 1990.

Chapter 6

Note 6.1. I have assumed throughout the book that the reader is familiar with the concepts of 'standard deviation' and 'statistical significance'. In Chapter 19 I also assume familiarity with the concepts of correlation and regression and in Chapter 26 the concept of 'explained variance'. Otherwise statistical technicalities are mentioned only in end-of-chapter notes.

Chapter 7

Note 7.1. It is, of course, widely accepted that if a scientific theory is not to be mere 'wind of words' (William James' phrase: see *Varieties of Religious Experience*, London: Longman's Green & Co., 1902, p.443) it must be capable in principle of being falsified. 'Confirmations', says Sir Karl Popper, 'should count only if they are the result of *risky predictions*' (his italics). See K. Popper, *Conjectures and Refutations*, London: Routledge and Kegan Paul, 1963, p.36.

Note 7.2. I am grateful to Ian Pollard for collecting control data for subjects aged 9 to 12 and to Barbara Large and Celia Hopkinson for their help in administering the dyslexia test to subjects aged 7–8 and aged 13–18.

Note 7.3. J. C. Raven, *Standard Progressive Matrices*, London: H. K. Lewis & Co., 1938.

Note 7.4. Although the matching was only approximate it was not wholly arbitrary, since use was made of the percentile rankings given in the manual for the Raven Progressive Matrices (Note 7.3) and also of the fact that the WISC is standardised so as to give a mean of 10 and a standard deviation of 3. It should be noted that the control subjects, like the dyslexic subjects, were appreciably above average in general intelligence level and that their results on the dyslexia test are not therefore an accurate indication of the norm for their particular age.

Note 7.5. See Chapter 2.

Note 7.6. As with the dyslexic subjects (Note 8.1), no attempt was made to take into account the months of the subject's age since the gain in precision by so doing would have been minimal.

Note 7.7. The appropriate 'pairs' among the dyslexic subjects are marked with the letter (m) (= 'match') in the Summary Chart.

Note 7.8. It should be noted that in the scoring of the Digits Reversed and Polysyllables items the subject's age is taken into account and that a *history* of early difficulty contributes to a 'plus' in the case of the Left–Right and the Tables items. In these cases, therefore, comparison of the number of 'pluses' at different age-levels is illegitimate (compare also Note 19.1).

Note 7.9. Ages 7–8: $t = 4.02$, $p < 0.001$; ages 9–12: $t = 14.50$, $p < 0.001$; ages 13–18: $t = 10.07$, $p < 0.001$.

Note 7.10. I am grateful to Andriana Kasviki and Maria Theodorakakou for their help in extracting the relevant information from the files.

Note 7.11. For safety I have included only those with significant retardation at spelling (at least 12 months at age 7, at least 18 months at age 8, and at least 24 months at ages 9 and over). To ensure the exclusion of those of limited intellectual ability I selected only those who (a) had at least two WISC sub-test scores of 10 or more, or (b) had a pass on a Terman–Merrill item at least one year above their chronological age or, in the case of those aged 15 and over, at least one pass at the first grade of Superior Adult, or (c) had a score of at least 15 on the Raven Advanced Matrices.

Chapter 8

Note 8.1. To save complications the earlier Schonell norms were used (Note 2.3) and subjects were assigned to an age-level in years, with months discounted. It follows that the range for any 8-year-old is a score of between 30 and 40, and 80% of the bottom point of the range therefore comes to 24. In what follows I shall speak of the 'top' and 'bottom' points of the range, and I shall also have occasion to refer to those who were below the bottom point of the range but above 80% of it. In the case of the 8-year-olds this would comprise those with scores between 24 and 29, in the case of the 9-year-olds those with scores between 32 and 39, and so on.

Note 8.2. Where the criterion was not satisfied the reading score in the Summary Chart has been underlined.

Note 8.3. Since a score of 100 gives a 'reading age' of 15 it is impossible for the notion of 'above-the-range' to be applicable in the case of any one aged 15 or over. This means that the eight subjects who were classified as 'above' were drawn from a pool of 164, not 223.

Note 8.4. For further discussion of this point see in particular W. Yule, M. Rutter, M. Berger and J. Thompson, 'Over- and under-achievement in reading: distribution in the general population', *British Journal of Educational Psychology*, 44, 1974, 1–12.

Note 8.5. Although I believe this argument could be valid in the present case, it is one which should be used sparingly, since in some contexts it may be difficult to specify the difference between a 'potential' problem which has been overcome and no problem at all. To take an extreme case, if a left-hander, for constitutional reasons, has a weak backhand at lawn tennis which improves as a result of constant practice, does one say that he has 'compensated for a disability' or simply that his backhand has improved? I owe this example to my former colleague, Dr N. M. Cheshire.

Note 8.6. See C. Spring and C. Capps, 'Encoding speed, rehearsal, and probed recall of dyslexic boys', *Journal of Educational Psychology*, 65, 5, 1974, 780–786.

Note 8.7. See N. C. Ellis and T. R. Miles, 'Visual information processing in dyslexic children', in M.M. Gruneberg, P. E. Morris and R. N. Sykes (eds), *Practical Aspects of Memory*, London: Academic Press, 1978.

Chapter 9

Note 9.1. See T. R. Miles, *Understanding Dyslexia*, Bath: Amethyst Books, 1987.

Note 9.2. For detailed evidence on this point see B. Hornsby and T. R. Miles, 'The effects of a dyslexia-centred teaching programme', *British Journal of Educational Psychology*, 50, 1980, 236–242.

Note 9.3. In the 1970s few of the children whom I assessed had received any specialist dyslexia teaching before the time of the assessment. The fact that the older subjects spelled more words correctly on the S_1 test than did the younger ones (see Chapter 19) is evidence that some degree of improvement is possible without such teaching. At all ages, however, the great majority were severely retarded.

Note 9.4. See, for example, M. Peters, *Spelling: Caught or Taught?*, London: Routledge and Kegan Paul, 1967.

Note 9.5. See Elaine Miles, 'A study of dyslexic weaknesses and the consequences for teaching', in G. Th. Pavlidis and T. R. Miles (eds), *Dyslexia Research and its Applications to Education*, Chichester: John Wiley & Sons, 1981.

Note 9.6. In this connection I should like to report an incident of which I was told during my schooldays. A boy who had been asked to write down the French for 'they are' wrote 'ils ont' (when the answer should, of course, have been 'ils sont'). When asked what he had written he said, 'Please, sir, I left out the "s" in "sont"'. This was literally true; but his chosen form of words has the effect (as he no doubt intended) of making the mistake seem more trivial than it was, namely the careless omission of a single letter. A better account of the error would have been to say that he had muddled up 'avoir' with 'être'. I owe this story to that most stimulating of pedagogues, the late Geoffrey Bolton.

Note 9.7. The only two misspellings I have met which would have been unsuitable for the Victorian drawing room are this one and S136's spelling of *would* as 'whored'. I cannot at this point forebear to mention a story told to me by a headmaster's wife who had been using the Kathleen Hickey cards with a young teenage boy. When he reached the card with the digraph 'ff' he duly said 'ff' and turned the card over so as to see the full word, accompanied by the appropriate picture, of which 'ff' was a component. The word is in fact 'cuff', but dyslexic children are sometimes known to read from right to left instead of from left to right, and, slightly abashed, he said to the headmaster's wife, 'That's a naughty word!' (For the latest version of the Kathleen Hickey system see J. Augur and S. Briggs, London: Whurr, 1992.)

Note 9.8. See in particular R. Conrad, 'Acoustic confusion in immediate memory', *British Journal of Psychology*, **55**, 1964, 75–84.

Note 9.9. See Note 1.11.

Note 9.10. Elaine Miles, 'A study of dyslexic weaknesses and the consequences for teaching', in G.Th. Pavlidis and T. R. Miles (eds), *Dyslexia Research and its Applications to Education*, Chichester: John Wiley & Sons, 1981, p.253.

Note 9.11. Compare their tendency to 'lose the place' in reciting tables, see Chapter 16.

Note 9.12. The question of consistency in spelling has been studied in detail by Caroline Dobson, who in fact suggests that it could be a more advantageous topic for spelling research than is correctness. See C. J. Dobson, *The Use of Instability as the Dependent Variable in the Study of Young Children's Spellings*, PhD thesis, University of Wales, 1978.

Note 9.13. See, for instance, D. J. Done and T. R. Miles, 'Learning, memory and dyslexia', in M. M. Gruneberg, P. E. Morris and R. N. Sykes (eds), *Practical Aspects of Memory*, London: Academic Press, 1978.

Note 9.14. For example I might all too easily have written 'from time to time to time' in the above sentence. It is also of interest that on some of the occasions when I have cited dyslexic misspellings for illustration purposes typists have inadvertently 'corrected' what I wrote to something more like the normal spelling. For example I once wrote that a dyslexic student had written 'corelatated' for *correlated*, and in the typed version it said that he had written 'corelated' for *correlated* – a much less spectacular mistake.

Note 9.15. See Note 1.11.

Note 9.16. The following 'translation' was given by this subject's mother: 'And all the time that he worked, the little butterfly sat on the brim of his hat, just above the left eye. At nightfall when the miller went tired to bed the butterfly folded its wings and slept by the leg of the miller's chair.'

Chapter 10

Note 10.1. See T. R. Miles and N. C. Ellis, 'A lexical encoding deficiency II', in G. Th. Pavlidis and T. R. Miles (eds), *Dyslexia Research and Its Applications to Education*, Chichester: John Wiley & Sons, 1981.

Note 10.2. C. Spring and C. Capps, 'Encoding speed, rehearsal, and probed recall of dyslexic boys', *Journal of Educational Psychology*, 66, 5, 1974, p.782.

Note 10.3. T. R. Miles and N. C. Ellis, 'A lexical encoding deficiency II', in G. Th. Pavlidis and T. R. Miles (eds), *Dyslexia Research and Its Applications to Education*, Chichester: John Wiley & Sons, 1981.

Note 10.4. $\chi^2 = 23.05$, $p < 0.001$. In all calculations of chi-squared Yates' correction has been applied.

Chapter 12

Note 12.1. In a few cases parents brought school exercise books which contained b–d confusions. When this happened it was scored as 'plus', even though the mistakes could have been made a year or two before the assessment.

Note 12.2. I received at the same time a letter from this subject's mother saying that he had just been accepted to read Physics at

Oxford University. This seems to me a remarkable triumph in view of his earlier struggles.

Note 12.3. See T. Bottomley (1980), *An Analysis of Spelling Errors in Dyslexic and Non-Dyslexic Boys* (unpublished). Bottomley was in fact analysing data which had been collected at the Word Blind Centre in London and used in Sandhya Naidoo's book, *Specific Dyslexia*, London: Pitman, 1972. Naidoo reports that her controls were 'unselected for reading and spelling ability', and the possibility that a few of these were in fact dyslexic is not totally ruled out. I am grateful to the Invalid Children's Aid Association for making these spellings available.

Note 12.4. Ian Pollard, personal communication.

Note 12.5. She was also known to have had a quite remarkable pattern of eye-movements in reading. See also Note 5.1.

Note 12.6. For further discussion of this point see T. R. Miles and N. C. Ellis, 'A lexical encoding deficiency II', in G. Th. Pavlidis and T. R. Miles (eds), *Dyslexia Research and Its Applications to Education*, Chichester: John Wiley & Sons, 1981.

Note 12.7. It is a matter of familiar experience that any of us can have had a 'bad day' or be 'off form' in respect of a variety of skills. A possible way of talking about this situation is in the language of signal detection theory. (For a readable account see Chapter 2 of *Sensation and Perception*, by S. Coren, C. Porac and L. M. Ward. New York: Academic Press, 1978.) One could say that on a 'bad day' there is extra 'noise' in the nervous system and hence less reduction of uncertainty.

Chapter 13

Note 13.1. This is true, for example, when we represent time by the angular distance travelled by the hands of a clock. As Kant points out, we 'represent the course of time by a line progressing to infinity'. See his *Critique of Pure Reason*, Transcendental Aesthetic, **ii**, 7.

Note 13.2. I have heard it suggested that the famous Spooner, who was Warden of New College, Oxford, was in fact dyslexic. The evidence from a recent study, however, seems to me to make this suggestion unlikely, and there is reason to believe that many reports of 'Spoonerisms' are in fact apocryphal. See J. M. Potter, 'What was the matter with Dr. Spooner?', in V. A. Fromkin (ed.), *Errors in Linguistic Performance*, New York: Academic Press, 1980.

Chapter 14

Note 14.1. For the pool of 132 dyslexic subjects and 132 controls: $\chi^2 = 36.95, p < 0.001$.

Note 14.2. Tulving and Pearlstone have suggested that a word can be 'available' without necessarily being accessible. See E. Tulving and Z. Pearlstone, 'Availability versus accessibility of information in memory for words', *Journal of Verbal Learning and Verbal Behaviour*, **5**, 1966, 381–391.

Note 14.3. I noted that both S69 and S90 ended 'months reversed' with 'March, February, July' (though S90 immediately corrected to 'January'); one can perhaps legitimately ask why, if a wrong month is to be given, it should be the same month on both occasions. It seems to me possible that acoustic confusion may be the explanation of the error, since both months begin with 'J' and end in 'y', though admittedly the y-sounds are somewhat different in the two cases. (Compare the reference to Conrad's work; Note 9.8.)

Note 14.4. This point should of course be considered in conjunction with the evidence cited in Chapter 19 . Months Forwards and Months Reversed were more susceptible to 'learning overlay' than Digits Forwards and Digits Reversed, but there were plenty of older subjects who still displayed difficulty. By adulthood, however, it seems that the difficulty is largely outgrown (see Chapter 31).

Note 14.5. Some of my subjects also reported uncertainty over the alphabet. Thus S257, a successful business man who came to me at the age of 38, reported that he had never been able to learn the alphabet, and this was also reported of S214. S95 said, 'No, I don't know my alphabet – ABC...DE...GHIJKLMNOPQRST...W X Y Z'; and in reply to 'Do you use a dictionary?' he said, 'Yes, it's horrible, I can hardly do it at all'. S244 recited the alphabet correctly as far as R, after which he said, S W X Y Z. S193 used the well-known mnemonic of chanting: 'It took me a long time to learn the alphabet until I discovered a song'. I did not investigate knowledge of the alphabet systematically, but one would certainly expect dyslexic subjects to have difficulty with it since it involves arranging a long series of symbols in the correct order. The problems experienced by dyslexic subjects in looking words up in a dictionary are, of course, widely known.

Chapter 15

Note 15.1. For further evidence of the errors and uncertainties of dyslexics in the area of mathematics see the various chapters in

T.R. and E. Miles (eds), *Dyslexia and Mathematics*, London: Routledge, 1992.

Note 15.2. There would, of course, be advantages for the dyslexic if instead of the 'teens' (thirteen, fourteen etc.) we spoke of 'one-ty three', 'one-ty four' etc. I am grateful to my colleague, J.M. Griffiths, for calling my attention to this point.

Note 15.3. See J.M. Griffiths, *Basic Arithmetic Processes in the Dyslexic Child*, MEd dissertation, University of Wales, 1980.

Note 15.4. In a widely read paper G. A. Miller has cited evidence which suggests that for a typical adult in a variety of tasks there is an upper limit of about seven items which can be handled instantly without resort to 'working out' or counting (see G. A. Miller, 'The magic number seven, plus or minus two. Some limits on our capacity for processing information', *Psychological Review*, 63, 1956, 81–97). It is possible, therefore, that in certain tasks this limit is somewhat lower in dyslexics.

Note 15.5. For further discussion of this point see Chapter 25.

Note 15.6. The subject is required to bring back 13 pints of water using a 5-pint-can and a 9-pint-can and is told that he must begin by filling the 9-pint-can.

Note 15.7. In this item the subject is given four items of increasing complexity in which he has to give the total number of boxes when specified numbers of boxes are placed inside each other.

Note 15.8. In this item the subject is told the heights of a tree at the time of planting and at yearly intervals for the next three years. He is then required to work out its height at the end of the fourth year. This involves finding a pattern in its rate of growth over successive years.

Chapter 16

Note 16.1. This mistake appears to be similar to that reported in connection with 'months reversed' (Note 14.3). Just as in that case the j-sound appears to have suggested the wrong month, so in the present case the similar sounding 'sixty' is substituted for 'six'. All such confusions presumably arise because the difficulty of the task puts the subject under pressure.

Note 16.2. See Note 16.1, above.

Note 16.3. For the two matched groups: $\chi^2 = 43.26, p < 0.001$.

Chapter 17

Note 17.1. For a discussion of the evidence see T. R. Miles and N. C. Ellis, 'A lexical encoding deficiency II', in G. Th. Pavlidis and T. R. Miles (eds), *Dyslexia Research and Its Applications to Education*, Chichester: John Wiley & Sons, 1981. The main sources for this discussion were G. D. Spache, *Investigating the Issues of Reading Disabilities*, Boston: Allyn & Bacon, 1976, and R. P. Rugel, 'WISC subtest scores of disabled readers', *Journal of Learning Disabilities*, 7, 1974, 48–55.

Note 17.2. Many of the records were only marginally incomplete, and since all the subjects in this group were dyslexic it seemed justifiable to increase the size of this particular sample from 40 to 42.

Note 17.3. Two different tachistoscopes were used, one 3-field, one 2-field, both having been made by Electronic Developments Ltd. Digits were printed on cards by means of Letraset, about 1 cm high. Each exposure followed the preceding one without a break except for the time required for me to write the subject's answer down and insert the next card. Choice of digits was determined on the basis of a random number table but with the additional stipulation that no digit should appear more than once in any array. Zero was included.

Note 17.4. According to this method of scoring, which I owe to Ian Pollard, each correctly named digit scores a point if and only if it is in the correct directional relationship to another correctly named digit. Thus if the stimulus was 4 3 2 8 5 1 and the subject responded 4 3 2 8 1 5 this would score 5 out of 6, since the 1 and the 5 are not both in the correct directional relationship and only one of them (it does not matter which) satisfies the criterion. If the subject responded 4 8 7 6 0 5, this would score 3 out of 6 since the 4, 8 and 5 all satisfy the criterion, whereas if he replied 4 5 8 7 6 0 this would score only 2 out of 6 since only one of the 8 and the 5 is in the correct directional relationship to the 4. In practice this procedure is easier to operate than it sounds!

Note 17.5. I am not, of course, suggesting that this represents a prediction as to what the subject would in fact do at an exposure-time of 1000 ms, since the relationship between exposure-time and number of digits correctly identified is not necessarily linear or at any rate cannot be assumed to be so. The figure is simply a mathematical device to aid comparisons.

Note 17.6. In the auditory condition a score of 7 or more for 'Digits Forwards was counted as 'high', a score of 6 as 'medium', a score of 5 as 'low' and a score of 4 or less as 'very low'. In the visual condition a comparison ratio of 5 or more was counted as 'high', one between 4.00 and 4.99 as 'medium', one between 2.00 and 3.99 as 'low', one under 2.00 as 'very low'.

Note 17.7. These relate to 133 children in the Manchester area who were within 80% of their age-level on the Schonell S_1 test. Seven digits were exposed for 800 ms, and the mean number of digits correct, with scoring as described in Note 17.4 above, was 4.99. The comparison ratio is obtained by multiplying this figure by 10/8.

Note 17.8. See N. C. Ellis and T. R. Miles, 'Dyslexia as a limitation in the ability to process information', *Bulletin of the Orton Society*, **27**, 1977, 72–81. The conditions of this experiment were different from those described here, since only five digits were presented and a measure was taken of the minimum time needed for correct responding. For 41 control subjects aged 10–14 the figure was 289 ms, s.d. 156; for 41 dyslexic subjects the figure was 1331 ms, s.d. 585. There is also evidence that dyslexic subjects are slower than controls in identifying visual arrays of letters (see G. Stanley and R. Hall, 'A comparison of dyslexics and normals in recalling letter arrays after brief presentation', *British Journal of Educational Psychology*, **43**, 1973, 301–304).

Note 17.9. I re-examined this subject's file but saw no grounds for revising my view that he was dyslexic.

Note 17.10. For further discussion of this point see Elaine Miles, 'A study of dyslexic weaknesses and the consequences for teaching', in G. Th. Pavlidis and T. R. Miles (eds), *Dyslexia Research and its Applications to Education*, Chichester: John Wiley & Sons, 1981. See also Elaine Miles, 'Visual dyslexia–auditory dyslexia: is this a valuable distinction?', in M.Snowling and M.Thomson (eds), *Dyslexia: Integrating Theory and Practice*, London: Whurr, 1991.

Note 17.11. If Table 17.2 is 'telescoped' into a 4-cell table with pooling of 'high' and 'medium' and pooling of 'low' and 'very low', the value of chi-squared comes to 0.80, which is non-significant.

Note 17.12. It seems to me possible, though this is admittedly speculative, that the occasional successes, for example S49 in the visual condition and S34 and S174 in the auditory condition, are task specific and do not imply that their speed of processing is higher in general than for most dyslexics. Certainly S49 was not a fast processer in general since he could repeat no more than four digits in the auditory condition. What I have in mind is, for instance, strong eidetic imagery in the visual condition and a clever strategy of grouping in the auditory condition; there is no reason why a dyslexic subject should not use these or other personal idiosyncrasies to help him with one or other task.

Chapter 18

Note 18.1. It seems to me unlikely that this was simply a case of 'not hearing what I said' in the popular sense, but was probably a memorising error similar to those described by Conrad (Note 9.8).

Note 18.2. T. R. Miles, *Understanding Dyslexia*, Bath: Amethyst Books, 1987. Oliver, described on pp.116–119, found the word 'red' as a rhyme for 'head' by spelling out both words to himself and noting that both ended in '-ed'. He recognised the 'a' in 'head' as being irrelevant.

Note 18.3. See L. Bradley and P. Bryant, 'Difficulties in auditory organisation as a possible cause of reading backwardness', *Nature*, **270**, 1978, 746–747.

Note 18.4. S. Naidoo, *Specific Dyslexia*, London: Pitman, 1972.

Note 18.5. Perhaps even more compelling is the fact that two recent postgraduate students whom 1 know very well personally are both extremely talented musicians despite their dyslexia. Two of the subjects described in Chapter 31 were professional musicians.

Note 18.6. A leaflet, *Music and Dyslexia*, is now available from the British Dyslexia Association, 98 London Road, Reading, and various papers have been published. These include: M.Hubicki, 'Learning Difficulties in Music', in G.Hales (ed.), *Meeting Points in Dyslexia*, British Dyslexia Association, 1990; M.Hubicki, 'A multisensory approach to reading music', in M.Thomson and M.Snowling (eds), *Dyslexia: Integrating Theory and Practice*, London, Whurr, 1991; M.Hubicki and T.R.Miles, 'Musical notation and multisensory learning', *Child Language Teaching and Therapy*, 7, 5, 1991, 61–78.

Chapter 19

Note 19.1. Some of the other items were unsuitable because of the method of scoring: in the case of Left–Right, Tables, and b–d confusion

a *history* of earlier difficulty contributed to a 'plus' score; familial incidence is clearly unrelated to age, and in the case of polysyllables the
method of scoring took age into account. In scoring the two digits tests
the figure used was the highest series-length at which the subject
responded correctly.

Note 19.2. Because their ages were appreciably beyond those of all
other subjects the scores for S221, S222 and S223 have been omitted
from all calculations in this chapter.

Note 19.3. I am grateful to Dr J. Y. Kassab for his considerable help with
the statistics that are presented in this chapter.

Note 19.4. The proportion of the total variability in each test pre-
dictable from age is given by the value of r squared. Expressed as percentages these values were: Reading, 61; Spelling, 53; Months
Forwards, 14; Months Reversed, 12; Digits Reversed, 9; Digits
Forwards, 7.

Note 19.5. The existence of a linear relationship was checked in each
case. Analysis of residuals showed no serious departure from the
underlying assumption, namely that true errors are independent and
normally distributed and have constant variance.

Note 19.6. Compare the larger number of trials needed by dyslexic subjects in order to match arbitrarily chosen names with particular shapes.
See D.J. Done and T. R. Miles, 'Learning, memory, and dyslexia', in
M. M. Gruneberg, P. E. Morris and R. N. Sykes (eds), *Practical Aspects
of Memory*, London: Academic Press, 1987.

Note 19.7. As an example of what a dyslexic child can achieve by hard
practice the following experience is perhaps worth recording. Some
years ago (too early for the results to be included in the present book)
I assessed a boy who scored a solitary 'minus' on months of the year
despite a whole series of 'pluses' on other parts of the dyslexia test.
When I said to his mother that I was surprised that he could do the
months of the year so well, she replied: 'We have spent *hours and
hours* working on them!'

Note 19.8. A minor adjustment was necessary to take account of the fact
that in the two Schonell tests an increased score of 10 words represents an increase in reading or spelling age of 12 months. The difference between the 'numbers of words correct' on the two occasions had
therefore to be modified so as to represent differences in reading and
spelling age. The figures in both the final two columns are, of course,
ratios, and therefore decimals, since they were obtained by dividing the

reading and spelling gains in years and months by the time-interval between the two assessments also in years and months. The loss of accuracy arising from the use of the earlier Schonell R_1 norms (Note 8.1) was considered to be minimal.

Note 19.9. The figures for rate of gain given in Table 19.7 are in many ways unsatisfactory. In particular they take no account of the fact that if there were relatively high scores on the first testing then even a fully adequate performance on the re-test necessarily gives a relatively small rate of gain; the figure becomes even more misleading if there is a long time-interval between assessments, as there was in the case of S202. The figure of 0.2 for reading gain in the case of S118 is also an example where both these factors were at work and certainly does not reflect slow progress. Similarly S143 has a 'rate of gain' at spelling of only 0.4, yet an advance from 61 words correct at age 13 to 75 words correct at 17 is by no means a failure. In spite of these seemingly low figures, however, there is still evidence for considerable improvement. The rates of gain are not, of course, as large as those reported by Hornsby and Miles (see 'The effects of a dyslexia-centred teaching programme', *British Journal of Educational Psychology*, **50**, 1980, 236–242); but the children in that study were known to have received tuition from dyslexia specialists, whereas in the case of the subjects mentioned in this chapter the possibilities of skilled help may have been more variable. Part of the difference, of course, must be accounted for by the fact that the children in the Hornsby and Miles study would certainly have been discharged when their progress was adequate, and hence the time-interval between assessments would have been less. It should also be noted that, of the 21 subjects who were re-assessed, one had an intelligence rating of V, three a rating of W, and the remaining 17 a rating of X or above. Although improvement is possible if the child is only of average ability, as the Hornsby and Miles study shows, the high intelligence of the present group of subjects may well have been an important factor in their successes. Certainly 'high IQ' is cited by Dr Critchley as one of the 'pentagon' of factors which contribute to a good prognosis. See M. Critchley, 'Dyslexia: an overview', in G. Th. Pavlidis and T. R. Miles (eds), *Dyslexia Research and Its Applications to Education*, Chichester: John Wiley & Sons, 1981, p.9.

Note 19.10. It should again be borne in mind that events in the subject's past history can contribute to the number of 'pluses' and that this information is available regardless of whether it is the first assessment or a later one.

Note 19.11. She was therefore assigned to Group II (see Chapter 4). I had wondered at one stage whether to assign S190 to Group II also, but the re-testing showed enough residual difficulties to justify assigning him to Group I.

Note 19.12. These are the 'formes frustes' of dyslexia described by Dr Critchley and his wife. See M. and E. A. Critchley, *Dyslexia Defined*, London: Heinemann Medical Books, 1978, Chapter 9. Compare Note 4.2 of this book.

Note 19.13. It is not always easy, of course, to convince unsympathetic listeners of this point of view. For example, I was told by the mother of S34 that she had failed to convince a particular official that there was anything wrong with her son and had therefore had to arrange teaching help without any assistance from him. Fortunately the boy made striking progress. However, when the official came to hear of this he asked her disparagingly what she had been worrying about! Her good-humoured comment was, 'Sometimes you can't win!'

Chapter 20

Note 20.1. It is worth recording that S259 was the sister of S6 and S110, while S260 was the brother of S234. These two cases have not been included in the statistics in this chapter since the degree of handicap seemed insufficiently severe.

Note 20.2. The five earlier assessments took place before 1972, the four later ones after 1978. They therefore fell outside the period of time chosen for the case studies reported in this book .

Note 20.3. She in fact achieved a university degree late in life after her dyslexia was recognised. The mother of S97 was also dyslexic, but had nevertheless achieved a degree in mathematics.

Note 20.4. Throughout the chapter I have used my 'full' number of 257 cases, not the 223 assigned to Group I. The records all contained the necessary information on sex and on familial incidence, and since a larger sample of cases was available it seemed appropriate to make use of it.

Note 20.5. In one case (S86) a report of an earlier assessment mentioned that there was 'a suspicious family history' of dyslexia; but this evidence seemed to me insufficient to justify a 'zero'.

Note 20.6. T. R. Miles, *Understanding Dyslexia*, Bath: Amethyst Books, 1987, pp.74–75.

Note 20.7. For sources see Note 24.25.

Note 20.8. For further discussion see J.M.Finucci and B.Childs, 'Are there really more dyslexic boys than girls?', in A. Ansara, N. Geschwind, A. Galaburda, M. Albert and N. Gartrell (eds), *Sex Differences in Dyslexia*, Towson, Maryland: Orton Dyslexia Society, 1981. It has recently been argued that there is no major preponderance of boys if properly conducted population studies are carried out. (See S.E. Shaywitz, B.A. Shaywitz, J.M. Fletcher and M.D. Escobar, 'Prevalence of reading disability in boys and girls – results of the Connecticut longitudinal study', *Journal of the American Medical Association*, 264, 1990, 998–1002.) The subjects in this study, however, were selected simply on the basis of poor reading in relation to intelligence; it is therefore not clear how many were dyslexic in the strict sense. In a population study in which items from the Bangor Dyslexia Test were used there was a preponderance of boys in the ratio of about 4 to 1; see T.R. Miles and M.N. Haslum, 'Dyslexia: anomaly or normal variation?', *Annals of Dyslexia*, 36, 1986, 103–117. It is possible the ratio is even higher; see T.R. Miles, 'On determining the prevalence of dyslexia', in M. Snowling and M. Thomson (eds), *Dyslexia: Integrating Theory and Practice*, London: Whurr, 1991. The population study by MacMeeken in 1939 (Note 1. 8) also found a preponderance of boys.

Chapter 21

Note 21.1. $\chi^2 = 0.09, p > 0.05$.

Note 21.2. $\chi^2 = 1.95, p > 0.05$.

Note 21.3. For sources see M.Thomson, *Developmental Dyslexia*, London: Whurr, 1990.

Note 21.4. For a comprehensive review of the evidence see D.L.Molfese and S.J. Segalowitz (eds), *Brain Lateralisation in Children*, New York: Guildford Press, 1988.

Note 21.5. $\chi^2 = 3.70$. A value of 3.84 is needed for significance at the 5% level.

Note 21.6. $\chi^2 = 0.08, p > 0.05$.

Note 21.7. $\chi^2 = 0.79, p > 0.05$.

Note 21.8. $\chi^2 = 1.24, p > 0.05$.

Note 21.9. $\chi^2 = 0.58, p > 0.05$.

Chapter 22

Note 22.1. For an account of the way in which methods of teaching dyslexics have evolved over the years, see Chapter 10 of T.R. and E. Miles, *Dyslexia: 100 Years On*, Milton Keynes: Open University Press, 1990.

Chapter 23

Note 23.1. Those with a psychodynamic orientation might say that I was doing 'family therapy'. I accept this description, provided two important qualifications are made. In the first place my 'interpretations' were far more restricted in their range than those commonly offered by psychotherapists, since they were usually limited to remarks such as, 'You must have found it extremely frustrating' or 'No wonder you felt discouraged'. Secondly, most therapists tend to avoid giving direct advice or making practical suggestions, whereas I regularly made clear by word and gesture that I was on the parents' side in their struggles to obtain help. Indeed, I often made a point of encouraging parents to back their own judgement, particularly if others had implied that they were being neurotic or over-fussy.

Note 23.2. I am sometimes asked, 'This is all very well with bright children, but how can you be similarly encouraging with slower children?' Even here, however, it is perfectly possible to be constructive, for example in making suggestions as to how the child might be taught or given other kinds of help; and over the years I have met very few parents indeed who have had unrealistic expectations about their child's future.

Note 23.3. In this connection I should like to quote from Dr Gerald Hales' paper, delivered to the second international conference of the British Dyslexia Association held in Oxford in 1991. See also Note 32.3. The full title of the paper was: 'Are dyslexics real people? Interacting with the personal aspects of dyslexia: counselling and helping'. The following passage reveals in a remarkable way the thoughts and feelings of a 9-year-old dyslexic:

> John was nine years old when his parents decided that they wanted to know why he was not progressing at school. A full diagnostic assessment was carried out, and John was found to be dyslexic. His mother, a teacher, made the decision that she should impart the diagnosis to him, and so explained to him, in suitable words, what she thought was the problem. John listened to this carefully, and then asked, 'Do you mean I've *got* something?' Mother thought that this was not a bad description for a nine-year-old, and so said

yes. John then replied, in all seriousness, 'Oh, that's OK then. If I've got something I can cope. I thought I was going round the bend'.

Note 23.4. I hope that in this part of the chapter I do not give the impression of flaunting all the bouquets which I have received! The point is quite an impersonal one, namely that suitable explanations of what dyslexia is are likely to be quite striking in their effects.

Chapter 24

Note 24.1. These techniques include EEG ('electroencephalography'), the BEAM method ('brain electrical activity mapping'), PET scan ('positron emission tomography') and MRI ('magnetic resonance imaging'). For more details the reader is referred to the first volume of G.Th. Pavlidis (ed.), *Perspectives on Dyslexia*, Chichester: John Wiley & Sons, 1990; to D. Duane, 'Neurobiological correlates of learning disorders', *Journal of the American Academy of Child and Adolescent Psychiatry*, 1989, **28**, 3, 314–318; and to D. Duane, 'Neurobiological issues in dyslexia', in M. Snowling and M. Thomson (eds), *Dyslexia: Integrating Theory and Practice*, London: Whurr, 1991.

Note 24.2. See in particular A.M. Galaburda, J. Corsiglia, G.D. Rosen, and G.F. Sherman, 'Planum temporale asymmetry: reappraisal since Geschwind and Levitsky', *Neuropsychologia*, **28**, 6, 1987, 853–868. Also G.F. Sherman, G.D. Rosen and A.M. Galaburda, 'Neuroanatomical findings in developmenmtal dyslexia', in C. Von Euler, I. Lundberg and G.Lennerstrand (eds), *Brain and Reading*, Wenner-Gren International Symposium Series, **54**, 1989, London: Macmillan. Also A.M. Galaburda, G.D. Rosen and G.F. Sherman, 'The neural origin of developmental dyslexia: implications for medicine, neurology, and cognition', in A.M.Galaburda (ed.) *From Reading to Neurons*, Cambridge, Mass.: MIT Press, 1989.

Note 24.3. Dr Galaburda was kind enough to let me see a set of case notes on a patient who had been examined *post mortem*. Using the criteria set out in this book I had no hesitation in saying that this patient was dyslexic.

Note 24.4. Neuropsychologia, 1987. See Note 24.2.

Note 24.5. See M.S. Livingstone, G.D. Rosen, F.W. Drislane and A.M. Galaburda, 'Physiological and anatomical evidence for a magnocellular defect in developmental dyslexia', *Proceedings of the National Academy of Science of the USA*, **88**, September 1991, 7943–7947.

Note 24.6. See W. Lovegrove, 'Visual deficits in dyslexia: evidence and implications', to be published in A.J. Fawcett and R.I. Nicolson (eds), *Skills and their Development in Dyslexic Children*, forthcoming.

Note 24.7. See P. Tallal, 'Auditory temporal perception, phonics, and reading disabilities in children', *Brain and Language*, 9, 1980, 182–198.

Note 24.8. From P. Tallal, 'Language and reading: some perceptual requisites', *Bulletin of the Orton Society* (now *Annals of Dyslexia*), 30, 1980, 170–178.

Note 24.9. F.R. Vellutino, 'Dyslexia', *Scientific American*, 256, 3, 1987, 20–27.

Note 24.10. In some of my earlier papers I have spoken of a 'lexical encoding deficiency' (see the references made on various occasions in this book to the two papers by Nick Ellis and myself in G.Th. Pavlidis and T.R. Miles, (eds), *Dyslexia Research and Its Applications to Education*, Chichester: John Wiley & Sons, 1981); more recently I have followed current practice and spoken of 'phonological difficulties' (see T.R. and E. Miles, *Dyslexia: 100 Years On*, Milton Keynes: Open University Press, 1990). Without wishing to change the basic arguments in these earlier publications, I am now inclined to favour the expression 'deficiency in verbal labelling'. This makes clear that there need be no deficiency in verbal *reasoning* and avoids unnecessary technicality.

Note 24.11. See H.W. Catts, 'Phonological processing deficits and reading disabilities', in A.G. Kamhi and H.W. Catts (eds), *Reading Difficulties: A Developmental Language Perspective*, Boston: Little Brown, 1989. At this point I should like to pay tribute to the pioneering work of the late Isabel Liberman at the Haskins Laboratories, Connecticut, who was one of the earliest researchers to emphasise that dyslexia was primarily a problem of language. See, for instance, I.Y. Liberman, D. Shankweiler, C. Orlando, K. Harris and F. Bell-Berti, 'Letter confusions and reversals of sequence in the beginning reader: implications for Orton's theory of developmental dyslexia', *Cortex*, 7, 127–142.

Note 24.12. Phonemes are the individual units of sounds. Sometimes they are represented by individual letters of the alphabet, as when, in the present example, the three phonemes in the word 'cat' are represented by the letters 'c', 'a', and 't'. This one-to-one correspondence, however, is not invariable. Thus the word 'six' contains four phonemes, the letter 'x' standing for two of them, while the word 'shop' contains three phonemes, the combination 'sh' standing for a single phoneme.

Note 24.13. For an interesting discussion of the evidence in this area see U.Goswami and P.E.Bryant, *Phonological Skills and Learning to Read*, Hove: Lawrence Erlbaum, 1990.

Note 24.14. For a recent discussion see L.L. Bradley, 'Rhyming connections in learning', in P.D. Pumfrey and C.D. Elliott (eds), *Children's Difficulties in Reading, Spelling and Writing*, Basingstoke: Falmer Press, 1990.

Note 24.15. See M. Snowling, N. Goulandris, M. Bowlby and P. Howell, 'Segmentation and speech perception in relation to reading skill: a developmental analysis', *Journal of Experimental Child Psychology*, **41**, 1986, 489–507.

Note 24.16. See U. Frith, 'Beneath the surface of developmental dyslexia', in K.E. Patterson, J.C. Marshall and M. Coltheart (eds), *Surface Dyslexia. Neuropsychological and Cognitive Studies of Phonological Reading*, Hove: Lawrence Erlbaum, 1985.

Note 24.17. See E. Miles and T.R. Miles, 'The interface between research and remediation', to be published in G.D.A. Brown and N.C. Ellis (eds), *Handbook of Normal and Disturbed Spelling*, Chichester: John Wiley & Sons, forthcoming.

Note 24.18. See F.R. Vellutino, J.A. Steger, C. Harding and F. Phillips, 'Verbal vs. non-verbal paired associates learning in poor and normal readers, *Neuropsychologia*, **13**, 1975, 75–82. Also D.J. Done and T.R. Miles, 'Learning, memory, and dyslexia', in M.M. Gruneberg, P.E. Morris and R.N. Sykes (eds), *Practical Aspects of Memory*, London: Academic Press, 1978.

Note 24.19. For some interesting evidence on this point see S. Naidoo, *Specific Dyslexia*, London: Pitman, 1972, pp.59–62

Note 24.20. See J.B. Carroll and M.N. White, 'Word frequency and age-of-acquisition as determinants of picture-naming latency', *Quarterly Journal of Experimental Psychology*, **25**, 1973, 85–95.

Note 24.21. See D.J. Done and T.R. Miles, 'Age of word-acquisition in developmental dyslexics as determined by response latencies in a picture naming task', in M.M. Gruneberg, P.E. Morris and R.N. Sykes (eds), *Practical Aspects of Memory: Current Research and Issues*, vol.2, Chichester: John Wiley & Sons, 1988.

Note 24.22. See C. Hulme, N. Thomson, C. Muir and A. Lawrence, 'Speech rate and the development of short-term memory', *Journal of Experimental Child Psychology*, **38**, 1984, 241–253.

Note 24.23. See N.C. Ellis and T.R. Miles, 'Dyslexia as a limitation in the ability to process information', *Bulletin of the Orton Society* (now *Annals of Dyslexia*), **27**, 1977, 72–81.

Note 24.24. See in particular R.I.Nicolson and A.J.Fawcett, 'Automaticity: a new framework for dyslexia research', *Cognition*, **35**, 1990, 159–182.

Note 24.25. For a recent review of the evidence see J.C. DeFries, 'Genetics and dyslexia: an overview', in M.Snowling and M.Thomson (eds), *Dyslexia: Integrating Theory and Practice*, London: Whurr, 1991. See also Chapter 4 of T.R. and E. Miles, *Dyslexia: A Hundred Years On*, Milton Keynes: Open University Press, 1990.

Note 24.26. For further information in this area and some very pertinent comments, see S.P. Springer and G. Deutsch, *Left Brain, Right Brain*, New York: W.H. Freeman, 1984.

Note 24.27. T.G. West, *In the Mind's Eye: Visual Thinkers, Gifted People with Learning Difficuilties, Computer Images, and the Ironies of Creativity*, Buffalo, New York: Prometheus Books, 1991.

Note 24.28. See Jean Augur, 'Is three too young to know?', *Dyslexia Contact*, 9, 1, June 1990, 10–11.

Chapter 25

Note 25.1. This problem was, of course, a difficulty for Pooh Bear, as is shown by the following passage: 'Pooh looked at his two paws. He knew that one of them was the right, and he knew that when you had decided which one of them was the right, then the other one was the left, but he could never remember how to begin'. From A.A. Milne, *The House at Pooh Corner*, London: Methuen, 1928, Chapter 7.

Note 25.2. This point is discussed further in T.R. Miles and N.C. Ellis, 'A lexical encoding deficiency II', in G.Th. Pavlidis and T.R. Miles (eds), *Dyslexia Research and Its Applications to Education*, Chichester: John Wiley & Sons, 1981.

Note 25.3. I am grateful to Claudia de Wall and Dr Michelle Aldridge for their help with this section.

Note 25.4. On various occasions I have sat alongside dyslexic adults who were themselves administering the Bangor Dyslexia Test. This is no easy task for them, particularly in the case of the Left–Right and Polysyllables items. On one occasion the dyslexic tester solved his problem by saying the word 'preliminary' somewhat slowly, syllable by syllable – not so slowly that it sounded absurd but not fast enough to cause him to lose his way.

Note 25.5. For evidence on this point see R.A. Pritchard, T.R. Miles, S.J. Chinn and A.T. Taggart, 'Dyslexia and knowledge of number facts', *Links*, **14** (3), 1989, 17–20.

Note 25.6. 'Reaction time patterns suggested that third grade is a transitional stage with respect to memory structure for addition – half of these children seemed to be counting and half retrieving from memory'. See M.H. Ashcraft and B.A. Fierman, 'Mental addition in third, fourth, and sixth graders', *Journal of Experimental Child Psychology*, **33**, 1982, 216–234.

Note 25.7. See Note 24.24.

Note 25.8. Although this point has not, to my knowledge, been adequately researched in English-speaking countries, there is evidence that dyslexics in Japan have difficulty with recall of the syllabary which is a string of syllables which all Japanese children are made to learn. For details see Chapter 30.

Note 25.9. See T.R. Miles, 'On the persistence of dyslexic difficulties into adulthood', in G.T. Pavlidis and D.F. Fisher (eds), *Dyslexia: Its Neuropsychology and Treatment*, Chichester: John Wiley & Sons, 1986.

Note 25.10. For sources see Note 24.25.

Chapter 26

Note 26.1. The data came from the Ten Year Follow-Up of the Child Health and Education Study which was funded by the Departments of Health and of Education and Science, the Joseph Rowntree Memorial Trust, and the Institutes of Mental Health in the USA.

Note 26.2. The Edinburgh Reading test is published by Hodder & Stoughton, Sevenoaks, Kent. The shortened version for the survey was published in 1985.

Note 26.3. See C.D. Elliott, D.J. Murray and L.S. Pearson, *The British Ability Scales*, Windsor: NFER-Nelson, 1983.

Note 26.4. We of course had no right to *assume* that responses of a specified kind to these four test items were evidence for dyslexia; this assumption is not made in the arguments which follow. It was rather that we were exploring what could be achieved by defining dyslexia in a particular way using responses to these four items as part of the definition. Since other researchers had already asked for the Recall of Digits item from the British Ability Scales to be included in the battery of tests there was no point in also including the Digits Forwards and Digits Reversed items from the Bangor Dyslexia Test. The Left–Right, Months Forwards and Months Reversed items were chosen on the grounds that they were relatively easy for teachers to administer and did not require an excessive amount of time.

Note 26.5. There is evidence that, at least for the most part, dyslexics are able to perform adequately, in relation to their other skills, at 'Similarities' items. For sources see T.R. Miles and N.C. Ellis, 'A lexical encoding deficiency II', in G.Th. Pavlidis and T.R. Miles (eds), *Dyslexia Research and Its Applications to Education*, Chichester: John Wiley & Sons, 1981. Dr Michael Thomson's research confirms both this point and the relative strength of dyslexics at matrices tests; see M.E.Thomson, 'The assessment of children with specific reading difficulties (dyslexia) using the British Ability Scales', *British Journal of Psychology*, 73, 1982, 461–478. Dr Joyce Steeves has also reported considerable success on the part of dyslexics at the Raven Standard Progressive Matrices; see K.J. Steeves, 'Memory as a factor in the computational efficiency of dyslexic children with high abstract reasoning ability', *Annals of Dyslexia*, 33, 1983, 141–152

Note 26.6. Scores on the word recognition and spelling tests were each regressed on the combined score for the Similarities and Matrices tests. In an effort to find a better fit for the regression equation outliers beyond 1.5 s.d. from the mean were excluded; the equations were recalculated on the remainder and then refitted to the entire population. Residual scores (observed–predicted) were then calculated; any child whose residual score on either word recognition or spelling was 1.5 or more standard deviations below prediction in either case was classified as 'discrepant' (or 'underachieving').

Note 26.7. Norms will be found in the British Ability Scales (Note 26.2) and in the Wechsler Intelligence Scale for Children, National Foundation for Educational Research, Slough, 1976.

Note 26.8. The issue of test validation is problematic at the best of times. Examples from other fields are interesting in this connection. Thus it is arguable that one might validate a test of intelligence by checking if the results in individual cases were in agreement with teachers' estimates; or, again, one might arguably validate a test for schizophrenia by checking if those who came out as schizophrenic on the test were also those whom psychiatrists judged to be schizophrenic on the basis of clinical assessment. This procedure is legitimate, however, only if we assume that teachers are in agreement as to how to rate people as 'intelligent' and that psychiatrists are in agreement as to how to diagnose schizophrenia. Those who work regularly with dyslexics are now arguably in a position where they can make comparable judgments as to whether someone is dyslexic, but validating in this way would not necessarily command general acceptance.

Note 26.9. See in particular M.J. Norusis, *Introductory Statistics Guide*, Chicago, SPSS Inc., 1983.

Chapter 27

Note 27.1. See S.A. Ellis, *Dyslexia and the Speed of Multiplication* (in preparation).

Note 27.2. This is true of many of the cases described in this book. It is interesting in this connection that Sandhya Naidoo found it necessary to distinguish those dyslexics who were retarded at both reading and spelling from those who were retarded at spelling only. See S. Naidoo, *Specific Dyslexia*, London: Pitman, 1972.

Note 27.3. See F.J. Schonell and F.E. Schonell, *Diagnostic and Attainment Testing*, Edinburgh: Oliver and Boyd, 1952, p.71.

Note 27.4. J.C. Raven, *Standard Progressive Matrices*, London: H.K. Lewis & Co., 1938.

Note 27.5. J.C. Raven, *Coloured Progressive Matrices*, London: H.K. Lewis & Co., 1962.

Note 27.6. This result is not altogether surprising since the boy was aged only 7 and a half.

Note 27.7. For the test group and the CA controls $U = 0$, $p<0.001$; for the test group and the SA controls $U = 7$, $p<0.001$, one-tailed tests.

Note 27.8. In both cases $U = 0$, $p<0.001$, one-tailed tests.

Chapter 28

Note 28.1. See A. Kasviki, *The Diagnosis of Developmental Dyslexia in Greece*, MPhil. dissertation, University of Wales.

Note 28.2. J.C.Raven, *Standard Progressive Matrices*, London: H.K. Lewis & Co., 1938.

Note 28.3. The three sentences were each three words long and comprised verb, article and noun. The five non-words were taken from real words but had changed consonants either at the beginning or in the middle. nine of the 42 words were of two syllables, seven of three syllables, 15 of four syllables and 11 of five or more syllables. Thirty of the words were 'irregular' in the sense that they were based on inconsistencies of pronunciation of both vowels and consonants.

Note 28.4. For the test group and the CA controls $t = 13.79$, $p<0.001$; for the test group and the SA controls $t = 10.34$, $p<0.001$.

Note 28.5. Further details will be found in A. Kasviki, *The Diagnosis of Developmental Dyslexia in Greece*, MPhil. dissertation, University of Wales.

Chapter 29

Note 29.1. Like 'dyslexia', 'legasthenie' is derived from the Greek. 'Leg' is connected with 'logos', 'lexis' etc.; 'a' = 'not', and 'sthenos' = 'strength'.

Note 29.2. The *Kaufman-Assessment Battery for Children* (K-ABC) has recently been translated into German (Peter Melchers and Ulrich Preuss, 1991).

Note 29.3. See A.D. Baddeley, N. Thomson and M. Buchanan, 'Word length and the structure of short-term memory', *Journal of Verbal Learning and Verbal Behaviour*, **14**, 1975, 575–589.

Note 29.4. See C. Hulme, N. Thomson, C. Muir and A. Lawrence, 'Speech rate and the development of short-term memory', *Journal of Experimental Child Psychology*, **38**, 1984, 241–253. Compare Note 24.25.

Note 29.5. For instance the Wechsler Intelligence Scale for Children (see Note 2.9) and the British Ability Scales (C.D. Elliott, D.J. Murray and L.S. Pearson, 1983, Windsor: NFER-Nelson).

Note 29.6. We should like to thank the Institut für Legastheniker Therapie und Deutsche Orthographie, as well as the headmasters and all the staff of the Waldschule, the Albert Einstein Gymnasium, the Carl-Arnold-Kortum Schule and the Hans-Böckler Realschule (especially

Frau Fründ) for their support with this research. We should also like to thank Bernhard Schmidt for his helpful comments.

Note 29.7. In Germany the system is different from that in Britain. After four years at primary school the children go either to a Gymnasium (grammar school), to a Realschule (O-level high school), or to a Hauptschule (nine-year elementary school). The final awards differ in each case. Besides these there are some comprehensive schools and some 'free schools' which work with a particular philosophical background such as the Walldorf Schule.

Note 29.8. An interesting incident in this study deserves mention. On one occasion the teachers 'smuggled' a boy into the control group whom they knew to have severe reading and writing problems in order to see if the tester (C de W) would detect this. On the seven BLT items he scored four 'pluses', one 'zero' and two 'minuses'!

Note 29.9. J.C.Raven, *Standard Progressive Matrices,* London: H.K. Lewis & Co., 1938.

Note 29.10. Rudolf Meis, *Diagnosticher Rechtschreibtest für Klasses 4 und 5 (DRT 4–5)*, Weinheim und Berlin: Verlag Julius Beltz, 1970.

Note 29.11. The original norms are recorded in terms of number of errors. 'Spelling score' is therefore 'number of errors' subtracted from 100.

Note 29.12. $U = 2, p < 0.001$ (one-tailed test).

Note 29.13. $U = 16.5, p < 0.06$ (one-tailed test).

Chapter 30

Note 30.1. A morpheme is a grammatical unit such as a noun or verb, or in some cases that part of a word which indicates a grammatical function, such as the suffixes '-ing' and '-ed' in English.

Note 30.2. It had earlier been claimed by Makita that reading problems in Japan were very infrequent (see K. Makita, 'The rarity of reading disability in Japanese children', *American Journal of Orthopsychiatry*, **38**, 1968, 599–614. More recently, however, this claim has been disputed (see H.W. Stevenson, J.W. Stigler, G.W. Lucker, S. Lee, C. Hau and S. Kitamura, 'Reading disabilities in the case of Chinese, Japanese, and English', *Child Development*, **53**, 1982, 1164–1181.

Note 30.3. According to a classroom teacher one of the eight was 'often' absent from school. Even in this case, however, it does not seem as though the absences were sufficiently frequent to have deprived him of the opportunity to learn to read and spell.

Note 30.4. For references on the male–female ratio in dyslexia see Note 20.8.

Note 30.5. The figures in the literature for the incidence of dyslexia are extremely varied. An interesting discussion of this issue will be found in M. Thomson, *Developmental Dyslexia*, 3rd edn, London: Whurr, 1989. It seems likely that different researchers were using different criteria for who was or was not dyslexic.

Note 30.6. In the future we propose to describe the test as *The Bangor Hiroshima Dyslexia Test*.

Note 30.7. One way of solving the problem of translating the Polysyllables item into Japanese would be to present the *English* words ('preliminary' etc.) as they stand. To a Japanese child the resultant stimuli would be nonsense words and therefore a suitable test. We hope that it will be possible to explore this idea further.

Note 30.8. $p < 0.004$ (median test).

Chapter 31

Note 31.1. Intelligence scores were missing in five cases (see Table 31.1). S289 was a graduate; S296 was a highly successful joiner; S306 was a business man in the meat trade; S309 was reading for a degree and S311 had been a grade 5 technician. In the 17 cases where spelling scores were either missing or above 80 I satisfied myself that the evidence for dyslexia was unambiguous. The main criteria used were, first, a history of reading or spelling difficulty at an earlier age and, secondly, indicators during the assessment (other than those supplied by the Bangor Dyslexia Test) of slow processing and other typical dyslexic manifestations. S312 was so disgusted with his spelling performance that he tore the sheet up and would not let me keep it! He had very clear recollections of failure at school, however, and mentioned in particular his difficulty in remembering messages.

Note 31.2. The entry 'WAIS' for S291 indicates a reported WAIS full-scale IQ of 142, though I did not test this subject myself. The entry 'SPM' for S311 indicates a score on the Standard Progressive Matrices (Note 7.3) of 46. The Polysyllables item was not given to S306 because he had a severe stammer.

Note 31.3. 'University' in this chapter refers to those institutions which were universities before 1992.

Note 31.4. In the case of adults it did not seem appropriate to use the very stringent criteria which I set in the case of younger subjects. A clear report of b–d confusion was sufficient for a 'plus' and if the response was hesitant (e.g. 'Yes, I think I may have done') it was scored as 'zero'.

Note 31.5. These are the subjects referred to in the postscript to Chapter 7.

Note 31.6. The view is still held in some quarters that a preferable term to 'dyslexia' is 'specific learning difficulty' (or 'disability'). This term seems an absurd description of the adult dyslexic, and in particular of dyslexics with academic interests. Their ability to *learn* is not in question. I am grateful to my colleague, Dr Rod Nicolson, for calling my attention to this absurdity.

Note 31.7. While I was preparing this chapter I received a letter from a 26-year-old adult. She wrote: 'There are a number of whole words I always seem to get wrong...A recent and embarassing (sic) one was on a work report writing "contraception" instead of "conception" – Well what would Freud have said about that?'

Note 31.8. This comment reminds me of the insightful remarks of the 19th-century neurologist J. Hughlings Jackson, who wrote: 'Written and printed words, strictly, have no meaning. They are merely arbitrary signs of words. They require translation into words and into an order of words'. From J. Taylor (ed.), *Selected Writings of John Hughlings Jackson*, London: Staples Press, 1931.

Note 31.9. For an interesting review of investigations into the personal and social consequences of dyslexia, see J.H. and T. Bryan, 'Social factors in learning disabilities: attitudes and interactions', in G.Th. Pavlidis (ed.), *Perspectives on Dyslexia*, vol. II, Chichester: John Wiley & Sons, 1990. For a discussion of the needs of dyslexic students in tertiary education, see T.R. Miles and D.E. Gilroy, *Dyslexia at College*, London: Routledge, 1986.

Chapter 32

Note 32.1. In this connection I should like to refer again to T.G. West's book, *In the Mind's Eye* (Note 24.27).

Note 32.2. For some telling arguments in this area, see K. Stanovich, 'The theoretical and practical consequences of discrepancy definitions of dyslexia', in M. Snowling and M. Thomson (eds), *Dyslexia: Integrating Theory and Practice*, London: Whurr, 1991. See also various papers in *Journal of Learning Disabilities*, **22**, 8, October 1989, 465–528.

Note 32.3. I am grateful to my friend and colleague Dr Gerald Hales for calling attention to this somewhat overlooked area of research. See in particular his 'Are dyslexics real people? Interacting with the personal aspects of dyslexia: counselling and helping'. Paper delivered at the Second International Conference of the British Dyslexia Association, Oxford, 1991. A further very striking example of this 'personal' approach to dyslexia is a book written by Marion Fenwick Stuart entitled *Personal Insights into the World of Dyslexia*, obtainable from Educators Publishing Service Inc., 75 Moulton St., Cambridge, Mass., 02138, USA.

Author Index

Subject Index